Table of Contents

Preface

The main purpose of this book is to provide the reader with information about the possibility that a prescription drug will harm the fetus and cause a major birth defect. Put differently, the book attempts to help answer the question: Is this drug safe for unborn babies?

Some birth defects are minor, while a major birth defect is one that threatens a child's health, often requiring surgery to correct it. In order to get a feeling for just how often drugs consumed by pregnant moms might cause birth defects, let's list the broad causes under the following headings:

- Genetic
- Environmental (drugs, infections, radiation, and chemicals)
- Multifactorial Inheritance (a combination of genetic and environmental factors)
- Unknown

Now, which heading contains the most birth defects? If you answered "unknown," that's correct. We don't know the cause for 50%–60% of all major birth defects. Are you surprised?

From the other end of the spectrum: which heading contains the fewest birth defects? If you answered "environmental factors," that's also correct. Environmental factors account for 7%–10% of all major birth defects. But, if we focus in on the role drugs play in causing birth defects, we find that roughly .5%–1.0% of all major birth defects are caused by drugs.

So, how many birth defects are caused by drugs? There are 4.4 million births annually in this country. Studies show that roughly 3%, or 132,000, of those babies will have a major birth defect. If drugs account for approximately .5%–1.0% of those defects, that's 660 to 1,320 major birth defects each year possibly caused by drugs. It is not an insignificant number, especially if it's your baby.

We also know drugs may harm the fetus in ways that don't show up as birth defects. For instance, parents may not get suspicious until six, twelve, or eighteen months after birth when their child fails to reach certain developmental milestones, like sitting up, walking, or talking on time. Mental retardation, cerebral palsy, and behavioral problems come to mind. Puzzled and often frustrated, those parents and their doctors will always wonder if the child's problem is linked to a drug mom took while pregnant.

One of the things you will notice in this book is how often we say there are no controlled studies of pregnant women taking a particular drug. The reason for this is simple: as a society, we don't "experiment" on pregnant women. Moreover, it's also true that studies using a particular drug on pregnant mice, rats, or rabbits often tell us little about how that drug might affect the human fetus. After all, thalidomide did not cause birth defects in all pregnant animals. Yet it raised havoc for the human fetus, causing thousands upon thousands of major birth defects in babies born around the world.

While pregnant moms should be prudent about the drugs they take, this doesn't necessarily mean they should refuse to take an antidepressant just because the drug might harm their unborn babies. After all, depression itself harms unborn babies, too.

Clinicians should also be prudent, weighing the potential benefit for mom's health versus the potential harms for her unborn baby—even though we often know less than we would like to about those potential harms—before we pick up a prescription pad and start to write. Hopefully, pregnant moms and their clinicians will make those decisions together.

D. Gary Benfield, M.D.

Introduction

Many women of childbearing age take one or more prescription drugs for a variety of health disorders, such as diabetes, high blood pressure, and obesity. Whether planning a pregnancy or already pregnant, these women are anxious to know if the drugs they are already taking—or may take when pregnant—are safe for unborn babies. Ideally, they would like to know before discovering they are pregnant. But the reality is more than 50% of all pregnancies in this country are unplanned.

This book contains up-to-date information about fetal risk for hundreds of commonly prescribed drugs. If a drug seems unsafe in pregnancy, this book will help you and your clinician decide if the benefit of taking the drug outweighs the risk for your unborn baby or not. On the other hand, if a drug seems safe for unborn babies, this information can help allay your concerns.

Currently, the U.S. Food and Drug Administration (FDA) assigns a Pregnancy Risk Category: A, B, C, D, or X to each prescription drug. Moreover, some 12% of prescription drugs are assigned two Pregnancy Risk Categories, depending on which trimester of pregnancy the drug is taken. We will explain the five categories follow-ing this introduction.

Specifically, this book lists alphabetically, by generic name, the following information about more than 300 prescription drugs:

- Brand name
- Drug use
- FDA Pregnancy Risk Category: A, B, C, D, or X
- Explanation of Pregnancy Risk Category
- Studies in pregnant animals
- Studies in pregnant women
- Helpful hints

In addition, the book lists alphabetically, by generic name, the FDA Pregnancy Risk Category for hundreds of less-commonly prescribed drugs.

Lastly, the appendix contains six must-read articles:

- **ACE Inhibitor Drugs in Pregnancy** ACE inhibitors are used mainly for the treatment of high blood pres-sure. For quite a while, the FDA has included a Black Box Warning for pregnant women that they should avoid exposing the fetus to these drugs in the second and third trimesters of pregnancy. Now, a more recent study has raised doubt about the safety of these drugs even when taken during the first trimester. For more information and a list of drugs within this family, be sure to read this article.

- **Antidepressants in Pregnancy** While antidepres-sants may potentially pose some risk to an unborn baby, depression in a pregnant woman is also a real cause for concern. Refer to this article for information to help weigh the risks and benefits, including the most recent warnings from the FDA and the drugs involved in their proposed labeling changes.

- **Folic Acid Antagonist Drugs in Pregnancy** Drugs in this family impact the effectiveness of folic acid, a supplemental form of a B complex vitamin, important for the role it plays in cell growth and development. Women taking these type of drugs should be informed about the possible need to increase the normal recommended daily dose of folic acid while pregnant. Read this article for important information to discuss with your physician.

- **Grapefruit Juice–Drug Interactions Can Make You Sick** Fortunately, most drugs don't interact with grapefruit juice in a clinically important way. But, unfortunately, some do. In some of those cases, the interaction has resulted in serious, sometimes life-threatening, toxic effects on the patient. To understand how grapefruit juice might interact with a drug you are taking and make you sick, be sure to read this informative article.

- **Non-Steroidal, Anti-Inflammatory Drugs (NSAIDS) in Pregnancy** This family of drugs is commonly used to reduce inflammation and pain associated with arthritis. Read this article for more information and a list of commonly used drugs in this family, as well as their potentially life-threatening effects on the unborn fetus.

- **Taking Acetaminophen: The Good and the Ugly** Most clinicians consider acetaminophen as the drug of choice for pain relief and fever control in pregnancy. They also rely on its safety for unborn babies, having a Pregnancy Risk Category of "B." However, since

acetaminophen is found in more than 90 prescription
and non-prescription medications, some pregnant women
have unintentionally taken more than one medication
at a time containing acetaminophen. When this happens,
pregnant or not, patients risk acute liver failure and even
death from the toxic effects of this normally safe drug.
To understand how this might happen and how to avoid
it, don't miss this valuable article.

Now, let's turn the page for the FDA's Pregnancy Risk
Categories.

FDA Pregnancy Risk Categories: A, B, C, D, & X

Category A: The FDA assigns a drug to Category A when controlled studies using the drug in pregnant women do not show harmful fetal effects throughout pregnancy. Approximately 1% of prescription drugs fall in this category.

Category B: The FDA assigns a drug to Category B for one of two reasons: (1) Studies show no evidence of fetal harm when using the drug in pregnant animals, but no controlled studies have been done using the drug in pregnant women, or (2) Studies show evidence of fetal harm when using the drug in pregnant animals, but controlled studies using the drug in pregnant women do not show evidence of fetal harm. Approximately 21% of prescription drugs fall in this category.

Category C: The FDA assigns a drug to Category C for one of two reasons: (1) Studies show evidence of fetal harm when using the drug in pregnant animals, but no controlled studies have been done using the drug in pregnant women, or (2) Studies using the drug in pregnant animals have not been done, and studies of pregnant women using the drug are insufficient to reach a conclusion. Thus, the drug should only be used if the potential benefit for mom is greater than the potential risk of fetal harm, which, in many cases, is unknown. (Yes, it is confusing!) Approximately 50% of prescription drugs fall in this category.

Category D: The FDA assigns a drug to Category D when studies of pregnant women using the drug show evidence of fetal harm. Rarely, however, the potential benefit of using the drug in some life-threatening situations for mom may outweigh the potential risk of fetal harm. For example, the drug may be used when mom requires cancer treatment or when she has a serious disease for which safer drugs cannot be used or are less effective. Approximately 11% of prescription drugs fall in this category.

Category X: The FDA assigns a drug to Category X when studies have shown the risk of fetal harm clearly outweighs any potential maternal benefit from the drug. **Drugs in this category should not be used by pregnant women.** Approximately 5% of prescription drugs fall in this category.

Two-Category Drugs: Approximately 12% of prescription drugs are assigned two pregnancy risk categories, depending on which trimester of pregnancy the drug is used. For example, a drug may be assigned to Category B if used in the first trimester, but reassigned to Category D if used in the second and third trimesters, suggesting the drug should not be used in the second and third trimesters unless mom faces a life-threatening situation, and the potential benefit of using the drug outweighs the potential risk to her unborn baby.

The FDA's New Proposal for Labeling Prescription Drugs in Pregnancy and Lactation

In 2008, the FDA proposed a new rule to eliminate the current Pregnancy Risk Categories A, B, C, D, and X in favor of a more informative method of labeling prescription drugs for pregnancy and lactation.

One of the concerns was that the five categories, A, B, C, D, and X might mislead healthcare providers and the women they counsel into believing that fetal risk simply increases from category A to B to C to D to X. This may oversimplify the process of weighing potential fetal harm versus potential maternal benefit, especially for drugs that fall in category C.

Take, for example, the Varicella (Chicken Pox) Vaccine. This vaccine is assigned Pregnancy Risk Category C, suggesting to many that the vaccine is safe in pregnancy. But since the vaccine has not been tested in pregnant animals or in pregnant women, its effect on the fetus is unknown. Therefore, the manufacturer, the American Academy of Pediatrics, and the American College of OB-GYN have all recommended that pregnant women should not receive the vaccine.

So, yes, assigning Pregnancy Risk Category C to this vaccine might be misleading. But healthcare providers also have a responsibility to dig deeper before prescribing any medication in pregnancy. Unfortunately, the information needed from drug studies in pregnant animals and in pregnant women for estimating potential fetal harm is often woefully inadequate. That's unlikely to change much, regardless of which method the FDA endorses for labeling prescription drugs in the future.

Based on the FDA's progress to date, the sweeping changes proposed in its new rule may take several more years before they are published in final form. After that, it will likely take five to ten years to fully implement those changes, according to the timetable outlined in the proposal.

Meanwhile, you can count on this handy guide to help answer your questions about fetal risk. And when the time comes, a revised edition will keep you up-to-date.

Acknowledgments

This book is dedicated to my lovely wife, Cathy.

Thank you, Malia Lane, for your technical assistance; Dan Weimer and Ted Stevens for your creative photography; Ryan Feasal for your outstanding cover; Laura Weimer, my daughter, for sharing a special moment of your pregnancy for the cover; and Cynthia S. Kelley, D.O., my ever-smiling, always optimistic, fun-to-work-with, co-author and daughter.

D. Gary Benfield, M.D.

* * * *

I would like to thank my dad, D. Gary Benfield, for the opportunity to co-author this book and share this journey with him.

Cynthia S. Kelley, D.O.

A

ACARBOSE

Brand Names: Glucobay, Precose

Drug Use: Acarbose is approved by the FDA for oral use in treating diabetes.

Pregnancy Risk Category: B

> **Category B rating:** The FDA assigns a drug to Category **B** for one of two reasons: (1) Studies show no evidence of fetal harm when using the drug in pregnant animals, but no controlled studies have been done using the drug in pregnant women, or (2) Studies show evidence of fetal harm when using the drug in pregnant animals, but controlled studies using the drug in pregnant women do not show evidence of fetal harm. Approximately 21% of prescription drugs fall in this category.

Animal Studies: Researchers found no evidence of fetal harm when this drug was used in pregnant animals.

Human Studies: Controlled studies using this drug in pregnant women have not been done.

Helpful Hints: The American College of Obstetricians and Gynecologists (ACOG) recommends using insulin to treat Types I and II diabetes during pregnancy. For gestational diabetes, or diabetes that develops during pregnancy, ACOG recommends using insulin to treat it if diet therapy alone is not successful.

Remember: All pregnancies have a background risk of about 3% for a major birth defect, even when mom doesn't take a drug of any kind. If you are pregnant or planning a pregnancy, always let your doctor know before taking any drug, prescription or non-prescription, or herbal remedy.

. . . .

ACEBUTOLOL

Brand Name: Sectral

Drug Uses: Acebutolol is approved by the FDA for the treatment of hypertension (high blood pressure) or to prevent an irregular heart rate. This drug belongs to the family of beta-blocker drugs.

Pregnancy Risk Categories: This drug has been assigned two pregnancy risk categories: a **B** rating when used in the first trimester (first 12 weeks of pregnancy), and a **D** rating when used in the second or third trimesters. Approximately 12% of prescription drugs are assigned two pregnancy risk categories, depending on which trimester of pregnancy the drug is used.

> **Category B rating:** The FDA assigns a drug to Category **B** for one of two reasons: (1) Studies show no evidence of fetal harm when using the drug in pregnant animals, but no controlled studies have been done using the drug in pregnant women, or (2) Studies show evidence of fetal harm when using the drug in pregnant animals, but controlled studies using the drug in pregnant women do not show evidence of fetal harm. Approximately 21% of prescription drugs fall in this category.

> **Category D rating:** The FDA assigns a drug to Category **D** when studies of pregnant women using the drug show evidence of fetal harm. Rarely, however, the potential benefit of using the drug in some life-threatening situations for mom may outweigh the potential risk of fetal harm. For example, the drug may be used when mom requires cancer treatment or when she has a serious disease for which safer drugs cannot be used or are less effective. Approximately 11% of prescription drugs fall in this category.

Animal Studies: Researchers found no evidence of fetal harm when this drug was used in pregnant animals.

Human Studies: A limited number of studies using this drug have been done in pregnant women. However, some drugs in this beta-blocker family of drugs are associated with decreased fetal and placental weight when taken during the second and third trimesters. That is mainly why this drug has been assigned a Category **D** rating if used in the second or third trimesters.

Helpful Hints:

1. This drug should only be taken during the second and third trimesters after consulting with your doctor to see if the benefits of using the drug may outweigh the potential risk of fetal harm.

2. This drug weakly interacts with grapefruit and grapefruit juice, which can cause harmful, and even life-threatening, side effects. Before taking this drug with grapefruit juice, or before consuming grapefruit or grapefruit juice during the day while taking this drug, first read the section "Grapefruit Juice–Drug Interactions Can Make You Sick" in the appendix of this book. Then discuss this with your pharmacist or the healthcare provider who prescribed this drug.

Remember: All pregnancies have a background risk of about 3% for a major birth defect. If you are pregnant or planning a pregnancy, always let your doctor know before taking any drug, prescription or non-prescription, or herbal remedy.

· ·

ACETAMINOPHEN

Brand Names: Acetaminophen is used for non-prescription purposes and in combination with other drugs for prescription purposes. Tylenol and Excedrin Extra-Strength tablets are examples of non-prescription brands, while Darvocet, Percocet, and Vicodin are examples of prescription brands of acetaminophen.

Drug Uses: This drug is used to relieve pain for headaches, muscle aches, menstrual periods, colds and sore throats, toothaches, backaches, reactions to vaccine shots, and to reduce fever. Acetaminophen may also be used to relieve the pain of osteoarthritis.

Pregnancy Risk Category: B

Category B rating: The FDA assigns a drug to Category **B** for one of two reasons: (1) Studies show no evidence of fetal harm when using the drug in pregnant animals, but no controlled studies have been done using the drug in pregnant women, or (2) Studies show evidence of fetal harm when using the drug in pregnant animals, but controlled studies using the drug in pregnant women do not show evidence of fetal harm. Approximately 21% of prescription drugs fall in this category.

Animal Studies: No birth defects have been reported in pregnant animals treated with acetaminophen.

Human Studies: Most experts feel that this drug is the analgesic of choice for pregnant women. No birth defects have been reported in pregnant women.

Helpful Hints:

1. When used according to directions, acetaminophen is considered safe for pregnancy as long as the daily dose does not exceed 4,000 mg in patients with normal liver function. For example, taking two-500 mg tablets every six hours would be a typical maximum daily dose. Thus, if one were to take a second drug that contained acetaminophen, one would be exceeding the maximum of 4,000 mg daily and cross over into the higher risk area for liver toxicity and liver failure if the toxic dose were to exceed more than a few days. See "Taking Acetaminophen: The Good and the Ugly" in the appendix of this book for further information.

2. This drug weakly interacts with grapefruit and grapefruit juice, which can cause harmful, and even life-threatening, side effects. Before taking this drug with grapefruit juice, or before consuming grapefruit or grapefruit juice during the day while taking this drug, first read the section "Grapefruit Juice–Drug Interactions Can Make You Sick" in the appendix of this book. Then discuss this with your pharmacist or the healthcare provider who prescribed this drug.

Remember: All pregnancies have a background risk of about 3% for a major birth defect, even when mom doesn't take a drug of any kind. If you are pregnant or planning a pregnancy, always let your doctor know before taking any drug, prescription or non-prescription, or herbal remedy.

. . . .

ACETAZOLAMIDE

Brand Name: Diamox

Drug Uses: Acetazolamide is approved by the FDA for use as a diuretic (fluid pill) and as an anticonvulsant.

Pregnancy Risk Category: C

> **Category C rating:** The FDA assigns a drug to Category **C** for one of two reasons: (1) Studies show evidence of fetal harm when using the drug in pregnant animals, but no controlled studies have been done using the drug in pregnant women, or (2) Studies using the drug in pregnant animals have not been done, and studies of pregnant women using the drug are insufficient to reach a conclusion. Thus, the drug should only be used if the potential benefit for mom is greater than the potential risk of fetal harm, which, in many cases, is unknown. Approximately 50% of prescription drugs fall in this category.

Animal Studies: Fetal limb defects have been found in rodents exposed to the drug during pregnancy, but not in monkeys.

Human Studies: Studies of pregnant women who have used this drug have shown no evidence of fetal harm. Acetazolamide has been widely used for many years and no reports linking it with birth defects have been found.

Remember: All pregnancies have a background risk of about 3% for a major birth defect, even when mom doesn't take a drug of any kind. If you are pregnant or planning a pregnancy, always let your doctor know before taking any drug, prescription or non-prescription, or herbal remedy.

• •

ACETOHEXAMIDE

Brand Name: Dymelor

Drug Use: This drug is approved by the FDA for the oral treatment of adult onset diabetes.

Pregnancy Risk Category: C

> **Category C rating:** The FDA assigns a drug to Category **C** for one of two reasons: (1) Studies show evidence of fetal harm when using the drug in pregnant animals, but no controlled studies have been done using the drug in pregnant women, or (2) Studies using the drug in pregnant animals have not been done, and studies of pregnant women using the drug are insufficient to reach a conclusion. Thus, the drug should only be used if the potential benefit for mom is greater than the potential risk of fetal harm, which, in many cases, is unknown. Approximately 50% of prescription drugs fall in this category.

Animal Studies: This drug has been reported to cause birth defects when used in pregnant animals.

Human Studies: Uncontrolled studies using this drug in pregnant women have shown no evidence of fetal harm.

Helpful Hints: The American College of Obstetricians and Gynecologists (ACOG) recommends using insulin to treat Types 1 and 2 diabetes during pregnancy. If diet therapy alone is not successful for treating gestational diabetes, which is diabetes that develops during pregnancy, ACOG recommends using insulin to treat it, also.

Remember: All pregnancies have a background risk of about 3% for a major birth defect, even when mom doesn't take a drug of any kind. If you are pregnant or planning a pregnancy, always let your doctor know before taking any drug, prescription or non-prescription, or herbal remedy.

• •

ACETOPHENAZINE

Brand Name: Tindal

Drug Use: The FDA has approved this drug for use as a tranquilizer. It is a member of the phenothiazine family of drugs.

Pregnancy Risk Category: C

> **Category C rating:** The FDA assigns a drug to Category C for one of two reasons: (1) Studies show evidence of fetal harm when using the drug in pregnant animals, but no controlled studies have been done using the drug in pregnant women, or (2) Studies using the drug in pregnant animals have not been done, and studies of pregnant women using the drug are insufficient to reach a conclusion. Thus, the drug should only be used if the potential benefit for mom is greater than the potential risk of fetal harm, which, in many cases, is unknown. Approximately 50% of prescription drugs fall in this category.

Animal Studies: No relevant information is available from studies in pregnant animals.

Human Studies: No relevant information is available from studies in pregnant women. According to most experts, the bulk of evidence suggests that members of this family of drugs are safe for pregnant women and their unborn babies.

Remember: All pregnancies have a background risk of about 3% for a major birth defect, even when mom doesn't take a drug of any kind. If you are pregnant or planning a pregnancy, always let your doctor know before taking any drug, prescription or non-prescription, or herbal remedy.

• •

ACETYLCYSTEINE

Brand Names: Acetadote, Mucomyst

Drug Uses: The FDA has approved this drug for use to reduce the thickness of secretions and as an antidote for acetaminophen overdose.

Pregnancy Risk Category: B

> **Category B rating:** The FDA assigns a drug to Category **B** for one of two reasons: (1) Studies show no evidence of fetal harm when using the drug in pregnant animals, but no controlled studies have been done using the drug in pregnant women, or (2) Studies show evidence of fetal harm when using the drug in pregnant animals, but controlled studies using the drug in pregnant women do not show evidence of fetal harm. Approximately 21% of prescription drugs fall in this category.

Animal Studies: No birth defects were found in pregnant animals when exposed to this drug.

Human Studies: Limited data is available from studies in pregnant women. There are no reports of fetal harm from using this drug in pregnant women.

Remember: All pregnancies have a background risk of about 3% for a major birth defect, even when mom doesn't take a drug of any kind. If you are pregnant or planning a pregnancy, always let your doctor know before taking any drug, prescription or non-prescription, or herbal remedy.

• •

ACITRETIN

Brand Name: Soriatane

Drug Uses: This oral drug is used to treat severe psoriasis and other skin disorders in adults.

Pregnancy Risk Category: **X**

> **Category X rating:** The FDA assigns a drug to Category **X** when studies have shown the risk of fetal harm clearly outweighs any potential maternal benefit from the drug. **Drugs in this category should not be used by pregnant women.** Approximately 5% of prescription drugs fall in this category.

Animal Studies: This drug causes birth defects in the offspring of several animals, including mice, rats, and rabbits. It also causes testicular changes in male dogs.

Human Studies: This drug is a potent cause of serious birth defects in pregnant women. It has also been shown that the drug may be stored in maternal fat tissue for three years or more after the drug has been discontinued.

Helpful Hints:

1. Two types of contraception must be used for at least one month before beginning this drug, throughout the course of treatment, and for at least three years after treatment has stopped. Women of childbearing age who are considering treatment with this drug should be told about the drug's very slow elimination and the possibility of an adverse pregnancy outcome if they conceive within three years after stopping treatment.

2. Do not consume alcohol while using this drug and for two months after stopping it. This is because alcohol causes acitretin to linger in the body longer.

3. Because this drug can cause dry eyes, contact lens wearers may become uncomfortable while taking this drug.

4. Acitretin may make you more sensitive to sunlight. Users should avoid prolonged exposure

to the sun, tanning booths, and sunlamps. It is also wise to use a sunscreen and wear protective clothing when outdoors.

5. Users should not donate blood while taking acitretin and for at least three years after treatment is stopped. This will avoid the possibility of your blood being given to a pregnant woman.

Remember: All pregnancies have a background risk of about 3% for a major birth defect, even when mom doesn't take a drug of any kind. If you are pregnant or planning a pregnancy, always let your doctor know before taking any drug, prescription or non-prescription, or herbal remedy.
• •

ACYCLOVIR

Brand Name: Zovirax

Drug Uses: This antiviral drug has been used to treat herpes simplex, herpes zoster, and chicken pox infections.

Pregnancy Risk Category: B

Category B rating: The FDA assigns a drug to Category **B** for one of two reasons: (1) Studies show no evidence of fetal harm when using the drug in pregnant animals, but no controlled studies have been done using the drug in pregnant women, or (2) Studies show evidence of fetal harm when using the drug in pregnant animals, but controlled studies using the drug in pregnant women do not show evidence of fetal harm. Approximately 21% of prescription drugs fall in this category.

Animal Studies: Researchers found no evidence of fetal harm when this drug was used in pregnant rats, mice, and rabbits.

Human Studies: Researchers have found no evidence of fetal harm when this drug was used during pregnancy. This drug has been used in more pregnant women than any other antiviral drug. Since this experience has not shown evidence of fetal harm, most experts consider it safe for use in pregnancy.

Helpful Hints: The sun may cause a skin reaction when using this drug. Avoid prolonged sun exposure and wear sunscreen during treatment.

Remember: All pregnancies have a background risk of about 3% for a major birth defect, even when mom doesn't take a drug of any kind. If you are pregnant or planning a pregnancy, always let your doctor know before taking any drug, prescription or non-prescription, or herbal remedy.

ADENOSINE

Brand Name: Adenocard

Drug Use: Adenosine is approved for the treatment of paroxysmal, supraventricular tachycardia, a specific type of heart rate irregularity.

Pregnancy Risk Category: C

> **Category C rating:** The FDA assigns a drug to Category **C** for one of two reasons: (1) Studies show evidence of fetal harm when using the drug in pregnant animals, but no controlled studies have been done using the drug in pregnant women, or (2) Studies using the drug in pregnant animals have not been done, and studies of pregnant women using the drug are insufficient to reach a conclusion. Thus, the drug should only be used if the potential benefit for mom is greater than the potential risk of fetal harm, which, in many cases, is unknown. Approximately 50% of prescription drugs fall in this category.

Animal Studies: A study using adenosine in pregnant chicks showed that the drug is not associated with birth defects.

Human Studies: A number of case reports have described the safe use of adenosine to treat maternal or fetal supraventricular tachycardia.

Remember: All pregnancies have a background risk of about 3% for a major birth defect, even when mom doesn't take a drug of any kind. If you are pregnant or planning a pregnancy, always let your doctor know before taking any drug, prescription or non-prescription, or herbal remedy.

• •

ALBUTEROL

Brand Names: Proventil, Bentolin, Bolmax

Drug Uses: Albuterol is used to treat wheezing and shortness of breath that may occur with asthma or chronic lung disease. It is also used to treat premature labor and chronic lung disease in infants.

Pregnancy Risk Category: C

> **Category C rating:** The FDA assigns a drug to Category C for one of two reasons: (1) Studies show evidence of fetal harm when using the drug in pregnant animals, but no controlled studies have been done using the drug in pregnant women, or (2) Studies using the drug in pregnant animals have not been done, and studies of pregnant women using the drug are insufficient to reach a conclusion. Thus, the drug should only be used if the potential benefit for mom is greater than the potential risk of fetal harm, which, in many cases, is unknown. Approximately 50% of prescription drugs fall in this category.

Animal Studies: Cleft palate has been reported in the offspring of pregnant mice treated with this drug. Skull defects have also been observed in the offspring of rabbits treated with extremely high doses of this drug.

Human Studies: There are no controlled studies using this drug in pregnant women. However, we could not find any reports linking albuterol to human birth defects.

One authority recommends avoiding this drug during the first trimester if possible. However, other experts might disagree.

Remember: All pregnancies have a background risk of about 3% for a major birth defect, even when mom doesn't take a drug of any kind. If you are pregnant or planning a pregnancy, always let your doctor know before taking any drug, prescription or non-prescription, or herbal remedy.

. . . .

ALENDRONATE

Brand Name: Fosamax

Drug Use: Alendronate is used to prevent or treat osteoporosis.

Pregnancy Risk Category: C

> **Category C rating:** The FDA assigns a drug to Category C for one of two reasons: (1) Studies show evidence of fetal harm when using the drug in pregnant animals, but no controlled studies have been done using the drug in pregnant women, or (2) Studies using the drug in pregnant animals have not been done, and studies of pregnant women using the drug are insufficient to reach a conclusion. Thus, the drug should only be used if the potential benefit for mom is greater than the potential risk of fetal harm, which, in many cases, is unknown. Approximately 50% of prescription drugs fall in this category.

Animal Studies: Studies in pregnant rats treated with alendronate have shown toxic effects on the mother as well as her fetus. However, the drug did not cause birth defects.

Human Studies: Controlled studies using this drug in pregnant women have not been done.

Helpful Hints: This drug did not cause birth defects in animals. However, in rats, it did cause toxic effects on the mother and her fetus. If this drug is used during pregnancy, doctors are encouraged to call the toll-free number (800-670-6126) for information about enrolling the patient in the Mother-Risk Study.

Remember: All pregnancies have a background risk of about 3% for a major birth defect, even when mom doesn't take a drug of any kind. If you are pregnant or planning a pregnancy, always let your doctor know before taking any drug, prescription or non-prescription, or herbal remedy.

• •

ALFENTANIL

Brand Name: Alfenta

Drug Use: This drug is approved by the FDA for use as a strong narcotic pain killer.

Pregnancy Risk Categories: This drug has been assigned two pregnancy risk categories: **C** when used throughout most of pregnancy, but **D** if used for prolonged periods or in high doses near the time of birth. Approximately 12% of prescription drugs are assigned two pregnancy risk categories, depending on which trimester of pregnancy the drug is used.

Category C rating: The FDA assigns a drug to Category **C** for one of two reasons: (1) Studies show evidence of fetal harm when using the drug in pregnant animals, but no controlled studies have been done using the drug in pregnant women, or (2) Studies using the drug in pregnant animals have not been done, and studies of pregnant women using the drug are insufficient to reach a conclusion. Thus, the drug should only be used if the potential benefit for mom is greater than the potential risk of fetal harm, which, in many cases, is unknown. Approximately 50% of prescription drugs fall in this category.

Category D rating: The FDA assigns a drug to Category **D** when studies of pregnant women using the drug show evidence of fetal harm. Rarely, however, the potential benefit of using the drug in some life-threatening situations for mom may outweigh the potential risk of fetal harm. For example, when mom requires cancer treatment or when she has a serious disease for which safer drugs cannot be used or are less effective. Approximately 11% of prescription drugs fall in this category.

Animal Studies: Animal studies in pregnant rats and rabbits treated with this drug showed no evidence of birth defects in the offspring.

Human Studies: Limited studies in pregnant women show no ill effects from using this drug. However, as with all narcotic pain killers, respiratory depression in the newborn immediately after birth is a potential complication. If a baby is depressed from the use of this drug, the effect can be quickly reversed with naloxone. The potential for respiratory depression is why this drug was assigned to a **D** category if used for prolonged periods or at term.

Helpful Hints: This drug weakly interacts with grapefruit and grapefruit juice, which can cause harmful, and even life-threatening, side effects. Before taking this drug with grapefruit juice, or before consuming grapefruit or grapefruit juice during the day while taking this drug, first read the section "Grapefruit Juice–Drug Interactions Can Make You Sick" in the appendix of this book. Then discuss this with your pharmacist or the healthcare provider who prescribed this drug.

Remember: All pregnancies have a background risk of about 3% for a major birth defect, even when mom doesn't take a drug of any kind. If you are pregnant or planning a pregnancy, always let your doctor know before taking any drug, prescription or non-prescription, or herbal remedy.

· ·

ALLOPURINOL

Brand Names: Lopurin, Zurinol, Zyloprin, Aloprin

Drug Use: Basically this drug is used to lower high levels of uric acid caused by one of several conditions, including gout, certain types of kidney stones, and patients receiving chemotherapy for cancer. Cancer cells that are destroyed with therapy release large amounts of uric acid into the bloodstream.

Pregnancy Risk Category: C

> **Category C rating:** The FDA assigns a drug to Category C for one of two reasons: (1) Studies show evidence of fetal harm when using the drug in pregnant animals, but no controlled studies have been done using the drug in pregnant women, or (2) Studies using the drug in pregnant animals have not been done, and studies of pregnant women using the drug are insufficient to reach a conclusion. Thus, the drug should only be used if the potential benefit for mom is greater than the potential risk of fetal harm, which, in many cases, is unknown. Approximately 50% of prescription drugs fall in this category.

Animal Studies: Studies in pregnant animals exposed to this drug have shown conflicting and inconclusive results. In studies done over 40 years ago, allopurinol produced cleft palate and skeletal defects in mice. However, in other animal studies, no fetal harm was found.

Human Studies: No fetal harm has been linked to the offspring of pregnant women using this drug. However, controlled studies have not been done.

Helpful Hints: According to one expert, this drug should be avoided during the first three months of pregnancy and only used during the last six months if clearly indicated. However, not all experts agree and use this drug throughout pregnancy. Thus, it becomes very important for you to discuss the potential risks and potential benefits of using this drug during pregnancy with your doctor.

Remember: All pregnancies have a background risk of about 3% for a major birth defect, even when mom doesn't take a drug of any kind. If you are pregnant or planning a pregnancy, always let your doctor know before taking any drug, prescription or non-prescription, or herbal remedy.

· ·

ALPRAZOLAM

Brand Name: Xanax

Drug Use: Alprazolam is used to treat anxiety and panic disorder and is a member of the benzodiazepine family of drugs.

Pregnancy Risk Category: D

> **Category D rating:** The FDA assigns a drug to Category **D** when studies of pregnant women using the drug show evidence of fetal harm. Rarely, however, the potential benefit of using the drug in some life-threatening situations for mom may outweigh the potential risk of fetal harm. For example, when mom requires cancer treatment or when she has a serious disease for which safer drugs cannot be used or are less effective. Approximately 11% of prescription drugs fall in this category.

Animal Studies: Although a limited amount of information is available from animal studies using this specific drug, a closely related member of the benzodiazepine family of drugs—diazepam—has been shown to cause cleft palate in mice and defects involving the skeleton in rats.

Human Studies: Controlled studies using alprazolam in pregnant women have not been done. However, some reports have suggested an association between diazepam and fetal cleft palate and heart defects. In addition, withdrawal symptoms after exposure to alprazolam throughout pregnancy have been reported in several newborns.

Helpful Hints:

1. Alprazolam is not recommended for use in pregnancy because it may cause significant birth defects, more by association with diazepam than anything else, and because it has been associated with withdrawal symptoms in newborns.

2. If this drug has been taken for a long time, do not stop it abruptly. Withdrawal symptoms, including seizures, may result. The dose should be gradually reduced to help prevent this kind of reaction.

3. The brand name **Xanax** is similar to the brand name **Zantac**, which is used to treat peptic ulcers and heartburn. Because the two brand names are similar, this can lead to serious medication errors.

4. This drug weakly interacts with grapefruit and grapefruit juice, which can cause harmful, and even life-threatening, side effects. Before taking this drug with grapefruit juice, or before consuming grapefruit or grapefruit juice during the day while taking this drug, first read the section "Grapefruit Juice–Drug Interactions Can Make You Sick" in the appendix of this book. Then discuss this with your pharmacist or the healthcare provider who prescribed this drug.

Remember: All pregnancies have a background risk of about 3% for a major birth defect, even when mom doesn't take a drug of any kind. If you are pregnant or planning a pregnancy, always let your doctor know

before taking any drug, prescription or non-prescription, or herbal remedy.
· ·

AMANTADINE

Brand Name: Symmetrel

Drug Uses: Amantadine is approved by the FDA for several uses: (1) to prevent or treat Influenza A; (2) to treat Parkinson's disease; (3) to treat certain side effects caused by drugs, chemicals, and other medical conditions.

Pregnancy Risk Category: C

> **Category C rating:** The FDA assigns a drug to Category C for one of two reasons: (1) Studies show evidence of fetal harm when using the drug in pregnant animals, but no controlled studies have been done using the drug in pregnant women, or (2) Studies using the drug in pregnant animals have not been done, and studies of pregnant women using the drug are insufficient to reach a conclusion. Thus, the drug should only be used if the potential benefit for mom is greater than the potential risk of fetal harm, which, in many cases, is unknown. Approximately 50% of prescription drugs fall in this category.

Animal Studies: Birth defects have been reported in the offspring of pregnant rats exposed to this drug, but not in the offspring of pregnant rabbits.

Human Studies: Since this drug is uncommonly used during pregnancy, there is very little information available about its use in pregnant women. In a survey study of pregnant women on Medicaid, a slightly greater number of babies of mothers who were taking this drug had birth defects than expected. However, no controlled studies of pregnant women using this drug have been done. Several experts believe this drug should not be used during the first 12 weeks of pregnancy.

Remember: All pregnancies have a background risk of about 3% for a major birth defect, even when mom doesn't take a drug of any kind. If you are pregnant or planning a pregnancy, always let your doctor know before taking any drug, prescription or non-prescription, or herbal remedy.

• •

AMIKACIN

Brand Name: Amikin

Drug Use: Amikacin is approved by the FDA for use as an antibiotic and is a member of the aminoglycoside antibiotic family of drugs.

Pregnancy Risk Category: C

Category C rating: The FDA assigns a drug to Category **C** for one of two reasons: (1) Studies show evidence of fetal harm when using the drug in pregnant animals, but no controlled studies have been done using the drug in pregnant women, or (2) Studies using the drug in pregnant animals have not been done, and studies of pregnant women using the drug are insufficient to reach a conclusion. Thus, the drug should only be used if the potential benefit for mom is greater than the potential risk of fetal harm, which, in many cases, is unknown. Approximately 50% of prescription drugs fall in this category.

Animal Studies: Amikacin has been shown to have a dose-related toxic effect on the kidneys in pregnant rats and their fetuses. However, other studies in pregnant mice and rats have shown no evidence of causing birth defects.

Human Studies: There have been no birth defects in pregnant women associated with the use of amikacin. Also, hearing toxicity, which is known to occur after amikacin treatment in humans, has not been reported as an effect of fetal exposure during pregnancy. However, exposure to other members of the aminoglycoside antibiotic family has resulted in fetal harm.

Helpful Hints: According to the drug's manufacturer, the amikacin pregnancy risk category should be D based primarily on the potential for hearing toxicity when using this drug before birth. Overall, however, human data suggests this drug has a low risk of causing fetal harm.

Remember: All pregnancies have a background risk of about 3% for a major birth defect, even when mom doesn't take a drug of any kind. If you are pregnant or planning a pregnancy, always let your doctor know before taking any drug, prescription or non-prescription, or herbal remedy.

. . . .

AMILORIDE

Brand Name: Midamor

Drug Uses: Amiloride is a diuretic (water pill) used to treat congestive heart failure and high blood pressure.

Pregnancy Risk Categories: This drug has been assigned to two pregnancy risk categories: **B** because studies in pregnant animals did not show a risk for fetal birth defects, but data from controlled studies in pregnant women was not available. However, the drug has also been assigned a risk category of **D** if used to treat gestational hypertension because maternal hypovolemia (low blood volume) is typical of this condition, making the use of a "water pill" unnecessary and even dangerous for mother and baby. Thus, this drug should only be used when clearly needed in pregnancy. Approximately 12% of prescription drugs are assigned two pregnancy risk categories, depending on which trimester of pregnancy the drug is used.

> **Category B rating:** The FDA assigns a drug to Category **B** for one of two reasons: (1) Studies show no evidence of fetal harm when using the drug in pregnant animals, but no controlled studies have

been done using the drug in pregnant women, or (2) Studies show evidence of fetal harm when using the drug in pregnant animals, but controlled studies using the drug in pregnant women do not show evidence of fetal harm. Approximately 21% of prescription drugs fall in this category.

Category D rating: The FDA assigns a drug to Category **D** when studies of pregnant women who use the drug show evidence of fetal harm. Rarely, however, the potential benefit of using the drug in some life-threatening situations for mom may outweigh the potential risk of fetal harm. For example, when mom requires cancer treatment or when she has a serious disease for which safer drugs cannot be used or are less effective. Approximately 11% of prescription drugs fall in this category.

Animal Studies: No birth defects have been reported in pregnant mice and rabbits treated with this drug.

Human Studies: Limited data is available for pregnant women treated with amiloride.

Remember: All pregnancies have a background risk of about 3% for a major birth defect, even when mom doesn't take a drug of any kind. If you are pregnant or planning a pregnancy, always let your doctor know before taking any drug, prescription or non-prescription, or herbal remedy.

AMINOCAPROIC ACID

Brand Name: Amicar

Drug Use: This drug is used to treat excessive bleeding caused by problems with blood clotting.

Pregnancy Risk Category: C

Category C rating: The FDA assigns a drug to Category **C** for one of two reasons: (1) Studies show evidence of fetal harm when using the drug in pregnant animals, but no controlled studies have been done using the drug in pregnant women, or (2) Studies using the drug in pregnant animals have not been done, and studies of pregnant women using the drug are insufficient to reach a conclusion. Thus, the drug should only be used if the potential benefit for

mom is greater than the potential risk of fetal harm, which, in many cases, is unknown. Approximately 50% of prescription drugs fall in this category.

Animal Studies: Controlled studies in pregnant animals have not been done.

Human Studies: Controlled studies using this drug in pregnant women have not been done. In one case report, however, no fetal toxicity was observed.

Helpful Hints: Since this drug has not been formally studied in animals or pregnant women, we don't know what risk it poses for the fetus. This makes it extremely difficult to assess the risk versus the potential benefit before prescribing this drug.

Remember: All pregnancies have a background risk of about 3% for a major birth defect, even when mom doesn't take a drug of any kind. If you are pregnant or planning a pregnancy, always let your doctor know before taking any drug, prescription or non-prescription, or herbal remedy.

AMINOPHYLLINE

Brand Name: Aminophyllin

Drug Use: Aminophylline is approved by the FDA for the treatment of asthma. Since it is actually 79% theophylline, we will use the theophylline profile for further details.

Pregnancy Risk Category: C

Category C rating: The FDA assigns a drug to Category C for one of two reasons: (1) Studies show evidence of fetal harm when using the drug in pregnant animals, but no controlled studies have been done using the drug in pregnant women, or (2) Studies using the drug in pregnant animals have not been done, and studies of pregnant women using the drug are insufficient to reach a conclusion. Thus, the drug should only be used if the potential benefit for mom is greater than the potential risk of fetal harm, which, in many cases, is unknown. Approximately 50% of prescription drugs fall in this category.

Animal Studies: Studies performed on pregnant mice and rats using theophylline showed no evidence of fetal harm.

Human Studies: In the limited human studies that are available, no evidence was found for a link between this drug's use and fetal birth defects.

Helpful Hints: Theophylline crosses the placenta readily. As a result, previously exposed newborns may have significant levels of the drug in their blood at birth. This may create a rapid heart rate, irritability, and vomiting, explaining why the drug was assigned a pregnancy risk rating of **C**.

Remember: All pregnancies have a background risk of about 3% for a major birth defect, even when mom doesn't take a drug of any kind. If you are pregnant or planning a pregnancy, always let your doctor know before taking any drug, prescription or non-prescription, or herbal remedy.

AMIODARONE

Brand Names: Cardarone, Braxan, Pacerone

Drug Use: This drug is approved by the FDA for the treatment of cardiac arrhythmias (abnormal heart rhythms).

Pregnancy Risk Category: D

Category D rating: The FDA assigns a drug to Category **D** when studies of pregnant women using the drug show evidence of fetal harm. Rarely, however, the potential benefit of using the drug in some life-threatening situations for mom may outweigh the potential risk of fetal harm. For example, when mom requires cancer treatment or when she has a serious disease for which safer drugs cannot be used or are less effective. Approximately 11% of prescription drugs fall in this category.

Animal Studies: Studies in pregnant rats and rabbits have shown toxic maternal and fetal effects. These effects include spontaneous abortions, decreased live litter size, and growth retardation.

Human Studies: No controlled studies of pregnant women are available. However, various case reports of pregnant women treated with this drug reveal serious fetal effects including congenital goiter, hypothyroidism, and hyperthyroidism.

Helpful Hints:

1. This drug strongly interacts with grapefruit and grapefruit juice, which can cause harmful, and even life-threatening, side effects. Before taking this drug with grapefruit juice, or before consuming grapefruit or grapefruit juice during the day while taking this drug, first read the section "Grapefruit Juice–Drug Interactions Can Make You Sick" in the appendix of this book. Then discuss this with your pharmacist or the healthcare provider who prescribed this drug.

2. Since this drug takes a long time to be eliminated from the body, it should be discontinued several months before conception to avoid fetal exposure early in pregnancy.

3. Newborns who have been exposed to this drug during pregnancy may need to have thyroid studies performed after birth.

Remember: All pregnancies have a background risk of about 3% for a major birth defect, even when mom

doesn't take a drug of any kind. If you are pregnant or planning a pregnancy, always let your doctor know before taking any drug, prescription or non-prescription, or herbal remedy.

. . . .

AMITRIPTYLINE

Brand Names: Amitid, Amitril, Elavil

Drug Uses: This drug is approved by the FDA for the treatment of depression. It is also used to treat anxiety, bipolar disorder, certain types of pain, chronic fatigue, panic disorder, and post-traumatic stress.

Pregnancy Risk Category: C

> **Category C rating:** The FDA assigns a drug to Category C for one of two reasons: (1) Studies show evidence of fetal harm when using the drug in pregnant animals, but no controlled studies have been done using the drug in pregnant women, or (2) Studies using the drug in pregnant animals have not been done, and studies of pregnant women using the drug are insufficient to reach a conclusion. Thus, the drug should only be used if the potential benefit for mom is greater than the potential risk of fetal harm, which, in many cases, is unknown. Approximately 50% of prescription drugs fall in this category.

Animal Studies: Extremely high doses of this drug in pregnant mice, hamsters, rats, and rabbits have caused birth defects in their offspring.

Human Studies: Birth defects have been found in babies born to pregnant women using this drug, but not significantly more than expected in the untreated population. Controlled studies in pregnant women have not been done.

Helpful Hints:

   1. Studies show that antidepressants increase the risk of suicidal thinking and behavior in children,

adolescents, and young adults. Anyone considering the use of this drug or any other antidepressant in these patients must balance that risk with the clinical need.

2. Almost all antidepressants carry some risk to the developing fetus. However, we also know depression in a pregnant woman carries potential risk for her and her unborn baby's health. For example, a higher percentage of depressed pregnant women tend to have low birth weight and premature babies than non-depressed pregnant women. The risks and benefits of medications and untreated depression must be weighed carefully. If you are pregnant and think you may have depression, or if you already know you do, talk with your doctor so the two of you can create the right plan for you and your unborn baby. (See "Antidepressants in Pregnancy" in the appendix for more details.)

Remember: All pregnancies have a background risk of about 3% for a major birth defect, even when mom doesn't take a drug of any kind. If you are pregnant or planning a pregnancy, always let your doctor know before taking any drug, prescription or non-prescription, or herbal remedy.

· ·

AMLODIPINE

Brand Names: Norvasc, Lotrel

Drug Uses: This drug is approved by the FDA for the treatment of high blood pressure and chest pain. This drug is a member of the calcium channel blocker family of drugs.

Pregnancy Risk Category: C

Category C rating: The FDA assigns a drug to Category C for one of two reasons: (1) Studies show evidence of fetal harm when using the drug in pregnant animals, but no controlled studies have been done using the drug in pregnant women, or (2) Studies using the drug in pregnant animals have not been done, and studies of pregnant women using the drug are insufficient to reach a conclusion. Thus, the drug should only be used if the potential benefit for mom is greater than the potential risk of fetal harm, which, in many cases, is unknown. Approximately 50% of prescription drugs fall in this category.

Animal Studies: When very high doses were given to rats for 14 days before mating and throughout pregnancy, litter size was reduced and the number of fetal deaths was increased.

Human Studies: There are no reports of controlled studies using this drug in pregnant women.

Helpful Hints:

1. One expert recommends avoiding this drug during the first trimester or 12 weeks of pregnancy and only using it during the last six months if clearly needed. Other experts, however, are not so cautious in their assessment.

2. Excessive exposure to the sun while taking this drug has resulted in several case reports of phototoxicity.

3. This drug weakly interacts with grapefruit and grapefruit juice, which can cause harmful, and even life-threatening, side effects. Before taking this drug with grapefruit juice, or before consuming grapefruit or grapefruit juice during the day while taking this drug, first read the section "Grapefruit Juice–Drug Interactions Can Make You Sick" in the appendix of this book. Then

discuss this with your pharmacist or the health-care provider who prescribed this drug.

Remember: All pregnancies have a background risk of about 3% for a major birth defect, even when mom doesn't take a drug of any kind. If you are pregnant or planning a pregnancy, always let your doctor know before taking any drug, prescription or non-prescription, or herbal remedy.

. . . .

AMOXAPINE

Brand Name: Asendin

Drug Use: This drug is approved by the FDA for the treatment of depression.

Pregnancy Risk Category: C

> **Category C rating:** The FDA assigns a drug to Category C for one of two reasons: (1) Studies show evidence of fetal harm when using the drug in pregnant animals, but no controlled studies have been done using the drug in pregnant women, or (2) Studies using the drug in pregnant animals have not been done, and studies of pregnant women using the drug are insufficient to reach a conclusion. Thus, the drug should only be used if the potential benefit for mom is greater than the potential risk of fetal harm, which, in many cases, is unknown. Approximately 50% of prescription drugs fall in this category.

Animal Studies: No birth defects were found in pregnant mice, rats, and rabbits treated with this drug.

Human Studies: Birth defects have been noted in some infants born to moms taking amoxapine. However, the number of exposures was too small to reach a definitive conclusion.

Helpful Hints:

1. Studies show that antidepressants increase the risk of suicidal thinking and behavior in children,

adolescents, and young adults. Anyone considering the use of this drug or any other antidepressant
in these patients must balance that risk with the
clinical need.

2. Almost all antidepressants carry some risk to the
    developing fetus. However, we also know de-
    pression in a pregnant woman carries potential
    risk for her health and for her unborn baby; for
    example, low birth weight and prematurity. The
    risks and benefits of medications and untreated
    depression must be weighed carefully. If you are
    pregnant and think you may have depression, or
    if you already know you do, talk with your doc-
    tor so the two of you can create the right plan for
    you and your unborn baby. (See "Antidepressants
    in Pregnancy" in the appendix for more details.)

Remember: All pregnancies have a background risk of
about 3% for a major birth defect, even when mom doesn't
take a drug of any kind. If you are pregnant or planning a
pregnancy, always let your doctor know before taking any
drug, prescription or non-prescription, or herbal remedy.

AMOXICILLIN

Brand Names: Amoxil, Trimox

Drug Use: This drug is approved by the FDA for the
treatment of a variety of bacterial infections. It is a member of the penicillin antibiotic family of drugs.

Pregnancy Risk Category: B

Category B rating: The FDA assigns a drug to Category **B** for one
of two reasons: (1) Studies show no evidence of fetal harm when
using the drug in pregnant animals, but no controlled studies have
been done using the drug in pregnant women, or (2) Studies show

evidence of fetal harm when using the drug in pregnant animals, but controlled studies using the drug in pregnant women do not show evidence of fetal harm. Approximately 21% of prescription drugs fall in this category.

Animal Studies: There have been no reports linking amoxicillin to birth defects in pregnant rats or mice.

Human Studies: A survey study of pregnant women taking this drug showed no increase in babies born with birth defects compared to pregnant women not taking the drug.

Helpful Hints: In general, this family of drugs is considered safe for use during pregnancy. However, amoxicillin may decrease the effectiveness of combination-type birth control pills, resulting in pregnancy. You may need to take an additional form of reliable birth control while using this drug.

Remember: All pregnancies have a background risk of about 3% for a major birth defect, even when mom doesn't take a drug of any kind. If you are pregnant or planning a pregnancy, always let your doctor know before taking any drug, prescription or non-prescription, or herbal remedy.

AMPHETAMINE

Brand Name: Adderall

Drug Uses: This drug is approved by the FDA for the treatment of attention deficit-hyperactivity disorder (ADHD). Amphetamines have also been used for appetite suppression and to treat narcolepsy. The drug is also used for illicit purposes.

Pregnancy Risk Category: C

Category C rating: The FDA assigns a drug to Category C for one of two reasons: (1) Studies show evidence of fetal harm when using the drug in pregnant animals, but no controlled studies have been done using the drug in pregnant women, or (2) Studies using the drug in pregnant animals have not been done, and studies of pregnant women using the drug are insufficient to reach a conclusion. Thus, the drug should only be used if the potential benefit for mom is greater than the potential risk of fetal harm, which, in many cases, is unknown. Approximately 50% of prescription drugs fall in this category.

Animal Studies: Studies using this drug in pregnant mice revealed no evidence of fetal harm in the offspring.

Human Studies: There is no data from controlled studies in pregnant women. Although the use of amphetamines for medical purposes does not seem to pose a risk in pregnant women for birth defects in their babies, mild withdrawal symptoms have been reported in their newborns after birth. The relatively few follow-up studies of these babies have not shown long-term adverse effects.

Helpful Hints: The illicit use of amphetamines during pregnancy is another story. Some of these babies have been under grown, premature, and at risk for long-term health problems. These babies are often exposed to multiple drugs during pregnancy and poor maternal health.

Remember: All pregnancies have a background risk of about 3% for a major birth defect, even when mom doesn't take a drug of any kind. If you are pregnant or planning a pregnancy, always let your doctor know before taking any drug, prescription or non-prescription, or herbal remedy.

AMPHOTERICIN B

Brand Names: Amphocin, Amphoteric B, Fungizone

Drug Use: This drug is approved by the FDA for treating serious fungal infections.

Pregnancy Risk Category: **B**

Category B rating: The FDA assigns a drug to Category **B** for one of two reasons: (1) Studies show no evidence of fetal harm when using the drug in pregnant animals, but no controlled studies have been done using the drug in pregnant women, or (2) Studies show evidence of fetal harm when using the drug in pregnant animals, but controlled studies using the drug in pregnant women do not show evidence of fetal harm. Approximately 21% of prescription drugs fall in this category.

Animal Studies: Researchers have found no evidence of major fetal birth defects when this drug was used in pregnant animals.

Human Studies: There are no controlled studies using this drug in pregnant women. Follow-up studies have shown no evidence of harmful fetal effects when this drug was used in pregnancy.

Remember: All pregnancies have a background risk of about 3% for a major birth defect, even when mom doesn't take a drug of any kind. If you are pregnant or planning a pregnancy, always let your doctor know before taking any drug, prescription or non-prescription, or herbal remedy.

· ·

AMPICILLIN

Brand Names: Principen, Ampicil, Omnipen

Drug Use: This antibiotic is approved by the FDA for the treatment of bacterial infections. It is a member of the penicillin family of antibiotics.

Pregnancy Risk Category: **B**

Category B rating: The FDA assigns a drug to Category **B** for one of two reasons: (1) Studies show no evidence of fetal harm when using the drug in pregnant animals, but no controlled studies have been done using the drug in pregnant women, or (2) Studies show evidence of fetal harm when using the drug in pregnant animals, but controlled studies using the drug in pregnant women do not show evidence of fetal harm. Approximately 21% of prescription drugs fall in this category.

Animal Studies: There are no reports of significant birth defects in pregnant animals treated with this drug.

Human Studies: Studies in pregnant women have not shown a relationship between taking this drug during pregnancy and birth defects.

Remember: All pregnancies have a background risk of about 3% for a major birth defect, even when mom doesn't take a drug of any kind. If you are pregnant or planning a pregnancy, always let your doctor know before taking any drug, prescription or non-prescription, or herbal remedy.

· ·

ANAKINRA

Brand Name: Kineret

Drug Use: The FDA has approved this drug for use alone or in combination with other drugs to reduce the pain and swelling of rheumatoid arthritis.

Pregnancy Risk Category: B

Category B rating: The FDA assigns a drug to Category **B** for one of two reasons: (1) Studies show no evidence of fetal harm when using the drug in pregnant animals, but no controlled studies have been done using the drug in pregnant women, or (2) Studies show evidence of fetal harm when using the drug in pregnant animals, but controlled studies using the drug in pregnant women do not show evidence of fetal harm. Approximately 21% of prescription drugs fall in this category.

Animal Studies: Studies in pregnant rats and rabbits treated with this drug showed no evidence of fetal harm.

Human Studies: There are no reported controlled studies on pregnant women taking this drug.

Remember: All pregnancies have a background risk of about 3% for a major birth defect, even when mom doesn't take a drug of any kind. If you are pregnant or planning a pregnancy, always let your doctor know before taking any drug, prescription or non-prescription, or herbal remedy.

• •

ANASTROZOLE

Brand Name: Arimidex

Drug Use: This drug is approved by the FDA for treating breast cancer.

Pregnancy Risk Category: D

> **Category D rating:** The FDA assigns a drug to Category **D** when studies of pregnant women using the drug show evidence of fetal harm. Rarely, however, the potential benefit of using the drug in some life-threatening situations for mom may outweigh the potential risk of fetal harm. For example, when mom requires cancer treatment or when she has a serious disease for which safer drugs cannot be used or are less effective. Approximately 11% of prescription drugs fall in this category.

Animal Studies: No fetal harm was reported when this drug was used in pregnant animals.

Human Studies: There are no controlled studies using this drug in pregnant women.

Remember: All pregnancies have a background risk of about 3% for a major birth defect, even when mom doesn't take a drug of any kind. If you are pregnant or planning a pregnancy, always let your doctor know before taking any drug, prescription or non-prescription, or herbal remedy.

. . . .

ASPIRIN

Brand Names: Aspirin, Anacin, Bufferin, Darvon, Empirin, Excedrin

Drug Uses: This drug is approved by the FDA for the treatment of pain and symptoms and conditions characterized by inflammation and fever. It is also used in low doses to prevent the first heart attack. In addition, aspirin also has many unapproved uses. Aspirin is also a member of the non-steroidal anti-inflammatory (NSAIDs) family of drugs. (See Helpful Hint #2 on next page.)

Pregnancy Risk Categories: This drug has been assigned two pregnancy risk categories: Category **C** when used in the first two trimesters of pregnancy, and **D** when used in the third trimester of pregnancy. Approximately 12% of prescription drugs are assigned two pregnancy risk categories, depending on which trimester of pregnancy the drug is used.

> **Category C rating:** The FDA assigns a drug to Category **C** for one of two reasons: (1) Studies show evidence of fetal harm when using the drug in pregnant animals, but no controlled studies have been done using the drug in pregnant women, or (2) Studies using the drug in pregnant animals have not been done, and studies of pregnant women using the drug are insufficient to reach a conclusion. Thus, the drug should only be used if the potential benefit for mom is greater than the potential risk of fetal harm, which, in many cases, is unknown. Approximately 50% of prescription drugs fall in this category.

> **Category D rating:** The FDA assigns a drug to Category **D** when studies of pregnant women using the drug show evidence of fetal harm. Rarely, however, the potential benefit of using the drug in some life-threatening situations for mom may outweigh the potential risk of fetal harm. For example, when mom requires cancer treatment or when she has a serious disease for which safer drugs cannot be used or are less effective. Approximately 11% of prescription drugs fall in this category.

Animal Studies: Birth defects associated with aspirin treatment have been reported in pregnant animals.

Human Studies: Studies of pregnant women suggest no significant risk of birth defects in women taking aspirin. However, the regular use of aspirin in pregnancy, especially in high doses, should be avoided. The drug may affect both mothers' and babies' clotting ability, leading to increased risk of bleeding. When used in the third trimester of pregnancy, members of the non-steroidal anti-inflammatory family of drugs, including aspirin, have the potential to cause persistent pulmonary hypertension, which is another way of saying high blood pressure in the lungs. This can result in respiratory distress at birth and become a life-threatening condition. In addition, the use of non-steroidal anti-inflammatory drugs near the time of delivery has been associated with infection of the intestine, bleeding in the brain, and other complications. Therefore, when taken in the third trimester of pregnancy, especially near delivery, aspirin has been assigned a **D** rating.

Helpful Hints:

1. It is important to remember that aspirin should not be taken by children or even teenagers with a viral infection because of an increase of Reye's Syndrome, a sometimes fatal liver disease.

2. When taken in the third trimester of pregnancy, NSAIDs have seriously harmed the fetus, leading to life-threatening illness after birth and even death. These potential effects apply to all NSAIDs, whether purchased by prescription or over-the-counter without a prescription. They also explain why NSAIDs have been assigned a

> **D** pregnancy risk category. (See "Non-Steroidal,
> Anti-Inflammatory Drugs (NSAIDs) in Preg-
> nancy" in the appendix for more details.)

Remember: All pregnancies have a background risk of
about 3% for a major birth defect, even when mom doesn't
take a drug of any kind. If you are pregnant or planning
a pregnancy, always let your doctor know before taking any drug, prescription or non-prescription, or herbal
remedy.

• •

ATENOLOL

Brand Name: Tenormin

Drug Uses: Atenolol is approved by the FDA for the
treatment of the following: (1) angina pectorus (chest
pain); (2) high blood pressure, and; (3) following a heart
attack to reduce the risk of reoccurrence.

Pregnancy Risk Category: D

> **Category D rating:** The FDA assigns a drug to Category **D** when
> studies of pregnant women using the drug show evidence of fetal
> harm. Rarely, however, the potential benefit of using the drug in
> some life-threatening situations for mom may outweigh the poten-
> tial risk of fetal harm. For example, when mom requires cancer
> treatment or when she has a serious disease for which safer drugs
> cannot be used or are less effective. Approximately 11% of pre-
> scription drugs fall in this category.

Animal Studies: Although no birth defects have been
reported in pregnant animals treated with atenolol, several studies have shown an increased loss of pregnancy
in pregnant rats.

Human Studies: No birth defects have been associated
with pregnant women treated with atenolol. However, it
may cause reduced fetal growth and decreased placental

weight, accounting for the Category **D** rating in the second and third trimesters of pregnancy.

Helpful Hints: Newborns exposed to atenolol near the time of delivery should be observed closely for signs and symptoms of a low heart rate or low blood pressure during the first few days after birth.

Remember: All pregnancies have a background risk of about 3% for a major birth defect, even when mom doesn't take a drug of any kind. If you are pregnant or planning a pregnancy, always let your doctor know before taking any drug, prescription or non-prescription, or herbal remedy.

. . . .

ATOMOXETINE

Brand Name: Strattera

Drug Use: This drug is approved by the FDA for the treatment of attention deficit hyperactivity disorder (ADHD). It belongs to a family of drugs called selective norepinephrine reuptake inhibitors (SNRIs).

Pregnancy Risk Category: C

> **Category C rating:** The FDA assigns a drug to Category C for one of two reasons: (1) Studies show evidence of fetal harm when using the drug in pregnant animals, but no controlled studies have been done using the drug in pregnant women, or (2) Studies using the drug in pregnant animals have not been done, and studies of pregnant women using the drug are insufficient to reach a conclusion. Thus, the drug should only be used if the potential benefit for mom is greater than the potential risk of fetal harm, which, in many cases, is unknown. Approximately 50% of prescription drugs fall in this category.

Animal Studies: Studies in pregnant rats and rabbits treated with this drug have raised some concerns about pup weight and survival.

Human Studies: Since there are a limited number of studies using this drug in pregnant women, it makes it difficult to draw conclusions about fetal risk. If mom's condition requires treatment with this drug during pregnancy, it is prudent to use the lowest effective dose and to try to avoid first trimester use.

Remember: All pregnancies have a background risk of about 3% for a major birth defect, even when mom doesn't take a drug of any kind. If you are pregnant or planning a pregnancy, always let your doctor know before taking any drug, prescription or non-prescription, or herbal remedy.

ATORVASTATIN

Brand Name: Lipitor

Drug Use: This drug is approved by the FDA for the treatment of high cholesterol levels. Atorvastatin is a member of the "statin" family of drugs used to treat high levels of cholesterol.

Pregnancy Risk Category: X

> **Category X rating:** The FDA assigns a drug to Category **X** when studies have shown the risk of fetal harm clearly outweighs any potential maternal benefit from the drug. **Drugs in this category should not be used by pregnant women.** Approximately 5% of prescription drugs fall in this category.

Animal Studies: Studies in animals given this drug show no substantial increased risk of fetal harm.

Human Studies: Except for occasional case reports, there are no controlled studies of pregnant women treated with this drug. Because cholesterol and the products synthesized by cholesterol are important during fetal development, the use of this family of drugs is contraindicated in pregnancy. Interrupting the long-term treatment of elevated cholesterol for nine months should have no long-term detrimental effect on mom's health.

Helpful Hints:

1. Drugs that belong to the statin family of drugs, such as this one, should only be prescribed for women of childbearing age when they are highly unlikely to conceive and have been informed of the potential hazards, according to the FDA. Why? Because cholesterol is essential for normal fetal development, and anything that lowers the serum level of cholesterol—which is what statins do—might adversely affect fetal development. If a woman becomes pregnant while taking this drug, or any member of the statin family of drugs, it should be discontinued immediately and she should be told of the potential hazard to her unborn baby.

2. This drug moderately interacts with grapefruit and grapefruit juice, which can cause harmful, and even life-threatening, side effects. Before taking this drug with grapefruit juice, or before consuming grapefruit or grapefruit juice during the day while taking this drug, first read the section "Grapefruit Juice–Drug Interactions Can Make You Sick" in the appendix of this book. Then discuss this with your pharmacist or the healthcare provider who prescribed this drug.

Remember: All pregnancies have a background risk of about 3% for a major birth defect, even when mom doesn't take a drug of any kind. If you are pregnant or planning a pregnancy, always let your doctor know before taking any drug, prescription or non-prescription, or herbal remedy.

• •

ATROPINE

Brand Name: AtroPen

Drug Use: This drug is mainly used to treat abnormal heart rhythms, helping restore adequate circulation.

Pregnancy Risk Category: C

> **Category C rating:** The FDA assigns a drug to Category C for one of two reasons: (1) Studies show evidence of fetal harm when using the drug in pregnant animals, but no controlled studies have been done using the drug in pregnant women, or (2) Studies using the drug in pregnant animals have not been done, and studies of pregnant women using the drug are insufficient to reach a conclusion. Thus, the drug should only be used if the potential benefit for mom is greater than the potential risk of fetal harm, which, in many cases, is unknown. Approximately 50% of prescription drugs fall in this category.

Animal Studies: Adequate studies in animals are not available using atropine.

Human Studies: Human studies, as well, are limited. There are no controlled studies in pregnant women exposed to atropine.

Remember: All pregnancies have a background risk of about 3% for a major birth defect, even when mom doesn't take a drug of any kind. If you are pregnant or planning a pregnancy, always let your doctor know before taking any drug, prescription or non-prescription, or herbal remedy.

• •

AZATHIOPRINE

Brand Names: Imuran, Azasan

Drug Uses: This drug is primarily used to prevent rejection of kidney transplants. However, it is also used to treat inflammatory bowel disease by suppressing the patient's immune response.

Pregnancy Risk Category: **D**

Category D rating: The FDA assigns a drug to Category **D** when studies of pregnant women using the drug show evidence of fetal harm. Rarely, however, the potential benefit of using the drug in some life-threatening situations for mom may outweigh the potential risk of fetal harm. For example, when mom requires cancer treatment or when she has a serious disease for which safer drugs cannot be used or are less effective. Approximately 11% of prescription drugs fall in this category.

Animal Studies: This drug causes birth defects in pregnant rabbits but not in mice and rats.

Human Studies: This drug may interfere with the effectiveness of intrauterine contraceptive devices (IUDs).

Remember: All pregnancies have a background risk of about 3% for a major birth defect, even when mom doesn't take a drug of any kind. If you are pregnant or planning a pregnancy, always let your doctor know before taking any drug, prescription or non-prescription, or herbal remedy.

. . . .

AZITHROMYCIN

Brand Name: Zithromax

Drug Use: This antibiotic is used to treat bacterial infections.

Pregnancy Risk Category: **B**

Category B rating: The FDA assigns a drug to Category **B** for one of two reasons: (1) Studies show no evidence of fetal harm when using the drug in pregnant animals, but no controlled studies have been done using the drug in pregnant women, or (2) Studies show evidence of fetal harm when using the drug in pregnant animals, but controlled studies using the drug in pregnant women do not show evidence of fetal harm. Approximately 21% of prescription drugs fall in this category.

Animal Studies: Pregnant rats and mice treated with this drug showed no evidence of fetal harm.

Human Studies: Limited case reports of pregnant women taking this drug show no increased risk of fetal harm.

Remember: All pregnancies have a background risk of about 3% for a major birth defect, even when mom doesn't take a drug of any kind. If you are pregnant or planning a pregnancy, always let your doctor know before taking any drug, prescription or non-prescription, or herbal remedy.

• •

AZTREONAM

Brand Name: Azactam

Drug Use: This antibiotic is approved by the FDA for the treatment of bacterial infections.

Pregnancy Risk Category: B

Category B rating: The FDA assigns a drug to Category **B** for one of two reasons: (1) Studies show no evidence of fetal harm when using the drug in pregnant animals, but no controlled studies have been done using the drug in pregnant women, or (2) Studies show evidence of fetal harm when using the drug in pregnant animals, but controlled studies using the drug in pregnant women do not show evidence of fetal harm. Approximately 21% of prescription drugs fall in this category.

Animal Studies: No fetal harm has been found in pregnant rats and rabbits treated with this drug.

Human Studies: No controlled studies in pregnant women taking this drug have been done.

Remember: All pregnancies have a background risk of about 3% for a major birth defect, even when mom doesn't

take a drug of any kind. If you are pregnant or planning a pregnancy, always let your doctor know before taking any drug, prescription or non-prescription, or herbal remedy.

....

ADDITIONAL DRUGS AND THEIR FDA PREGNANCY RISK CATEGORIES

Since these additional drugs are uncommonly used in pregnancy, they are listed by generic name along with their FDA Pregnancy Risk Category without more detail:

Abacavir - C	**Alosetron** - B
Abatacept - C	**Alteplase** - C
Abciximab - C	**Amifostine** - C
Acamprosate - C	**Amprenavir** - C
Adalimumab - B	**Anthrax Vaccine** - C
Adapalene - C	**Aprepitant** - B
Adefovir - C	**Aprotinin** - B
Agalsidase Beta - B	**Argatroban** - B
Aldesleukin - C	**Aripiprazole** - C
Alefacept - B	**Asparaginase** - C
Alemtuzumab - C	**Atazanavir** - B
Almotriptan - C	**Azelastine** - C

B

BECLOMETHASONE

Brand Names: Vanceril, QVAR, Beconase AQ Nasal Spray, Beconase Nasal Inhaler

Drug Use: The FDA has approved beclomethasone for the treatment of asthma.

Pregnancy Risk Category: C

Category C rating: The FDA assigns a drug to Category C for one of two reasons: (1) Studies show evidence of fetal harm when using the drug in pregnant animals, but no controlled studies have been done using the drug in pregnant women, or (2) Studies using the drug in pregnant animals have not been done, and studies of pregnant women using the drug are insufficient to reach a conclusion. Thus, the drug should only be used if the potential benefit for mom is greater than the potential risk of fetal harm, which, in many cases, is unknown. Approximately 50% of prescription drugs fall in this category.

Animal Studies: Birth defects, such as cleft palate and small jaw, have occurred when this medication was injected into pregnant mice and rats.

Human Studies: Limited studies in pregnant women taking this medication have shown no increase in birth defects.

Helpful Hints: In 2000, the American College of Obstetricians and Gynecologists (ACOG) and the American College of Allergy, Asthma and Immunology (ACAAI) recommended beclomethasone and budesonide as two inhaled steroids of choice for the treatment of asthma in pregnancy.

Remember: All pregnancies have a background risk of about 3% for a major birth defect, even when mom doesn't take a drug of any kind. If you are pregnant or planning a pregnancy, always let your doctor know before taking any drug, prescription or non-prescription, or herbal remedy.

. . . .

BENAZEPRIL

Brand Name: Lotensin

Drug Uses: The FDA has approved benazepril for use in treating high blood pressure and congestive heart failure. This drug is a member of the ACE inhibitor family of drugs. (See Helpful Hint on next page.)

Pregnancy Risk Categories: This drug has been assigned two pregnancy risk categories: **C** when used in the first trimester, and **D** when used in the second and third trimesters. Approximately 12% of prescription drugs are assigned two pregnancy risk categories, depending on which trimester of pregnancy the drug is used.

Category C rating: The FDA assigns a drug to Category **C** for one of two reasons: (1) Studies show evidence of fetal harm when using the drug in pregnant animals, but no controlled studies have been done using the drug in pregnant women, or (2) Studies using the drug in pregnant animals have not been done, and studies of pregnant women using the drug are insufficient to reach a conclusion. Thus, the drug should only be used if the potential benefit for mom is greater than the potential risk of fetal harm, which, in many cases, is unknown. Approximately 50% of prescription drugs fall in this category.

Category D rating: The FDA assigns a drug to Category **D** when studies of pregnant women using the drug show evidence of fetal harm. Rarely, however, the potential benefit of using the drug in some life-threatening situations for mom may outweigh the potential risk of fetal harm. For example, when mom requires cancer treatment or when she has a serious disease for which safer drugs cannot be used or are less effective. Approximately 11% of prescription drugs fall in this category.

Animal Studies: No birth defects were found when pregnant mice, rats, or rabbits were given this drug.

Human Studies: Drugs in the ACE inhibitor drug family have been associated with birth defects and even death of the fetus when the drug was taken in the second and third trimesters of pregnancy. This is why benazepril has a pregnancy risk category **D** rating in the second and third trimesters.

Helpful Hints:

1. The FDA has issued the following Black Box Warning for benazepril: Do not take benazepril if you are pregnant. Benazepril can cause injury and possibly death to a fetus when used after the third month of pregnancy. Talk to your doctor at once if you think you are pregnant. (See "ACE Inhibitor Drugs in Pregnancy" in the appendix for more details.)

   A Black Box Warning is the most serious prescription drug warning the FDA can require a drug company to issue.

2. If you become pregnant while taking benazepril, contact your doctor immediately to discuss the benefits and risks of taking this medication during pregnancy.

Remember: All pregnancies have a background risk of about 3% for a major birth defect, even when mom doesn't take a drug of any kind. If you are pregnant or planning a pregnancy, always let your doctor know before taking any drug, prescription or non-prescription, or herbal remedy.

. . . .

BENZTROPINE

Brand Name: Cogentin

Drug Uses: The FDA has approved this drug for treating Parkinson's disease and tremors caused by other disorders or drugs.

Pregnancy Risk Category: C

> **Category C rating:** The FDA assigns a drug to Category C for one of two reasons: (1) Studies show evidence of fetal harm when using the drug in pregnant animals, but no controlled studies have been done using the drug in pregnant women, or (2) Studies using the drug in pregnant animals have not been done, and studies of pregnant women using the drug are insufficient to reach a conclusion. Thus, the drug should only be used if the potential benefit for mom is greater than the potential risk of fetal harm, which, in many cases, is unknown. Approximately 50% of prescription drugs fall in this category.

Animal Studies: No relevant studies in pregnant animals have been done.

Human Studies: Limited information available from reports about patients who took this drug in pregnancy suggests a possible association with birth defects.

Remember: All pregnancies have a background risk of about 3% for a major birth defect, even when mom doesn't take a drug of any kind. If you are pregnant or planning a pregnancy, always let your doctor know before taking any drug, prescription or non-prescription, or herbal remedy.

. . . .

BETAMETHASONE

Brand Name: Celestone (Betamethasone is also combined with other drugs to produce steroid creams and ointments. In this form, it has many other brand names, depending on which other drugs it is combined with). Celestone belongs to the corticosteroid family of drugs.

Drug Uses: The FDA has approved this drug for use in pregnant women who go into early labor to help stimulate fetal lung maturity. As a cream or lotion, it is used to treat various skin disorders.

Pregnancy Risk Categories: This drug has been assigned to a **D** category if used in the first trimester. The drug has been assigned to a **C** category when used in the second and third trimesters. Approximately 12% of prescription drugs are assigned two pregnancy risk categories, depending on which trimester of pregnancy the drug is used.

> **Category D rating:** The FDA assigns a drug to Category **D** when studies of pregnant women using the drug show evidence of fetal harm. Rarely, however, the potential benefit of using the drug in some life-threatening situations for mom may outweigh the potential risk of fetal harm. For example, when mom requires cancer treatment or when she has a serious disease for which safer drugs cannot be used or are less effective. Approximately 11% of prescription drugs fall in this category.

> **Category C rating:** The FDA assigns a drug to Category **C** for one of two reasons: (1) Studies show evidence of fetal harm when using the drug in pregnant animals, but no controlled studies have been done using the drug in pregnant women, or (2) Studies using the drug in pregnant animals have not been done, and studies of pregnant women using the drug are insufficient to reach a conclusion. Thus, the drug should only be used if the potential benefit for mom is greater than the potential risk of fetal harm, which, in many cases, is unknown. Approximately 50% of prescription drugs fall in this category.

Animal Studies: When given to pregnant animals, drugs in the corticosteroid family has been associated with smaller babies who have smaller heads, enlarged livers, and other changes in organ sizes.

Human Studies: Research has shown that when given to pregnant women who go into early labor, betamethasone reduces the incidence and severity of breathing problems in the baby and increases overall survival of these premature infants. No human studies have linked betamethasone to birth defects. However, studies have linked this family of drugs to cleft lip and cleft palate, two birth defects of the mouth and face, when the drugs were used in the first trimester.

Helpful Hints: Betamethasone, as well as certain other drugs in this corticosteroid family, is a medication that offers clear benefit to babies at risk of having breathing problems from immature lungs at birth. Betamethasone is a mainstay of treatment in helping to prevent these breathing problems. These benefits have been shown to clearly outweigh any risk to mom or her baby. But it is a different story if the drug is used in the first trimester of pregnancy.

Remember: All pregnancies have a background risk of about 3% for a major birth defect, even when mom doesn't take a drug of any kind. If you are pregnant or planning a pregnancy, always let your doctor know before taking any drug, prescription or non-prescription, or herbal remedy.

. . . .

BETAXOLOL

Brand Names: Kerlone, Betoptic

Drug Uses: This drug is approved for use in treating hypertension and topically to treat glaucoma. This drug is a member of the beta blocker family of drugs.

Pregnancy Risk Categories: This drug has been assigned to the **C** category when used in the first trimester and to the **D** category when used in the second and third trimesters. Approximately 12% of prescription drugs are assigned two pregnancy risk categories, depending on which trimester of pregnancy the drug is used.

> **Category C rating:** The FDA assigns a drug to Category **C** for one of two reasons: (1) Studies show evidence of fetal harm when using the drug in pregnant animals, but no controlled studies have been done using the drug in pregnant women, or (2) Studies using the drug in pregnant animals have not been done, and studies of pregnant women using the drug are insufficient to reach a conclusion. Thus, the drug should only be used if the potential benefit for mom is greater than the potential risk of fetal harm, which, in many cases, is unknown. Approximately 50% of prescription drugs fall in this category.

> **Category D rating:** The FDA assigns a drug to Category **D** when studies of pregnant women using the drug show evidence of fetal harm. Rarely, however, the potential benefit of using the drug in some life-threatening situations for mom may outweigh the potential risk of fetal harm. For example, when mom requires cancer treatment or when she has a serious disease for which safer drugs cannot be used or are less effective. Approximately 11% of prescription drugs fall in this category.

Animal Studies: This drug does cause birth defects in rats, especially when high enough doses that are toxic to the mother are used.

Human Studies: There are no studies using this drug in pregnant women. But other drugs in this family of drugs have been associated with decreased growth of the fetus and decreased placental weight. In addition, some of the drugs in this family have caused symptoms of bradycardia, or slow heart rate, in newborns within the first 48 hours after birth. For these reasons, the drug has a **D** rating for the second and third trimesters.

Remember: All pregnancies have a background risk of about 3% for a major birth defect, even when mom doesn't take a drug of any kind. If you are pregnant or planning a pregnancy, always let your doctor know

before taking any drug, prescription or non-prescription, or herbal remedy.

• •

BETHANECHOL

Brand Name: Urecholine

Drug Use: Bethanechol is approved by the FDA for use in treating several bladder disorders.

Pregnancy Risk Category: C

Category C rating: The FDA assigns a drug to Category C for one of two reasons: (1) Studies show evidence of fetal harm when using the drug in pregnant animals, but no controlled studies have been done using the drug in pregnant women, or (2) Studies using the drug in pregnant animals have not been done, and studies of pregnant women using the drug are insufficient to reach a conclusion. Thus, the drug should only be used if the potential benefit for mom is greater than the potential risk of fetal harm, which, in many cases, is unknown. Approximately 50% of prescription drugs fall in this category.

Animal Studies: There have been no studies using bethanechol in pregnant animals.

Human Studies: Bethanechol has seen limited use in pregnancy, so there is not enough information from which to draw conclusions.

Remember: All pregnancies have a background risk of about 3% for a major birth defect, even when mom doesn't take a drug of any kind. If you are pregnant or planning a pregnancy, always let your doctor know before taking any drug, prescription or non-prescription, or herbal remedy.

• •

BLEOMYCIN

Brand Name: Blenoxane

Drug Use: This drug is an antibiotic that is used only for its cancer-fighting abilities.

Pregnancy Risk Category: D

> **Category D rating:** The FDA assigns a drug to Category **D** when studies of pregnant women using the drug show evidence of fetal harm. Rarely, however, the potential benefit of using the drug in some life-threatening situations for mom may outweigh the potential risk of fetal harm. For example, when mom requires cancer treatment or when she has a serious disease for which safer drugs cannot be used or are less effective. Approximately 11% of prescription drugs fall in this category.

Animal Studies: This drug causes birth defects in rats and an increased incidence of spontaneous abortions in pregnant rabbits, but no birth defects in rabbits.

Human Studies: There have been several reports of normal babies born to mothers who received this drug during pregnancy, but no reports linking its use to birth defects in pregnant women.

Remember: All pregnancies have a background risk of about 3% for a major birth defect, even when mom doesn't take a drug of any kind. If you are pregnant or planning a pregnancy, always let your doctor know before taking any drug, prescription or non-prescription, or herbal remedy.

• •

BROMOCRIPTINE

Brand Names: Parlodel, Cycloset

Drug Uses: This drug is used for the treatment of infertility and other conditions, such as acromegaly, a condition in which there is too much growth hormone in the body, and Parkinson's disease.

Pregnancy Risk Category: B

> **Category B rating:** The FDA assigns a drug to Category **B** for one of two reasons: (1) Studies show no evidence of fetal harm

when using the drug in pregnant animals, but no controlled studies have been done using the drug in pregnant women, or (2) Studies show evidence of fetal harm when using the drug in pregnant animals, but controlled studies using the drug in pregnant women do not show evidence of fetal harm. Approximately 21% of prescription drugs fall in this category.

Animal Studies: No animal studies were located.

Human Studies: Various reports have not shown an increased risk of birth defects when compared to babies born to women not taking the drug.

Remember: All pregnancies have a background risk of about 3% for a major birth defect, even when mom doesn't take a drug of any kind. If you are pregnant or planning a pregnancy, always let your doctor know before taking any drug, prescription or non-prescription, or herbal remedy.

. . . .

BROMPHENIRAMINE

Brand Name: There is no stand-alone brand product for this generic drug. However, it is used as an active ingredient in multiple combination products such as Dimetapp and Bromadrine.

Drug Use: This antihistamine is used in combination with other drugs primarily for cough and cold medications.

Pregnancy Risk Category: **C**

Category C rating: The FDA assigns a drug to Category **C** for one of two reasons: (1) Studies show evidence of fetal harm when using the drug in pregnant animals, but no controlled studies have been done using the drug in pregnant women, or (2) Studies using the drug in pregnant animals have not been done, and studies of pregnant women using the drug are insufficient to reach a conclusion. Thus, the drug should only be used if the potential benefit for mom is greater than the potential risk of fetal harm, which, in many cases, is unknown. Approximately 50% of prescription drugs fall in this category.

Animal Studies: No animal studies are available.

Human Studies: Limited reports of pregnant women exposed to combination cough and cold products containing brompheniramine showed no increase in birth defects.

Helpful Hints: Some cough syrups contain ethanol (alcohol). Be sure to check the label on the bottle to see if ethanol is listed as an ingredient. Alcohol is known to cause birth defects in developing fetuses.

Remember: All pregnancies have a background risk of about 3% for a major birth defect, even when mom doesn't take a drug of any kind. If you are pregnant or planning a pregnancy, always let your doctor know before taking any drug, prescription or non-prescription, or herbal remedy.

BUDESONIDE

Brand Names: This drug comes in three forms and has three different brand names: (1) Rhinocort Aqua Nasal Spray, (2) Entocort EC, and (3) Pulmicort Respules.

Drug Uses: The nasal spray is used for nasal stuffiness and runny nose due to allergies. The oral form, which is Entocort EC, is used to treat Crohn's disease, and asthma. Budesonide is a member of the corticosteroid family of drugs.

Pregnancy Risk Categories: The inhaled products have a **B** rating; and the oral product has a **C** rating. Approximately 12% of prescription drugs are assigned two pregnancy risk categories, depending on which trimester of pregnancy the drug is used.

Category B rating: The FDA assigns a drug to Category **B** for one of two reasons: (1) Studies show no evidence of fetal harm when using the drug in pregnant animals, but no controlled studies have been done using the drug in pregnant women, or (2) Studies show evidence of fetal harm when using the drug in pregnant animals, but controlled studies using the drug in pregnant women do not show evidence of fetal harm. Approximately 21% of prescription drugs fall in this category.

Category C rating: The FDA assigns a drug to Category **C** for one of two reasons: (1) Studies show evidence of fetal harm when using the drug in pregnant animals, but no controlled studies have been done using the drug in pregnant women, or (2) Studies using the drug in pregnant animals have not been done, and studies of pregnant women using the drug are insufficient to reach a conclusion. Thus, the drug should only be used if the potential benefit for mom is greater than the potential risk of fetal harm, which, in many cases, is unknown. Approximately 50% of prescription drugs fall in this category.

Animal Studies: When given under the skin to pregnant rats and rabbits, budesonide has been associated with significant birth defects. However, the inhalation dose of budesonide in pregnant rats does not product birth defects.

Human Studies: No studies have been done in pregnant women taking the oral product. No significant increase in fetal risk when the inhaled product was taken has been found. Other members of the corticosteroid family of drugs have been associated with birth defects in humans when taken during the first trimester of pregnancy. Thus, the drug should only be used during the first trimester when the benefit of controlling maternal asthma, for example, outweighs any potential risk to her unborn baby.

Helpful Hints: This drug weakly interacts with grapefruit and grapefruit juice, which can cause harmful, and even life-threatening, side effects. Before taking this drug with grapefruit juice, or before consuming grapefruit or grapefruit juice during the day while taking this drug, first read the section "Grapefruit Juice–Drug Interactions Can Make You Sick" in the appendix of this book. Then discuss this with your pharmacist or the healthcare provider who prescribed this drug.

Remember: All pregnancies have a background risk of about 3% for a major birth defect, even when mom doesn't take a drug of any kind. If you are pregnant or planning a pregnancy, always let your doctor know before taking any drug, prescription or non-prescription, or herbal remedy.

∙ ∙

BUMETANIDE

Brand Name: Bumex

Drug Uses: This diuretic (water pill) is used to reduce swelling and fluid retention. It is also used to treat high blood pressure.

Pregnancy Risk Categories: This drug has a pregnancy risk rating of **C** except when used to treat hypertension if it develops during pregnancy. In that instance, the **C** rating changes to a **D**. Approximately 12% of prescription drugs are assigned two pregnancy risk categories. Since high blood pressure that develops during pregnancy is usually characterized by a low blood volume, and that is a contraindication for diuretic use, the pregnancy risk category shifts to a **D**.

Category C rating: The FDA assigns a drug to Category **C** for one of two reasons: (1) Studies show evidence of fetal harm when

using the drug in pregnant animals, but no controlled studies have been done using the drug in pregnant women, or (2) Studies using the drug in pregnant animals have not been done, and studies of pregnant women using the drug are insufficient to reach a conclusion. Thus, the drug should only be used if the potential benefit for mom is greater than the potential risk of fetal harm, which, in many cases, is unknown. Approximately 50% of prescription drugs fall in this category.

Category D rating: The FDA assigns a drug to Category **D** when studies of pregnant women using the drug show evidence of fetal harm. Rarely, however, the potential benefit of using the drug in some life-threatening situations for mom may outweigh the potential risk of fetal harm. For example, when mom requires cancer treatment or when she has a serious disease for which safer drugs cannot be used or are less effective. Approximately 11% of prescription drugs fall in this category.

Animal Studies: Pregnant rats, mice, hamsters, and rabbits all treated with this drug did not show an increased incidence of birth defects.

Human Studies: No published reports could be located for this drug's use in pregnant women.

Remember: All pregnancies have a background risk of about 3% for a major birth defect, even when mom doesn't take a drug of any kind. If you are pregnant or planning a pregnancy, always let your doctor know before taking any drug, prescription or non-prescription, or herbal remedy.

. . . .

BUPROPION

Brand Names: Wellbutrin, Zyban, Aplenzin

Drug Uses: Bupropion is approved by the FDA for the treatment of depression and to aid in smoking cessation.

Pregnancy Risk Category: B

Category B rating: The FDA assigns a drug to Category **B** for one of two reasons: (1) Studies show no evidence of fetal harm

when using the drug in pregnant animals, but no controlled studies have been done using the drug in pregnant women, or (2) Studies show evidence of fetal harm when using the drug in pregnant animals, but controlled studies using the drug in pregnant women do not show evidence of fetal harm. Approximately 21% of prescription drugs fall in this category.

Animal Studies: Studies in pregnant rats and rabbits show no harm to the developing fetus.

Human Studies: Based on the small number of pregnant women taking bupropion that researchers have been able to follow, no definitive conclusions have been reached about the safety of this drug in pregnancy. It appears, however, that the drug is not linked to causing fetal harm.

Helpful Hints:

1. Studies show that antidepressants increase the risk of suicidal thinking and behavior in children, adolescents, and young adults. Anyone considering the use of this drug or any other antidepressant in these patients must balance that risk with the clinical need.

2. Almost all antidepressants carry some risk to the developing fetus. However, we also know depression in a pregnant woman carries potential risk for her health and for her unborn baby; for example, low birth weight and prematurity. The risks and benefits of medications and untreated depression must be weighed carefully. If you are pregnant and think you may have depression, or if you already know you do, talk with your doctor so the two of you can create the right plan for you and your unborn baby. (See "Antidepressants in Pregnancy" in the appendix for more details.)

Remember: All pregnancies have a background risk of about 3% for a major birth defect, even when mom doesn't take a drug of any kind. If you are pregnant or planning a pregnancy, always let your doctor know before taking any drug, prescription or non-prescription, or herbal remedy.

. . . .

BUSPIRONE

Brand Name: BuSpar

Drug Use: The FDA has approved buspirone for treating anxiety disorders.

Pregnancy Risk Category: B

> **Category B rating:** The FDA assigns a drug to Category **B** for one of two reasons: (1) Studies show no evidence of fetal harm when using the drug in pregnant animals, but no controlled studies have been done using the drug in pregnant women, or (2) Studies show evidence of fetal harm when using the drug in pregnant animals, but controlled studies using the drug in pregnant women do not show evidence of fetal harm. Approximately 21% of prescription drugs fall in this category.

Animal Studies: Researchers have found no increase in birth defects in pregnant rats or rabbits treated with this drug.

Human Studies: Limited studies performed in pregnant women using this drug have not detected an increased risk of fetal harm.

Helpful Hints: This drug strongly interacts with grapefruit and grapefruit juice, which can cause harmful, and even life-threatening, side effects. Before taking this drug with grapefruit juice, or before consuming grapefruit or grapefruit juice during the day while taking this drug, first read the section "Grapefruit Juice–Drug Interactions

Can Make You Sick" in the appendix of this book. Then discuss this with your pharmacist or the healthcare provider who prescribed this drug.

Remember: All pregnancies have a background risk of about 3% for a major birth defect, even when mom doesn't take a drug of any kind. If you are pregnant or planning a pregnancy, always let your doctor know before taking any drug, prescription or non-prescription, or herbal remedy.

· ·

BUTALBITAL

Brand Names: Amaphen, Fioricet, Butace

Drug Use: Butalbital is a short-acting member of the barbiturate family of drugs. It is contained in a variety of pain-relieving mixtures such as Amaphen, Fioricet, and Butace.

Pregnancy Risk Categories: This drug is assigned to two pregnancy risk categories. If used for prolonged periods of time or in high doses at term, the drug has a risk rating of **D,** otherwise, its risk rating is **C.** Approximately 12% of prescription drugs are assigned two pregnancy risk categories, depending on which trimester of pregnancy the drug is used.

> **Category D rating:** The FDA assigns a drug to Category **D** when studies of pregnant women using the drug show evidence of fetal harm. Rarely, however, the potential benefit of using the drug in some life-threatening situations for mom may outweigh the potential risk of fetal harm. For example, when mom requires cancer treatment or when she has a serious disease for which safer drugs cannot be used or are less effective. Approximately 11% of prescription drugs fall in this category.

> **Category C rating:** The FDA assigns a drug to Category **C** for one of two reasons: (1) Studies show evidence of fetal harm when

using the drug in pregnant animals, but no controlled studies have been done using the drug in pregnant women, or (2) Studies using the drug in pregnant animals have not been done, and studies of pregnant women using the drug are insufficient to reach a conclusion. Thus, the drug should only be used if the potential benefit for mom is greater than the potential risk of fetal harm, which, in many cases, is unknown. Approximately 50% of prescription drugs fall in this category.

Animal Studies: No studies of this drug have been reported in pregnant animals.

Human Studies: Limited studies in pregnant women have shown no association between the drug and birth defects. However, neonatal withdrawal symptoms were found in one case report involving one baby.

Remember: All pregnancies have a background risk of about 3% for a major birth defect, even when mom doesn't take a drug of any kind. If you are pregnant or planning a pregnancy, always let your doctor know before taking any drug, prescription or non-prescription, or herbal remedy.

- -

BUTOCONAZOLE

Brand Names: Mycelex-3 and Gynazole-1 vaginal creams

Drug Use: The FDA has approved this drug for the treatment of vaginal yeast infections.

Pregnancy Risk Category: C

Category C rating: The FDA assigns a drug to Category **C** for one of two reasons: (1) Studies show evidence of fetal harm when using the drug in pregnant animals, but no controlled studies have been done using the drug in pregnant women, or (2) Studies using the drug in pregnant animals have not been done, and studies of pregnant women using the drug are insufficient to reach a conclusion.

Thus, the drug should only be used if the potential benefit for mom is greater than the potential risk of fetal harm, which, in many cases, is unknown. Approximately 50% of prescription drugs fall in this category.

Animal Studies: Birth defects have been found when large doses of this drug were given orally to pregnant animals.

Human Studies: When used vaginally during pregnancy, butoconazole has not been associated with an increased risk of birth defects or other forms of fetal harm.

Remember: All pregnancies have a background risk of about 3% for a major birth defect, even when mom doesn't take a drug of any kind. If you are pregnant or planning a pregnancy, always let your doctor know before taking any drug, prescription or non-prescription, or herbal remedy.

• •

BUTORPHANOL

Brand Name: Stadol

Drug Use: The FDA has approved butorphanol as a nasal spray or injection to treat moderate to severe pain. Butorphanol belongs to the family of narcotic medications.

Pregnancy Risk Categories: This drug has been assigned two risk categories: **C** and then **D** if used for prolonged periods or in high doses near the time of delivery. Approximately 12% of prescription drugs are assigned two pregnancy risk categories, depending on which trimester of pregnancy the drug is used.

> **Category C rating:** The FDA assigns a drug to Category **C** for one of two reasons: (1) Studies show evidence of fetal harm when using the drug in pregnant animals, but no controlled studies have

been done using the drug in pregnant women, or (2) Studies using the drug in pregnant animals have not been done, and studies of pregnant women using the drug are insufficient to reach a conclusion. Thus, the drug should only be used if the potential benefit for mom is greater than the potential risk of fetal harm, which, in many cases, is unknown. Approximately 50% of prescription drugs fall in this category.

Category D rating: The FDA assigns a drug to Category **D** when studies of pregnant women using the drug show evidence of fetal harm. Rarely, however, the potential benefit of using the drug in some life-threatening situations for mom may outweigh the potential risk of fetal harm. For example, when mom requires cancer treatment or when she has a serious disease for which safer drugs cannot be used or are less effective. Approximately 11% of prescription drugs fall in this category.

Animal Studies: No birth defects have been seen in studies on pregnant rats and rabbits. An increased risk of stillbirth, however, was seen in those same animals.

Human Studies: When pregnant women have taken this drug near the time of delivery, some of their babies have had difficulty breathing after birth. Also, if this drug is given during labor, there is an increased incidence of abnormal fetal heart rate tracings. These abnormal fetal heart rate tracings do not appear to reflect an adverse affect on the baby. Butorphanol can be addictive, both for the pregnant mother and her unborn baby. If used, it must be with extreme caution only under a doctor's careful care.

Remember: All pregnancies have a background risk of about 3% for a major birth defect, even when mom doesn't take a drug of any kind. If you are pregnant or planning a pregnancy, always let your doctor know before taking any drug, prescription or non-prescription, or herbal remedy.

. . . .

ADDITIONAL DRUGS AND THEIR FDA PREGNANCY RISK CATEGORIES

Since these additional drugs are uncommonly used in pregnancy, they are listed by generic name along with their FDA Pregnancy Risk Category without more detail:

Bacitracin - C

Baclofen - C

Balsalazide - B

Basiliximab - B

Bevacizumab - C

Bexarotene - X

Bicalutamide - X

Biperiden - C

Bisacodyl - C

Bisoprolol - C (first trimester use) - D (second and third trimester use)

Bivalirudin - B

Bortezomib - D

Bosentan - X

Botulinum Toxin Type A - C

Bromfenac - C

Buprenorphine - C

Busulfan - D

Butenafine - C

C

CAFFEINE

Brand Name: Caffeine is used in combination products often sold over the counter, such as Anacin tablets.

Drug Use: Caffeine is a central nervous system stimulant found in coffee and various over-the-counter medications which are used for the temporary relief of minor aches and pains.

Pregnancy Risk Category: B

Category B rating: The FDA assigns a drug to Category **B** for one of two reasons: (1) Studies show no evidence of fetal harm when using the drug in pregnant animals, but no controlled studies have been done using the drug in pregnant women, or (2) Studies show evidence of fetal harm when using the drug in pregnant animals, but controlled studies using the drug in pregnant women do not show evidence of fetal harm. Approximately 21% of prescription drugs fall in this category.

Animal Studies: Numerous studies in animals have shown that caffeine does cause fetal harm, but only when the dose was high enough to have toxic effects on their mothers. However, these findings have not been established in humans.

Human Studies: When used in moderation, caffeine has not been shown to cause birth defects in humans or reduce a woman's ability to become pregnant.

Helpful Hints: This drug weakly interacts with grapefruit and grapefruit juice, which can cause harmful, and even life-threatening, side effects. Before taking this drug with grapefruit juice, or before consuming grapefruit or grapefruit juice during the day while taking this drug, first read the section "Grapefruit Juice–Drug Interactions Can Make You Sick" in the appendix of this book. Then discuss this with your pharmacist or the healthcare provider who prescribed this drug.

Remember: All pregnancies have a background risk of about 3% for a major birth defect, even when mom doesn't take a drug of any kind. If you are pregnant or planning a pregnancy, always let your doctor know before taking any drug, prescription or non-prescription, or herbal remedy.

CALCITONIN SALMON

Brand Name: Miacalcin

Drug Uses: This drug is approved by the FDA for the treatment of osteoporosis and Paget's disease of bone.

Pregnancy Risk Category: C

> **Category C rating:** The FDA assigns a drug to Category C for one of two reasons: (1) Studies show evidence of fetal harm when using the drug in pregnant animals, but no controlled studies have been done using the drug in pregnant women, or (2) Studies using the drug in pregnant animals have not been done, and studies of pregnant women using the drug are insufficient to reach a conclusion. Thus, the drug should only be used if the potential benefit for mom is greater than the potential risk of fetal harm, which, in many cases, is unknown. Approximately 50% of prescription drugs fall in this category.

Animal Studies: Pregnant rabbits treated with this drug showed a decrease in fetal birth weights when they were treated with doses 14 to 56 times the recommended dose in humans.

Human Studies: This drug does not cross the placenta. There has been no link shown to birth defects in pregnant women.

Remember: All pregnancies have a background risk of about 3% for a major birth defect, even when mom doesn't take a drug of any kind. If you are pregnant or planning a pregnancy, always let your doctor know before taking any drug, prescription or non-prescription, or herbal remedy.

• •

CANDESARTAN

Brand Name: Atacand

Drug Use: This drug is approved by the FDA for the treatment of high blood pressure. Its mechanism of action is very similar to that of the ACE inhibitor family of drugs.

Pregnancy Risk Categories: This drug has been assigned two pregnancy risk categories: **C** when used in the first trimester and **D** when used in the second and third trimesters. Approximately 12% of prescription drugs are assigned two pregnancy risk categories, depending on which trimester of pregnancy the drug is used.

Category C rating: The FDA assigns a drug to Category **C** for one of two reasons: (1) Studies show evidence of fetal harm when using the drug in pregnant animals, but no controlled studies have been done using the drug in pregnant women, or (2) Studies using the drug in pregnant animals have not been done, and studies of pregnant women using the drug are insufficient to reach a conclusion. Thus, the drug should only be used if the potential benefit for mom is greater than the potential risk of fetal harm, which, in many cases, is unknown. Approximately 50% of prescription drugs fall in this category.

Category D rating: The FDA assigns a drug to Category **D** when studies of pregnant women using the drug show evidence of fetal harm. Rarely, however, the potential benefit of using the drug in some life-threatening situations for mom may outweigh the potential risk of fetal harm. For example, when mom requires cancer treatment or when she has a serious disease for which safer drugs cannot be used or are less effective. Approximately 11% of prescription drugs fall in this category.

Animal Studies: This drug has been studied in pregnant mice, rats, and rabbits. Rat offspring showed decreased survival and an increased incidence of kidney defects. Mice offspring showed no evidence of fetal harm. Rabbit offspring showed decreased body weight. There was also evidence of maternal toxicity.

Human Studies: The mechanism of action of this drug is very similar to that of the ACE inhibitor drug family, which is used to also treat high blood pressure. Since the mechanism of action is so similar, the FDA has issued a Black Box Warning regarding this drug:

"Do not take candesartan if you are pregnant or breast feeding. If you become pregnant while taking candesartan, call your doctor immediately."

A Black Box Warning is the most serious prescription drug warning the FDA can require a drug company to issue.

ACE inhibitors cause birth defects in the fetus and also neonatal toxicity. Fetal toxic effects may include lack of urine production, decrease in the amount of amniotic fluid, defect of the fetal skull, slow growth, prematurity, and underdevelopment of the lungs. As a result of a lack of amniotic fluid prior to birth, the fetus may develop limb contractures and deformities from crowding inside the uterus. In addition, after birth, lack of urine production and low blood pressure may occur. For all these reasons, this drug has a pregnancy risk category **D** rating for the second and third trimesters of pregnancy.

The FDA has issued another Black Box Warning for all drugs in the ACE inhibitor drug family: "When used in pregnancy during the second and third trimesters, ACE inhibitors can cause injury and even death to the developing fetus. When pregnancy is detected, this drug should be discontinued as soon as possible." (See "ACE Inhibitor Drugs in Pregnancy" in the appendix for more detail.)

A Black Box Warning is the most serious prescription drug warning the FDA can require a drug company to issue.

Helpful Hints: If you become pregnant while taking candesartan, contact your doctor immediately to discuss the benefits and risks of taking this medication during pregnancy.

Remember: All pregnancies have a background risk of about 3% for a major birth defect, even when mom doesn't take a drug of any kind. If you are pregnant or planning a pregnancy, always let your doctor know before taking any drug, prescription or non-prescription, or herbal remedy.

· ·

CAPTOPRIL

Brand Name: Captopen. This drug is a member of the ACE inhibitor family of drugs.

Drug Uses: This drug is approved by the FDA for the treatment of high blood pressure, congestive heart failure, for use after heart attacks, and for use in patients with diabetes who have kidney disease.

Pregnancy Risk Categories: This drug has been assigned two pregnancy risk categories: **C** when used in the first trimester (first 12 weeks of pregnancy), and **D** when used in the second and third trimesters. Approximately 12% of prescription drugs are assigned two pregnancy risk categories, depending on which trimester of pregnancy the drug is used.

Category C rating: The FDA assigns a drug to Category **C** for one of two reasons: (1) Studies show evidence of fetal harm when using the drug in pregnant animals, but no controlled studies have been done using the drug in pregnant women, or (2) Studies using the drug in pregnant animals have not been done, and studies of pregnant women using the drug are insufficient to reach a conclusion. Thus, the drug should only be used if the potential benefit for mom is greater than the potential risk of fetal harm, which, in many cases, is unknown. Approximately 50% of prescription drugs fall in this category.

Category D rating: The FDA assigns a drug to Category **D** when studies of pregnant women using the drug show evidence of fetal harm. Rarely, however, the potential benefit of using the drug in some life-threatening situations for mom may outweigh the potential risk of fetal harm. For example, when mom requires cancer treatment or when she has a serious disease for which safer drugs cannot be used or are less effective. Approximately 11% of prescription drugs fall in this category.

Animal Studies: This drug is toxic to embryos in animals and causes stillbirths in some species. In pregnant sheep and rabbits, captopril causes a decrease in blood flow to the placenta, resulting in decreased oxygen delivery to the fetus.

Human Studies: The FDA has issued a Black Box Warning for all ACE inhibitors when used in pregnancy as follows:

"When used in pregnancy during the second and third trimesters, ACE inhibitors can cause injury and even death to the developing fetus. When pregnancy is detected, captopril should be discontinued as soon as possible."

A Black Box Warning is the most serious prescription drug warning the FDA can require a drug company to issue.

Helpful Hints: If you become pregnant while taking captopril, contact your doctor immediately to discuss the benefits and risks of taking this medication during pregnancy.

Remember: All pregnancies have a background risk of about 3% for a major birth defect, even when mom doesn't take a drug of any kind. If you are pregnant or planning a pregnancy, always let your doctor know before taking any drug, prescription or non-prescription, or herbal remedy.

. . . .

CARBAMAZEPINE

Brand Names: Tegretol, Carbatrol, Epitol

Drug Uses: This drug is approved by the FDA for the treatment of seizures and as an analgesic for the treatment of the pain of trigeminal neuralgia. This drug is a member of the folic acid antagonist family of drugs. (See Helpful Hint on next page.)

Pregnancy Risk Category: D

> **Category D rating:** The FDA assigns a drug to Category **D** when studies of pregnant women using the drug show evidence of fetal harm. Rarely, however, the potential benefit of using the drug in some life-threatening situations for mom may outweigh the potential risk of fetal harm. For example, when mom requires cancer treatment or when she has a serious disease for which safer drugs cannot be used or are less effective. Approximately 11% of prescription drugs fall in this category.

Animal Studies: This drug causes birth defects in the offspring of pregnant rats.

Human Studies: Studies of pregnant women taking carbamazepine show a link between the drug and birth defects, including spina bifida (open spine).

Helpful Hints:

　　1. In pregnant women with epilepsy, the first priority is to prevent seizures. This can be difficult because many seizure medications do not work quite as well during pregnancy. Sometimes the dose has to be increased or other medications added just to prevent seizures. Regardless, the healthiest situation for both mom and unborn baby is to have the fewest seizures possible.

2. Folic acid antagonists are drugs that limit the effectiveness of folic acid, making it more likely that a baby born to a mom taking one of these drugs might have a serious birth defect, such as an open spine. If you are taking a folic acid antagonist and trying to become pregnant, discuss the possibility of increasing your folic acid intake with your clinician before becoming pregnant. (See "Folic Acid Antagonist Drugs in Pregnancy" in the appendix for more details.)

3. This drug moderately interacts with grapefruit and grapefruit juice, which can cause harmful, and even life-threatening, side effects. Before taking this drug with grapefruit juice, or before consuming grapefruit or grapefruit juice during the day while taking this drug, first read the section "Grapefruit Juice–Drug Interactions Can Make You Sick" in the appendix of this book. Then discuss this with your pharmacist or the healthcare provider who prescribed this drug.

Remember: All pregnancies have a background risk of about 3% for a major birth defect, even when mom doesn't take a drug of any kind. If you are pregnant or planning a pregnancy, always let your doctor know before taking any drug, prescription or non-prescription, or herbal remedy.

. . . .

CARBIMAZOLE

Brand Name: Neo-Merazole

Drug Use: This drug is approved by the FDA for the treatment of hyperthyroidism.

Pregnancy Risk Category: D

> **Category D rating:** The FDA assigns a drug to Category **D** when studies of pregnant women using the drug show evidence of fetal harm. Rarely, however, the potential benefit of using the drug in some life-threatening situations for mom may outweigh the potential risk of fetal harm. For example, when mom requires cancer treatment or when she has a serious disease for which safer drugs cannot be used or are less effective. Approximately 11% of prescription drugs fall in this category.

Animal Studies: No studies of this drug's use in pregnant animals were found.

Human Studies: Studies in pregnant women taking this drug for hyperthyroidism have shown an association with fetal birth defects.

Helpful Hints: Carbimazole is considered a second choice drug for the treatment of hyperthyroidism in pregnancy. Because the drug is converted in the body to methimazole, which is known to cause fetal birth defects, carbimazole has been assigned a category D rating.

Remember: All pregnancies have a background risk of about 3% for a major birth defect, even when mom doesn't take a drug of any kind. If you are pregnant or planning a pregnancy, always let your doctor know before taking any drug, prescription or non-prescription, or herbal remedy.

. . . .

CARISOPRODOL

Brand Names: Soma, Vanadom

Drug Use: This muscle relaxant is approved by the FDA to relax muscles and relieve pain and discomfort caused by strains, sprains, and other muscular injuries.

Pregnancy Risk Category: C

Category C rating: The FDA assigns a drug to Category **C** for one of two reasons: (1) Studies show evidence of fetal harm when using the drug in pregnant animals, but no controlled studies have been done using the drug in pregnant women, or (2) Studies using the drug in pregnant animals have not been done, and studies of pregnant women using the drug are insufficient to reach a conclusion. Thus, the drug should only be used if the potential benefit for mom is greater than the potential risk of fetal harm, which, in many cases, is unknown. Approximately 50% of prescription drugs fall in this category.

Animal Studies: This drug has not been studied in pregnant animals.

Human Studies: Limited studies in pregnant women have found no association of this drug with fetal birth defects.

Remember: All pregnancies have a background risk of about 3% for a major birth defect, even when mom doesn't take a drug of any kind. If you are pregnant or planning a pregnancy, always let your doctor know before taking any drug, prescription or non-prescription, or herbal remedy.

. . . .

CARTEOLOL

Brand Names: Cartrol, Ocupress

Drug Uses: This drug is approved by the FDA for the treatment of hypertension and glaucoma. The drug belongs to the beta-blocker family of drugs.

Pregnancy Risk Categories: This drug has been assigned two pregnancy risk categories: **C** when used in the first trimester, and **D** when used in the second and third trimesters. Approximately 12% of prescription drugs are assigned two pregnancy risk categories, depending on which trimester of pregnancy the drug is used.

Category C rating: The FDA assigns a drug to Category **C** for one of two reasons: (1) Studies show evidence of fetal harm when using the drug in pregnant animals, but no controlled studies have been done using the drug in pregnant women, or (2) Studies using the drug in pregnant animals have not been done, and studies of pregnant women using the drug are insufficient to reach a conclusion. Thus, the drug should only be used if the potential benefit for mom is greater than the potential risk of fetal harm, which, in many cases, is unknown. Approximately 50% of prescription drugs fall in this category.

Category D rating: The FDA assigns a drug to Category **D** when studies of pregnant women using the drug show evidence of fetal harm. Rarely, however, the potential benefit of using the drug in some life-threatening situations for mom may outweigh the potential risk of fetal harm. For example, when mom requires cancer treatment or when she has a serious disease for which safer drugs cannot be used or are less effective. Approximately 11% of prescription drugs fall in this category.

Animal Studies: No birth defects in the offspring of pregnant rats and rabbits were found.

Human Studies: Controlled studies using this drug in pregnant women have not been done.

Helpful Hints: This drug has received a **D** rating for the second and third trimesters of pregnancy because it belongs to the beta-blocker family of drugs, which, as a group, have been found to cause toxic fetal effects if taken during the second and third trimesters.

Remember: All pregnancies have a background risk of about 3% for a major birth defect, even when mom doesn't take a drug of any kind. If you are pregnant or planning a pregnancy, always let your doctor know before taking any drug, prescription or non-prescription, or herbal remedy.

· ·

CARVEDILOL

Brand Name: Coreg. This drug is a member of the alpha and beta-blocker family of drugs.

Drug Uses: This drug is approved by the FDA for the treatment of high blood pressure, heart failure, and for use following heart attack.

Pregnancy Risk Categories: This drug has been assigned two pregnancy risk categories: **C** when used in the first trimester, and **D** when used in the second and third trimesters. Approximately 12% of prescription drugs are assigned two pregnancy risk categories, depending on which trimester of pregnancy the drug is used.

> **Category C rating:** The FDA assigns a drug to Category **C** for one of two reasons: (1) Studies show evidence of fetal harm when using the drug in pregnant animals, but no controlled studies have been done using the drug in pregnant women, or (2) Studies using the drug in pregnant animals have not been done, and studies of pregnant women using the drug are insufficient to reach a conclusion. Thus, the drug should only be used if the potential benefit for mom is greater than the potential risk of fetal harm, which, in many cases, is unknown. Approximately 50% of prescription drugs fall in this category.

> **Category D rating:** The FDA assigns a drug to Category **D** when studies of pregnant women using the drug show evidence of fetal harm. Rarely, however, the potential benefit of using the drug in some life-threatening situations for mom may outweigh the potential risk of fetal harm. For example, when mom requires cancer treatment or when she has a serious disease for which safer drugs cannot be used or are less effective. Approximately 11% of prescription drugs fall in this category.

Animal Studies: Studies in pregnant rats and rabbits treated with this drug did cause fetal harm, but the doses used were approximately 25 to 50 times the maximum recommended human dose.

Human Studies: Studies in pregnant women taking this drug are quite limited. Most experts feel the risk of birth defects using this drug is quite low. Since this drug is a member of the alpha and beta-blocker family of drugs, drugs in this family have been shown to cause under grown development in the fetus and a decrease of placental weight when members of this family of drugs are used in the second or third trimester. This explains why this drug has been assigned to a **D** category in the second and third trimesters of pregnancy.

Remember: All pregnancies have a background risk of about 3% for a major birth defect, even when mom doesn't take a drug of any kind. If you are pregnant or planning a pregnancy, always let your doctor know before taking any drug, prescription or non-prescription, or herbal remedy.

CEFOTAXIME

Brand Name: Claforan. This drug is a member of the cephalosporin antibiotic family of drugs.

Drug Use: This oral antibiotic is approved by the FDA to treat various forms of bacterial infections.

Pregnancy Risk Category: B

Category B rating: The FDA assigns a drug to Category **B** for one of two reasons: (1) Studies show no evidence of fetal harm when using the drug in pregnant animals, but no controlled studies have been done using the drug in pregnant women, or (2) Studies show evidence of fetal harm when using the drug in pregnant animals, but controlled studies using the drug in pregnant women do not show evidence of fetal harm. Approximately 21% of prescription drugs fall in this category.

Animal Studies: Studies using this drug in pregnant animals show no evidence of fetal harm.

Human Studies: Limited studies in pregnant women taking this drug show no evidence of fetal birth defects.

Helpful Hints: This family of antibiotics may decrease the effectiveness of birth control pills in preventing conception and pregnancy.

Remember: All pregnancies have a background risk of about 3% for a major birth defect, even when mom doesn't take a drug of any kind. If you are pregnant or planning a pregnancy, always let your doctor know before taking any drug, prescription or non-prescription, or herbal remedy.

∙∙∙∙∙∙∙∙∙∙∙∙∙∙∙∙∙∙∙∙∙∙∙∙∙∙∙∙∙∙∙∙∙∙∙∙

CEFOXITIN

Brand Name: Mefoxin. This drug is a member of the cephalosporin antibiotic family of drugs.

Drug Use: This oral antibiotic is approved by the FDA to treat various forms of bacterial infections.

Pregnancy Risk Category: B

> **Category B rating:** The FDA assigns a drug to Category **B** for one of two reasons: (1) Studies show no evidence of fetal harm when using the drug in pregnant animals, but no controlled studies have been done using the drug in pregnant women, or (2) Studies show evidence of fetal harm when using the drug in pregnant animals, but controlled studies using the drug in pregnant women do not show evidence of fetal harm. Approximately 21% of prescription drugs fall in this category.

Animal Studies: Studies in pregnant animals exposed to this drug show no evidence of fetal harm.

Human Studies: Limited studies in pregnant women taking this drug show no evidence of fetal birth defects.

Helpful Hints: This family of antibiotics may decrease the effectiveness of birth control pills in preventing conception and pregnancy.

Remember: All pregnancies have a background risk of about 3% for a major birth defect, even when mom doesn't take a drug of any kind. If you are pregnant or planning a pregnancy, always let your doctor know before taking any drug, prescription or non-prescription, or herbal remedy.

. . . .

CEFTRIAXONE

Brand Name: Rocephin. This drug is a member of the cephalosporin antibiotic family of drugs.

Drug Use: This oral antibiotic is approved by the FDA to treat various forms of bacterial infections.

Pregnancy Risk Category: B

Category B rating: The FDA assigns a drug to Category **B** for one of two reasons: (1) Studies show no evidence of fetal harm when using the drug in pregnant animals, but no controlled studies have been done using the drug in pregnant women, or (2) Studies show evidence of fetal harm when using the drug in pregnant animals, but controlled studies using the drug in pregnant women do not show evidence of fetal harm. Approximately 21% of prescription drugs fall in this category.

Animal Studies: Studies in pregnant animals exposed to this drug show no evidence of fetal harm.

Human Studies: Limited studies in pregnant women taking this drug show no evidence of fetal defects.

Helpful Hints: This family of antibiotics may decrease the effectiveness of birth control pills in preventing conception and pregnancy.

Remember: All pregnancies have a background risk of about 3% for a major birth defect, even when mom doesn't take a drug of any kind. If you are pregnant or planning a pregnancy, always let your doctor know before taking any drug, prescription or non-prescription, or herbal remedy.

. . . .

CELECOXIB

Brand Name: Celebrex. This drug is a member of the non-steroidal anti-inflammatory (NSAID) family of drugs. (See Helpful Hint on next page.)

Drug Uses: This drug has been approved by the FDA to relieve pain, tenderness, swelling, and stiffness caused by osteoarthritis and rheumatoid arthritis.

Pregnancy Risk Categories: This drug has been assigned two pregnancy risk categories: **C** when used in the first and second trimesters, and **D** when used in the third trimester. Approximately 12% of prescription drugs are assigned two pregnancy risk categories, depending on which trimester of pregnancy the drug is used.

> **Category C rating:** The FDA assigns a drug to Category **C** for one of two reasons: (1) Studies show evidence of fetal harm when using the drug in pregnant animals, but no controlled studies have been done using the drug in pregnant women, or (2) Studies using the drug in pregnant animals have not been done, and studies of pregnant women using the drug are insufficient to reach a conclusion. Thus, the drug should only be used if the potential benefit for mom is greater than the potential risk of fetal harm, which, in many cases, is unknown. Approximately 50% of prescription drugs fall in this category.

> **Category D rating:** The FDA assigns a drug to Category **D** when studies of pregnant women using the drug show evidence of fetal harm. Rarely, however, the potential benefit of using the drug in some life-threatening situations for mom may outweigh the potential risk of fetal harm. For example, when mom requires cancer treatment or when she has a serious disease for which safer drugs cannot be used or are less effective. Approximately 11% of prescription drugs fall in this category.

Animal Studies: Studies in pregnant animals treated with this drug suggest a low-risk for fetal birth defects.

Human Studies: No reports have been located in which pregnant women were treated with this drug.

Helpful Hints:

1. If this drug is used in pregnancy to treat rheumatoid arthritis, doctors are encouraged to call the toll-free number (877-311-8972) to enroll their patient in the OTIS rheumatoid arthritis study.

2. When taken in the third trimester of pregnancy, NSAIDs have seriously harmed the fetus, leading to life-threatening illness after birth and even death. These potential effects apply to all NSAIDs, whether purchased by prescription or over the counter without a prescription. They also explain why NSAIDs have been assigned a **D** pregnancy risk category. (See "Non-Steroidal, Anti-Inflammatory Drugs (NSAIDs) in Pregnancy" in the appendix for more details.)

Remember: All pregnancies have a background risk of about 3% for a major birth defect, even when mom doesn't take a drug of any kind. If you are pregnant or planning a pregnancy, always let your doctor know before taking any drug, prescription or non-prescription, or herbal remedy.

CEPHALEXIN

Brand Names: Biocef, Cefanex, Keflex. This drug is a member of the cephalosporin antibiotic family of drugs.

Drug Use: This oral antibiotic is approved by the FDA to treat various forms of bacterial infections.

Pregnancy Risk Category: B

Category B rating: The FDA assigns a drug to Category **B** for one of two reasons: (1) Studies show no evidence of fetal harm when using the drug in pregnant animals, but no controlled studies have been done using the drug in pregnant women, or (2) Studies show evidence of fetal harm when using the drug in pregnant animals, but controlled studies using the drug in pregnant women do not show evidence of fetal harm. Approximately 21% of prescription drugs fall in this category.

Animal Studies: Studies in pregnant mice and rats reveal no evidence of fetal harm.

Human Studies: Published studies in which this drug was used by pregnant women showed no evidence of fetal defects or newborn toxicity.

Helpful Hints: This family of antibiotics may decrease the effectiveness of birth control pills in preventing conception and pregnancy.

Remember: All pregnancies have a background risk of about 3% for a major birth defect, even when mom doesn't take a drug of any kind. If you are pregnant or planning a pregnancy, always let your doctor know before taking any drug, prescription or non-prescription, or herbal remedy.

• •

CETIRIZINE

Brand Name: Zyrtec

Drug Use: This drug is an antihistamine approved for the treatment of allergic rhinitis and other allergic symptoms.

Pregnancy Risk Category: B

Category B rating: The FDA assigns a drug to Category **B** for one of two reasons: (1) Studies show no evidence of fetal harm when using the drug in pregnant animals, but no controlled studies have been done using the drug in pregnant women, or (2) Studies show evidence of fetal harm when using the drug in pregnant animals, but controlled studies using the drug in pregnant women do not show evidence of fetal harm. Approximately 21% of prescription drugs fall in this category.

Animal Studies: Studies in pregnant mice, rats, and rabbits show no evidence of fetal harm, including birth defects.

Human Studies: Studies of cetirizine taken by pregnant women show no harmful fetal effects.

Remember: All pregnancies have a background risk of about 3% for a major birth defect, even when mom doesn't take a drug of any kind. If you are pregnant or planning a pregnancy, always let your doctor know before taking any drug, prescription or non-prescription, or herbal remedy.

. . . .

CHLORAMBUCIL

Brand Name: Leukeran

Drug Use: This drug is approved by the FDA for the treatment of certain types of cancer, including leukemia and lymphoma.

Pregnancy Risk Category: D

Category D rating: The FDA assigns a drug to Category **D** when studies of pregnant women using the drug show evidence of fetal harm. Rarely, however, the potential benefit of using the drug in some life-threatening situations for mom may outweigh the potential risk of fetal harm. For example, when mom requires cancer treatment or when she has a serious disease for which safer drugs cannot be used or are less effective. Approximately 11% of prescription drugs fall in this category.

Animal Studies: Pregnant rats treated with chlorambucil showed defects of the central nervous system, palate, skeleton, and kidneys in the offspring.

Human Studies: Controlled studies using the drug in pregnant women are not available. However, case reports of pregnant women using the drug have shown babies born with birth defects.

Helpful Hints: This drug should be avoided during pregnancy, especially the first three months when early organ development occurs. A reliable contraceptive is advisable during treatment with this drug.

Remember: All pregnancies have a background risk of about 3% for a major birth defect, even when mom doesn't take a drug of any kind. If you are pregnant or planning a pregnancy, always let your doctor know before taking any drug, prescription or non-prescription, or herbal remedy.

CHLORAMPHENICOL

Brand Name: Chloromycetin

Drug Use: This antibiotic is approved by the FDA to treat bacterial infections.

Pregnancy Risk Category: C

> **Category C rating:** The FDA assigns a drug to Category **C** for one of two reasons: (1) Studies show evidence of fetal harm when using the drug in pregnant animals, but no controlled studies have been done using the drug in pregnant women, or (2) Studies using the drug in pregnant animals have not been done, and studies of pregnant women using the drug are insufficient to reach a conclusion. Thus, the drug should only be used if the potential benefit for mom is greater than the potential risk of fetal harm, which, in many cases, is unknown. Approximately 50% of prescription drugs fall in this category.

Animal Studies: No reports associating this drug with birth defects in animals are available.

Human Studies: No controlled studies have been done using this drug in pregnant women. There are also no case reports associating this drug with birth defects. However, this drug should be used with caution near the time of delivery. When used near the time of delivery or in newborns, it has caused the "gray baby" syndrome characterized by gray skin color, low body temperature, bleeding, shock, kidney failure, and even death. Some experts believe this drug should not be used in pregnancy.

Remember: All pregnancies have a background risk of about 3% for a major birth defect, even when mom doesn't take a drug of any kind. If you are pregnant or planning a pregnancy, always let your doctor know before taking any drug, prescription or non-prescription, or herbal remedy.

CHLORDIAZEPOXIDE

Brand Names: Librium, Librax, Limbitrol. This drug is a member of the benzodiazepine family of drugs.

Drug Uses: This drug is approved by the FDA to relieve anxiety and control agitation caused by withdrawal from alcohol. It is also used to treat irritable bowel syndrome.

Pregnancy Risk Category: D

> **Category D rating:** The FDA assigns a drug to Category **D** when studies of pregnant women using the drug show evidence of fetal harm. Rarely, however, the potential benefit of using the drug in some life-threatening situations for mom may outweigh the potential risk of fetal harm. For example, when mom requires cancer treatment or when she has a serious disease for which safer drugs cannot be used or are less effective. Approximately 11% of prescription drugs fall in this category.

Animal Studies: Studies in pregnant rats using moderate doses of this drug show no birth defects in the offspring. However, when higher doses were used, maternal toxicity and increased offspring death and low birth weight were thought to be caused by this drug.

Human Studies: Some studies of pregnant women taking drugs in the benzodiazepine family of drugs during the first trimester of pregnancy have shown an increased rate of birth defects, while other studies have not. Since many of the women in these studies were also abusing alcohol and other drugs, the resulting defects may not have been caused by exposure to drugs in the benzodiazepine family of drugs.

Helpful Hints: Newborn respiratory depression and poor feeding have occurred within hours of delivery in infants born to mothers receiving this drug.

Remember: All pregnancies have a background risk of about 3% for a major birth defect, even when mom doesn't take a drug of any kind. If you are pregnant or planning a pregnancy, always let your doctor know before taking any drug, prescription or non-prescription, or herbal remedy.

• •

CHLOROQUINE

Brand Name: Aralen

Drug Use: This drug is approved by the FDA for the treatment and prevention of malaria and amebiasis.

Pregnancy Risk Category: C

> **Category C rating:** The FDA assigns a drug to Category **C** for one of two reasons: (1) Studies show evidence of fetal harm when using the drug in pregnant animals, but no controlled studies have been done using the drug in pregnant women, or (2) Studies using the drug in pregnant animals have not been done, and studies of pregnant women using the drug are insufficient to reach a conclusion. Thus, the drug should only be used if the potential benefit for mom is greater than the potential risk of fetal harm, which, in many cases, is unknown. Approximately 50% of prescription drugs fall in this category.

Animal Studies: Pregnant rats treated with this drug have shown an increased number of fetal deaths and birth defects in surviving offspring.

Human Studies: Malaria itself is associated with an increased number of complications during pregnancy, for mother and for baby. Unless you are taking chloroquine to treat malaria, this drug is not recommended during pregnancy. However, when given in low doses (once a week) to prevent malaria, this drug has not been shown to cause birth defects or other problems in humans.

Helpful Hints: This drug weakly interacts with grapefruit and grapefruit juice, which can cause harmful, and even life-threatening, side effects. Before taking this drug with grapefruit juice, or before consuming grapefruit or grapefruit juice during the day while taking this drug, first read the section "Grapefruit Juice–Drug Interactions Can Make You Sick" in the appendix of this book. Then discuss this with your pharmacist or the healthcare provider who prescribed this drug.

Remember: All pregnancies have a background risk of about 3% for a major birth defect, even when mom doesn't take a drug of any kind. If you are pregnant or planning a pregnancy, always let your doctor know before taking any drug, prescription or non-prescription, or herbal remedy.

• •

CHLOROTHIAZIDE

Brand Name: Diuril

Drug Use: This drug is approved by the FDA for use as a "water pill" when treating high blood pressure. The drug is a member of the thiazide family of diuretics.

Pregnancy Risk Categories: This drug has been assigned two pregnancy risk categories: **C** when used throughout pregnancy, and **D** when used specifically to treat high blood pressure that develops during pregnancy. Approximately 12% of prescription drugs are assigned two pregnancy risk categories, depending on which trimester of pregnancy the drug is used.

> **Category C rating:** The FDA assigns a drug to Category **C** for one of two reasons: (1) Studies show evidence of fetal harm when using the drug in pregnant animals, but no controlled studies have been done using the drug in pregnant women, or (2) Studies using the drug in pregnant animals have not been done, and studies of pregnant women using the drug are insufficient to reach a conclusion. Thus, the drug should only be used if the potential benefit for mom is greater than the potential risk of fetal harm, which, in many cases, is unknown. Approximately 50% of prescription drugs fall in this category.

> **Category D rating:** The FDA assigns a drug to Category **D** when studies of pregnant women using the drug show evidence of fetal harm. Rarely, however, the potential benefit of using the drug in some life-threatening situations for mom may outweigh the potential risk of fetal harm. For example, when mom requires cancer treatment or when she has a serious disease for which safer drugs cannot be used or are less effective. Approximately 11% of prescription drugs fall in this category.

Animal Studies: Studies in pregnant mice, rats, and rabbits showed no increase in birth defects.

Human Studies: Limited studies in pregnant women showed no increase in birth defects.

Helpful Hints: Many experts believe diuretics are not helpful during pregnancy except to assist in the treatment of a patient's heart disease or chronic hypertension, that is, high blood pressure that starts before pregnancy. Thus, diuretics are not recommended for hypertension that develops during pregnancy because these patients already have a low blood volume and the use of a diuretic will further decrease that blood volume, leading to complications. Also, thiazide diuretics in general may inhibit labor. So the main reason this drug has a **D** rating at all is for when it is used to treat hypertension that develops during pregnancy.

Remember: All pregnancies have a background risk of about 3% for a major birth defect, even when mom doesn't take a drug of any kind. If you are pregnant or planning a pregnancy, always let your doctor know before taking any drug, prescription or non-prescription, or herbal remedy.

CHLORPROMAZINE

Brand Name: Thorazine

Drug Uses: This drug is approved by the FDA to treat psychotic disorders. It is also used to treat nausea and vomiting, behavioral problems in children, and to relieve severe hiccups.

Pregnancy Risk Category: C

> **Category C rating:** The FDA assigns a drug to Category C for one of two reasons: (1) Studies show evidence of fetal harm when using the drug in pregnant animals, but no controlled studies have been done using the drug in pregnant women, or (2) Studies using the drug in pregnant animals have not been done, and studies of pregnant women using the drug are insufficient to reach a conclusion. Thus, the drug should only be used if the potential benefit for mom is greater than the potential risk of fetal harm, which, in many cases, is unknown. Approximately 50% of prescription drugs fall in this category.

Animal Studies: Studies in pregnant animals exposed to this drug show inconsistent results with a potential for fetal defects.

Human Studies: This drug has been used safely for many years to treat nausea and vomiting in pregnancy during all stages of pregnancy, including labor. Its use during labor and delivery has shown a drop in maternal blood pressure that could be dangerous for mom and baby. Most studies have found this drug safe, for mother and her unborn baby, if used occasionally and in small doses.

Remember: All pregnancies have a background risk of about 3% for a major birth defect, even when mom doesn't take a drug of any kind. If you are pregnant or planning a pregnancy, always let your doctor know before taking any drug, prescription or non-prescription, or herbal remedy.

· ·

CHLORPROPAMIDE

Brand Name: Diabinese

Drug Use: This drug is approved by the FDA for the treatment of adult-onset diabetes. But it is not the treatment of choice for diabetes that starts during pregnancy.

Pregnancy Risk Category: C

> **Category C rating:** The FDA assigns a drug to Category C for one of two reasons: (1) Studies show evidence of fetal harm when using the drug in pregnant animals, but no controlled studies have been done using the drug in pregnant women, or (2) Studies using the drug in pregnant animals have not been done, and studies of pregnant women using the drug are insufficient to reach a conclusion. Thus, the drug should only be used if the potential benefit for mom is greater than the potential risk of fetal harm, which, in many cases, is unknown. Approximately 50% of prescription drugs fall in this category.

Animal Studies: In a study of mouse embryos exposed to this drug, chlorpropamide produced malformations and slow growth in the embryos.

Human Studies: Limited studies in human pregnancy do not appear to be associated with fetal birth defects.

Helpful Hints: The American College of Obstetricians and Gynecologists (ACOG) recommends using insulin to treat Types 1 and 2 diabetes during pregnancy. If diet therapy alone is not successful for treating diabetes that starts during pregnancy, ACOG recommends using insulin to treat it, also.

Remember: All pregnancies have a background risk of about 3% for a major birth defect, even when mom doesn't take a drug of any kind. If you are pregnant or planning a pregnancy, always let your doctor know before taking any drug, prescription or non-prescription, or herbal remedy.

CILOSTAZOL

Brand Name: Pletal

Drug Use: This drug is approved by the FDA for use in the treatment of intermittent claudication, meaning pain on walking.

Pregnancy Risk Category: C

Category C rating: The FDA assigns a drug to Category C for one of two reasons: (1) Studies show evidence of fetal harm when using the drug in pregnant animals, but no controlled studies have been done using the drug in pregnant women, or (2) Studies using the drug in pregnant animals have not been done, and studies of pregnant women using the drug are insufficient to reach a conclusion. Thus, the drug should only be used if the potential benefit for mom is greater than the potential risk of fetal harm, which, in many cases, is unknown. Approximately 50% of prescription drugs fall in this category.

Animal Studies: Pregnant rats treated with this drug showed kidney and skeletal birth defects in their offspring. In addition, pregnant rabbits treated with this drug also showed delayed development of the sternum.

Human Studies: Controlled human studies using this drug are not available. This lack of human data prevents a thorough assessment of the risk to the human fetus.

Helpful Hints:

1. This drug is contraindicated in all patients, pregnant or not, with heart failure since studies have shown that survival is shortened when taking this drug compared to a placebo.

2. This drug weakly interacts with grapefruit and grapefruit juice, which can cause harmful, and even life-threatening, side effects. Before taking this drug with grapefruit juice, or before consuming grapefruit or grapefruit juice during the day while taking this drug, first read the section "Grapefruit Juice–Drug Interactions Can Make You Sick" in the appendix of this book. Then discuss this with your pharmacist or the healthcare provider who prescribed this drug.

Remember: All pregnancies have a background risk of about 3% for a major birth defect, even when mom doesn't take a drug of any kind. If you are pregnant or planning a pregnancy, always let your doctor know before taking any drug, prescription or non-prescription, or herbal remedy.

· ·

CIMETIDINE

Brand Name: Tagamet

Drug Uses: This drug is approved by the FDA for the treatment of intestinal ulcers, prevention of intestinal ulcers, and the prevention of gastric bleeding in seriously ill patients. It works by reducing the amount of gastric acid produced by the stomach.

Pregnancy Risk Category: B

Category B rating: The FDA assigns a drug to Category **B** for one of two reasons: (1) Studies show no evidence of fetal harm

when using the drug in pregnant animals, but no controlled studies have been done using the drug in pregnant women, or (2) Studies show evidence of fetal harm when using the drug in pregnant animals, but controlled studies using the drug in pregnant women do not show evidence of fetal harm. Approximately 21% of prescription drugs fall in this category.

Animal Studies: Pregnant rats and rabbits treated with this drug showed no birth defects in their offspring.

Human Studies: Controlled studies of pregnant women using this drug have not been done. However, several case reports of pregnant women using this drug have not shown an increased risk of birth defects in their babies.

Remember: All pregnancies have a background risk of about 3% for a major birth defect, even when mom doesn't take a drug of any kind. If you are pregnant or planning a pregnancy, always let your doctor know before taking any drug, prescription or non-prescription, or herbal remedy.

· ·

CIPROFLOXACIN

Brand Names: Ciloxan, Cipro, Cipro XR

Drug Use: This antibiotic is approved for the treatment of susceptible strains of bacterial infections, especially those involving the lungs, the sinuses, and skin.

Pregnancy Risk Category: C

Category C rating: The FDA assigns a drug to Category C for one of two reasons: (1) Studies show evidence of fetal harm when using the drug in pregnant animals, but no controlled studies have been done using the drug in pregnant women, or (2) Studies using the drug in pregnant animals have not been done, and studies of pregnant women using the drug are insufficient to reach a conclusion. Thus, the drug should only be used if the potential benefit for mom is greater than the potential risk of fetal harm, which, in many cases, is unknown. Approximately 50% of prescription drugs fall in this category.

Animal Studies: Pregnant rats and mice given this drug did not show any evidence of fetal harm. In addition, when pregnant rabbits were treated with this drug, there was also no increase in the incidence of birth defects.

Human Studies: Although several studies of pregnant women exposed to ciprofloxacin have not shown an increase in birth defects when compared to pregnant women not exposed to this drug, these studies are not sufficient to draw reliable conclusions about the safety of this drug during pregnancy. In fact, some experts feel this drug should not be used in pregnancy since even safer alternatives are available.

Remember: All pregnancies have a background risk of about 3% for a major birth defect, even when mom doesn't take a drug of any kind. If you are pregnant or planning a pregnancy, always let your doctor know before taking any drug, prescription or non-prescription, or herbal remedy.

CISPLATIN

Brand Name: Platinol-AQ

Drug Use: This anti-cancer medication is approved by the FDA for use in the treatment of various cancers.

Pregnancy Risk Category: D

> **Category D rating:** The FDA assigns a drug to Category **D** when studies of pregnant women using the drug show evidence of fetal harm. Rarely, however, the potential benefit of using the drug in some life-threatening situations for mom may outweigh the potential risk of fetal harm. For example, when mom requires cancer treatment or when she has a serious disease for which safer drugs cannot be used or are less effective. Approximately 11% of prescription drugs fall in this category.

Animal Studies: This drug causes mutations in bacteria, chromosome damage in animal tissues, and causes birth defects in mice. It also causes cancer in rats.

Human Studies: This drug has been shown to be toxic for pregnant women and their unborn babies. However, healthy babies have been born to mothers who took this drug for cancer treatment during pregnancy.

Helpful Hints: This drug should not be used in pregnancy unless mom is seriously ill with a disorder that requires this life-saving drug in pregnancy.

Remember: All pregnancies have a background risk of about 3% for a major birth defect, even when mom doesn't take a drug of any kind. If you are pregnant or planning a pregnancy, always let your doctor know before taking any drug, prescription or non-prescription, or herbal remedy.

• •

CITALOPRAM

Brand Name: Celexa

Drug Use: This drug is approved by the FDA for the treatment of depression. It belongs to the selective serotonin reuptake inhibitor (SSRI) family of drugs.

Pregnancy Risk Categories: This drug has been assigned two pregnancy risk categories: **C** when used in the first half of pregnancy and **D** when taken in the second half of pregnancy. Approximately 12% of prescription drugs are assigned two pregnancy risk categories, depending on which trimester of pregnancy the drug is used.

> **Category C rating:** The FDA assigns a drug to Category **C** for one of two reasons: (1) Studies show evidence of fetal harm when using the drug in pregnant animals, but no controlled studies have

been done using the drug in pregnant women, or (2) Studies using the drug in pregnant animals have not been done, and studies of pregnant women using the drug are insufficient to reach a conclusion. Thus, the drug should only be used if the potential benefit for mom is greater than the potential risk of fetal harm, which, in many cases, is unknown. Approximately 50% of prescription drugs fall in this category.

Category D rating: The FDA assigns a drug to Category **D** when studies of pregnant women using the drug show evidence of fetal harm. Rarely, however, the potential benefit of using the drug in some life-threatening situations for mom may outweigh the potential risk of fetal harm. For example, when mom requires cancer treatment or when she has a serious disease for which safer drugs cannot be used or are less effective. Approximately 11% of prescription drugs fall in this category.

Animal Studies: This drug was associated with embryo and fetal growth retardation, reduced survival, and birth defects in pregnant rats.

Human Studies: There are no controlled studies using this drug in pregnant women. However, there are numerous case reports involving SSRIs which have led to the **D** pregnancy risk category for this family of drugs when used in the second half of pregnancy.

Newborns exposed to members of the SSRI family of drugs in the second half of pregnancy have developed complications immediately after birth. These complications have required hospitalization, respiratory support, and tube feeding. These features are consistent with either a direct toxic effect of the drug or, possibly, abrupt withdrawal from the drug which occurs at birth, once the umbilical cord is cut. When treating a woman with a SSRI during the second half of pregnancy, the physician should carefully weigh these potential risks to the baby and the benefits of treatment to the mother.

Helpful Hints:

1. Studies show that antidepressants increase the risk of suicidal thinking and behavior in children, adolescents, and young adults. Anyone considering the use of this drug or any other antidepressant in these patients must balance that risk with the clinical need.

2. Almost all antidepressants carry some risk to the developing fetus. However, we also know depression in a pregnant woman carries potential risk for her health and for her unborn baby; for example, low birth weight and prematurity. The risks and benefits of medications and untreated depression must be weighed carefully. If you are pregnant and think you may have depression, or if you already know you do, talk with your doctor so the two of you can create the right plan for you and your unborn baby. (See "Antidepressants in Pregnancy" in the appendix for more detail.)

Remember: All pregnancies have a background risk of about 3% for a major birth defect, even when mom doesn't take a drug of any kind. If you are pregnant or planning a pregnancy, always let your doctor know before taking any drug, prescription or non-prescription, or herbal remedy.

. . . .

CLARITHROMYCIN

Brand Names: Biaxin, Biaxin XL

Drug Use: This antibiotic is approved by the FDA for the treatment of a variety of bacterial infections.

Pregnancy Risk Category: C

Category C rating: The FDA assigns a drug to Category C for one of two reasons: (1) Studies show evidence of fetal harm when using the drug in pregnant animals, but no controlled studies have been done using the drug in pregnant women, or (2) Studies using the drug in pregnant animals have not been done, and studies of pregnant women using the drug are insufficient to reach a conclusion. Thus, the drug should only be used if the potential benefit for mom is greater than the potential risk of fetal harm, which, in many cases, is unknown. Approximately 50% of prescription drugs fall in this category.

Animal Studies: This drug has demonstrated harmful effects on the offspring of pregnant mice, rats, rabbits, and monkeys.

Human Studies: There are no controlled studies available in pregnant women treated with this drug. There are several case reports of pregnant women treated effectively with this drug for intestinal infections with no harmful effects on their unborn babies. According to the Physician's Desk Reference (PDR), clarithromycin should not be used in pregnant women except in clinical circumstances where no alternative therapy is appropriate. If pregnancy occurs while taking this drug, the patient should be warned of the potential hazard to the fetus.

Helpful Hints: This drug weakly interacts with grapefruit and grapefruit juice, which can cause harmful, and even life-threatening, side effects. Before taking this drug with grapefruit juice, or before consuming grapefruit or grapefruit juice during the day while taking this drug, first read the section "Grapefruit Juice–Drug Interactions Can Make You Sick" in the appendix of this book. Then discuss this with your pharmacist or the healthcare provider who prescribed this drug.

Remember: All pregnancies have a background risk of about 3% for a major birth defect, even when mom doesn't take a drug of any kind. If you are pregnant or planning a pregnancy, always let your doctor know before taking any drug, prescription or non-prescription, or herbal remedy.

· ·

CLINDAMYCIN

Brand Name: Cleocin

Drug Use: This antibiotic is approved by the FDA to treat various bacterial infections.

Pregnancy Risk Category: B

> **Category B rating:** The FDA assigns a drug to Category **B** for one of two reasons: (1) Studies show no evidence of fetal harm when using the drug in pregnant animals, but no controlled studies have been done using the drug in pregnant women, or (2) Studies show evidence of fetal harm when using the drug in pregnant animals, but controlled studies using the drug in pregnant women do not show evidence of fetal harm. Approximately 21% of prescription drugs fall in this category.

Animal Studies: Pregnant mice and rats treated with this drug have shown no increased risk of fetal harm in the offspring.

Human Studies: Controlled studies in pregnant women are unavailable. However, a survey study of Michigan Medicaid recipients between 1985 and 1992 showed no increase in the number of birth defects of babies born to mothers taking this drug.

Remember: All pregnancies have a background risk of about 3% for a major birth defect, even when mom doesn't take a drug of any kind. If you are pregnant or planning a pregnancy, always let your doctor know

before taking any drug, prescription or non-prescription,
or herbal remedy.

• •

CLOFIBRATE

Brand Names: Abitrate, Atromid-S

Drug Use: This drug is used to lower cholesterol and
other lipids levels in the blood.

Pregnancy Risk Category: C

> **Category C rating:** The FDA assigns a drug to Category C for
> one of two reasons: (1) Studies show evidence of fetal harm when
> using the drug in pregnant animals, but no controlled studies have
> been done using the drug in pregnant women, or (2) Studies using
> the drug in pregnant animals have not been done, and studies of
> pregnant women using the drug are insufficient to reach a conclu-
> sion. Thus, the drug should only be used if the potential benefit for
> mom is greater than the potential risk of fetal harm, which, in many
> cases, is unknown. Approximately 50% of prescription drugs fall
> in this category.

Animal Studies: Studies using this drug in pregnant animals are not available.

Human Studies: No controlled studies using this drug in
pregnant women are available. However, since this drug
is broken down by a process that is immature at birth,
this drug can build up to dangerous levels in unborn babies who do not have the ability to break the drug down.
Patients should not take this drug without first talking to
their doctor.

Remember: All pregnancies have a background risk of
about 3% for a major birth defect, even when mom doesn't
take a drug of any kind. If you are pregnant or planning a
pregnancy, always let your doctor know before taking any
drug, prescription or non-prescription, or herbal remedy.

. . . .

CLOMIPHENE

Brand Names: Clomid, Serophene

Drug Use: This drug is approved by the FDA for use in stimulating ovulation.

Pregnancy Risk Category: X

> **Category X rating:** The FDA assigns a drug to Category **X** when studies have shown the risk of fetal harm clearly outweighs any potential maternal benefit from the drug. **Drugs in this category should not be used by pregnant women.** Approximately 5% of prescription drugs fall in this category.

Animal Studies: Some studies using clomiphene in pregnant animals have shown fetal harm in mice and rats; but no birth defects resulted in monkeys.

Human Studies: There are no controlled studies of clomiphene in pregnant women.

This drug is contraindicated after conception has occurred. There is a chance that clomiphene may cause birth defects if it is taken after you become pregnant. Therefore experts advise that patients stop taking the drug and tell their doctor if they think they have become pregnant while taking this drug. Some experts warn patients not to start a new course of this drug until after pregnancy has been excluded.

Remember: All pregnancies have a background risk of about 3% for a major birth defect, even when mom doesn't take a drug of any kind. If you are pregnant or planning a pregnancy, always let your doctor know before taking any drug, prescription or non-prescription, or herbal remedy.

· ·

CLONAZEPAM

Brand Name: Klonopin. This drug is a member of the benzodiazepine family of drugs.

Drug Uses: This drug is approved by the FDA for use in treating several types of seizures. It is also used to treat anxiety disorders.

Pregnancy Risk Category: D

> **Category D rating:** The FDA assigns a drug to Category **D** when studies of pregnant women using the drug show evidence of fetal harm. Rarely, however, the potential benefit of using the drug in some life-threatening situations for mom may outweigh the potential risk of fetal harm. For example, when mom requires cancer treatment or when she has a serious disease for which safer drugs cannot be used or are less effective. Approximately 11% of prescription drugs fall in this category.

Animal Studies: Pregnant rabbits treated with this drug have produced offspring with cleft palate and limb defects, but this did not occur in pregnant mice or rats.

Human Studies: There are no controlled studies using this drug in pregnant women. Until more information is available, experts advise that the safest course is to avoid using the drug, especially in the first trimester of pregnancy. In addition, toxicity has been demonstrated in the newborn in situations where the medication was taken near the end of pregnancy, close to term. These babies showed evidence of shallow breathing, cyanosis, lethargy, and decreased tone. Moreover, many of the babies showed signs of weakness, low body temperature, and depressed breathing.

Helpful Hints:

1. In pregnant women with epilepsy, the first priority is to prevent seizures. This can be difficult because many seizure medications do not work

quite as well during pregnancy. Sometimes the dose has to be increased or other medications added just to prevent seizures. Regardless, the healthiest situation for both mom and unborn baby is to have the fewest seizures possible.

2. Patients are advised not to abruptly stop taking this medication. If the drug is discontinued, it should be tapered gradually.

Remember: All pregnancies have a background risk of about 3% for a major birth defect, even when mom doesn't take a drug of any kind. If you are pregnant or planning a pregnancy, always let your doctor know before taking any drug, prescription or non-prescription, or herbal remedy.

CLONIDINE

Brand Names: Catapress, Duraclon

Drug Use: This drug is approved by the FDA for the treatment of high blood pressure.

Pregnancy Risk Category: C

Category C rating: The FDA assigns a drug to Category C for one of two reasons: (1) Studies show evidence of fetal harm when using the drug in pregnant animals, but no controlled studies have been done using the drug in pregnant women, or (2) Studies using the drug in pregnant animals have not been done, and studies of pregnant women using the drug are insufficient to reach a conclusion. Thus, the drug should only be used if the potential benefit for mom is greater than the potential risk of fetal harm, which, in many cases, is unknown. Approximately 50% of prescription drugs fall in this category.

Animal Studies: In pregnant rabbits treated with this drug, there was no evidence of fetal harm. However, in rats and mice, a number of the embryos died and were reabsorbed.

Human Studies: There are no controlled studies using this drug in pregnant women.

Remember: All pregnancies have a background risk of about 3% for a major birth defect, even when mom doesn't take a drug of any kind. If you are pregnant or planning a pregnancy, always let your doctor know before taking any drug, prescription or non-prescription, or herbal remedy.

• •

CLOPIDOGREL

Brand Name: Plavix

Drug Use: This drug is approved by the FDA to reduce the incidence of heart attack, stroke, and vascular death in patients with atherosclerosis.

Pregnancy Risk Category: B

> **Category B rating:** The FDA assigns a drug to Category **B** for one of two reasons: (1) Studies show no evidence of fetal harm when using the drug in pregnant animals, but no controlled studies have been done using the drug in pregnant women, or (2) Studies show evidence of fetal harm when using the drug in pregnant animals, but controlled studies using the drug in pregnant women do not show evidence of fetal harm. Approximately 21% of prescription drugs fall in this category.

Animal Studies: No birth defects resulted in the offspring of pregnant rats and rabbits treated with this drug.

Human Studies: There are no controlled studies using this drug in pregnant women.

Helpful Hints: Although there is limited human data for the use of this drug in pregnancy, the animal data suggests there is a low risk for fetal harm.

Remember: All pregnancies have a background risk of about 3% for a major birth defect, even when mom

doesn't take a drug of any kind. If you are pregnant or planning a pregnancy, always let your doctor know before taking any drug, prescription or non-prescription, or herbal remedy.

. . . .

CLOTRIMAZOLE

Brand Names: Clotrimazole, Lotrimin, Lotrisone, Mycelex

Drug Use: This drug is approved by the FDA for the treatment of susceptible fungal infections of the skin and mouth.

Pregnancy Risk Category: B

> **Category B rating:** The FDA assigns a drug to Category **B** for one of two reasons: (1) Studies show no evidence of fetal harm when using the drug in pregnant animals, but no controlled studies have been done using the drug in pregnant women, or (2) Studies show evidence of fetal harm when using the drug in pregnant animals, but controlled studies using the drug in pregnant women do not show evidence of fetal harm. Approximately 21% of prescription drugs fall in this category.

Animal Studies: No birth defects were found in the off-spring of pregnant mice, rats, and rabbits treated with this drug.

Human Studies: Adequate studies in pregnant women using this drug are not available. There are no reports linking this medication to birth defects in infants born to pregnant women using this drug.

Remember: All pregnancies have a background risk of about 3% for a major birth defect, even when mom doesn't take a drug of any kind. If you are pregnant or planning a pregnancy, always let your doctor know before taking any drug, prescription or non-prescription, or herbal remedy.

• •

CLOXACILLIN

Brand Name: Cloxapen. This drug is a member of the penicillin family of antibiotics.

Drug Use: This drug is approved by the FDA for the treatment of bacterial infections.

Pregnancy Risk Category: B

> **Category B rating:** The FDA assigns a drug to Category **B** for one of two reasons: (1) Studies show no evidence of fetal harm when using the drug in pregnant animals, but no controlled studies have been done using the drug in pregnant women, or (2) Studies show evidence of fetal harm when using the drug in pregnant animals, but controlled studies using the drug in pregnant women do not show evidence of fetal harm. Approximately 21% of prescription drugs fall in this category.

Animal Studies: There are no published reports linking this drug to birth defects in pregnant animals exposed to the drug.

Human Studies: Studies in pregnant women using this specific drug or other members of the penicillin family of drugs have not shown an increase in risk of birth defects.

Helpful Hints: Members of this family of drugs are generally considered safe for use in pregnancy.

Remember: All pregnancies have a background risk of about 3% for a major birth defect, even when mom doesn't take a drug of any kind. If you are pregnant or planning a pregnancy, always let your doctor know before taking any drug, prescription or non-prescription, or herbal remedy.

. . . .

CLOZAPINE

Brand Name: Clozaril

Drug Use: This drug is approved for the treatment of schizophrenia. This drug is a member of the "atypical antipsychotic" family of drugs which are also folic acid antagonists, meaning they interfere with folic acid absorption or its metabolism. (See Helpful Hint below.)

Pregnancy Risk Category: B

> **Category B rating:** The FDA assigns a drug to Category **B** for one of two reasons: (1) Studies show no evidence of fetal harm when using the drug in pregnant animals, but no controlled studies have been done using the drug in pregnant women, or (2) Studies show evidence of fetal harm when using the drug in pregnant animals, but controlled studies using the drug in pregnant women do not show evidence of fetal harm. Approximately 21% of prescription drugs fall in this category.

Animal Studies: No birth defects have been reported in the offspring of pregnant rats and rabbits treated with this drug.

Human Studies: There are no controlled studies using this drug in pregnant women.

Helpful Hints: Folic acid antagonists like clozapine are drugs that limit the effectiveness of folic acid, making it more likely that a baby born to a mom taking one of these drugs might have a serious birth defect, such as an open spine. If you are taking a folic acid antagonist and trying to become pregnant, discuss the possibility of increasing your folic acid intake with your clinician before becoming pregnant. (See "Folic Acid Antagonist Drugs in Pregnancy" in the appendix for more details.)

Remember: All pregnancies have a background risk of about 3% for a major birth defect, even when mom doesn't take a drug of any kind. If you are pregnant or planning a pregnancy, always let your doctor know before taking any drug, prescription or non-prescription, or herbal remedy.

COCAINE

Brand Name: Cocaine

Drug Use: This drug is legally available as a topical anesthetic in the United States.

Pregnancy Risk Categories: This drug has been assigned two pregnancy risk categories: **C** when used legally, and **X** when used illegally. Approximately 12% of prescription drugs are assigned two pregnancy risk categories, usually depending on which trimester of pregnancy the drug is used. However, in this case, the drug has been assigned two categories to make the distinction between legal and illegal use of the drug.

> **Category C rating:** The FDA assigns a drug to Category **C** for one of two reasons: (1) Studies show evidence of fetal harm when using the drug in pregnant animals, but no controlled studies have been done using the drug in pregnant women, or (2) Studies using the drug in pregnant animals have not been done, and studies of pregnant women using the drug are insufficient to reach a conclusion. Thus, the drug should only be used if the potential benefit for mom is greater than the potential risk of fetal harm, which, in many cases, is unknown. Approximately 50% of prescription drugs fall in this category.

> **Category X rating:** The FDA assigns a drug to Category **X** when studies have shown the risk of fetal harm clearly outweighs any potential maternal benefit from the drug. **Drugs in this category should not be used by pregnant women.** Approximately 5% of prescription drugs fall in this category.

Animal Studies: When pregnant rats were treated with intravenous cocaine, their offspring demonstrated long-term deficits in attention and memory.

Human Studies: Widespread abuse of cocaine has caused major toxicity in the fetus, newborn, and mother, including increased risk of fetal growth retardation, still-birth, premature labor, separation of the placenta from the uterus, and developmental delay in these children.

Risk factor **X** has been assigned for the illicit, non-medical use of this drug, which means it is contraindicated during pregnancy for those purposes. However, topical use as an anesthetic is compatible with normal pregnancy.

The potential benefits of using a topical cocaine-based anesthetic in pregnancy may outweigh the potential risk in certain cases.

Remember: All pregnancies have a background risk of about 3% for a major birth defect, even when mom doesn't take a drug of any kind. If you are pregnant or planning a pregnancy, always let your doctor know before taking any drug, prescription or non-prescription, or herbal remedy.

CODEINE

Brand Name: Codeine

Drug Uses: This narcotic is used to treat mild to moderate pain and is also used as a cough suppressant in lower doses.

Pregnancy Risk Categories: This drug has been assigned two pregnancy risk categories: **C** when used throughout pregnancy, whereas it is assigned **D** if used for prolonged periods or in high doses at term. Approximately 12% of prescription drugs are assigned two pregnancy risk categories, depending on which trimester of pregnancy the drug is used.

Category C rating: The FDA assigns a drug to Category **C** for one of two reasons: (1) Studies show evidence of fetal harm when using the drug in pregnant animals, but no controlled studies have been done using the drug in pregnant women, or (2) Studies using the drug in pregnant animals have not been done, and studies of pregnant women using the drug are insufficient to reach a conclusion. Thus, the drug should only be used if the potential benefit for mom is greater than the potential risk of fetal harm, which, in many cases, is unknown. Approximately 50% of prescription drugs fall in this category.

Category D rating: The FDA assigns a drug to Category **D** when studies of pregnant women using the drug show evidence of fetal harm. Rarely, however, the potential benefit of using the drug in some life-threatening situations for mom may outweigh the potential risk of fetal harm. For example, when mom requires cancer treatment or when she has a serious disease for which safer drugs cannot be used or are less effective. Approximately 11% of prescription drugs fall in this category.

Animal Studies: In pregnant hamsters treated with codeine, skull defects were noted in some of the offspring.

Human Studies: Controlled studies of codeine in pregnant women are not available. The use of codeine during labor may produce respiratory depression in the newborn immediately after birth and signs of drug withdrawal.

Helpful Hints:

1. If codeine is used during labor around the time of birth, it is prudent for caregivers to have a skilled person available to respond to the baby's respiratory depression or symptoms of drug withdrawal should they occur.

2. Some cough syrups contain ethanol (alcohol). Be sure to check the label on the bottle to see if ethanol is listed as an ingredient. Alcohol is known to cause birth defects in developing fetuses.

Remember: All pregnancies have a background risk of about 3% for a major birth defect, even when mom doesn't take a drug of any kind. If you are pregnant or planning a pregnancy, always let your doctor know before taking any drug, prescription or non-prescription, or herbal remedy.

. . . .

COLCHICINE

Brand Name: Colchicine

Drug Use: This drug is approved by the FDA for the treatment of gout.

Pregnancy Risk Category: D

> **Category D rating:** The FDA assigns a drug to Category **D** when studies of pregnant women using the drug show evidence of fetal harm. Rarely, however, the potential benefit of using the drug in some life-threatening situations for mom may outweigh the potential risk of fetal harm. For example, when mom requires cancer treatment or when she has a serious disease for which safer drugs cannot be used or are less effective. Approximately 11% of prescription drugs fall in this category.

Animal Studies: Pregnant mice, rats, and rabbits exposed to colchicine produced harmful effects on their embryos and fetuses.

Human Studies: Controlled studies using colchicine in pregnant women have not been done.

Although no birth defects have been reported in the limited number of pregnant women taking colchicine during pregnancy, the drug should only be used for serious disease where safer drugs cannot be used for some reason.

Helpful Hints: This drug weakly interacts with grapefruit and grapefruit juice, which can cause harmful, and even life-threatening, side effects. Before taking this drug with grapefruit juice, or before consuming grapefruit or grapefruit juice during the day while taking this drug, first read the section "Grapefruit Juice–Drug Interactions Can Make You Sick" in the appendix of this book. Then discuss this with your pharmacist or the healthcare provider who prescribed this drug.

Remember: All pregnancies have a background risk of about 3% for a major birth defect, even when mom doesn't take a drug of any kind. If you are pregnant or planning a pregnancy, always let your doctor know before taking any drug, prescription or non-prescription, or herbal remedy.

COLESEVELAM

Brand Name: Welchol

Drug Use: This non-absorbed drug is approved by the FDA for use in lowering blood cholesterol.

Pregnancy Risk Category: B

Category B rating: The FDA assigns a drug to Category **B** for one of two reasons: (1) Studies show no evidence of fetal harm when using the drug in pregnant animals, but no controlled studies have been done using the drug in pregnant women, or (2) Studies show evidence of fetal harm when using the drug in pregnant animals, but controlled studies using the drug in pregnant women do not show evidence of fetal harm. Approximately 21% of prescription drugs fall in this category.

Animal Studies: Studies using this drug in pregnant rats and rabbits reveal no evidence of fetal harm.

Human Studies: Although controlled studies have not been done in pregnant women, because this drug is not absorbed from the intestine, it's unlikely that this drug will harm the embryo or fetus.

Remember: All pregnancies have a background risk of about 3% for a major birth defect, even when mom doesn't take a drug of any kind. If you are pregnant or planning a pregnancy, always let your doctor know before taking any drug, prescription or non-prescription, or herbal remedy.

. . . .

COLESTIPOL

Brand Names: Colestid, Lestid

Drug Use: This drug is approved by the FDA for lowering the blood level of cholesterol.

Pregnancy Risk Category: B

Category B rating: The FDA assigns a drug to Category **B** for one of two reasons: (1) Studies show no evidence of fetal harm when using the drug in pregnant animals, but no controlled studies have been done using the drug in pregnant women, or (2) Studies show evidence of fetal harm when using the drug in pregnant animals, but controlled studies using the drug in pregnant women do not show evidence of fetal harm. Approximately 21% of prescription drugs fall in this category.

Animal Studies: Studies using this drug in pregnant rats and rabbits showed no harmful fetal effects.

Human Studies: No studies using this drug in pregnant women have been reported. Most experts feel that this drug is safe to take during pregnancy.

Remember: All pregnancies have a background risk of about 3% for a major birth defect, even when mom doesn't take a drug of any kind. If you are pregnant or planning a pregnancy, always let your doctor know before taking any drug, prescription or non-prescription, or herbal remedy.

. . . .

CROMOLYN

Brand Name: Crolom

Drug Use: This drug is approved by the FDA for use in treating and preventing season allergic disorders.

Pregnancy Risk Category: B

> **Category B rating:** The FDA assigns a drug to Category **B** for one of two reasons: (1) Studies show no evidence of fetal harm when using the drug in pregnant animals, but no controlled studies have been done using the drug in pregnant women, or (2) Studies show evidence of fetal harm when using the drug in pregnant animals, but controlled studies using the drug in pregnant women do not show evidence of fetal harm. Approximately 21% of prescription drugs fall in this category.

Animal Studies: Studies using cromolyn in pregnant mice, rats, and rabbits revealed no birth defects due to this drug.

Human Studies: Controlled studies using this drug for pregnant women are not available. However, uncontrolled studies did not show an association with birth defects.

Remember: All pregnancies have a background risk of about 3% for a major birth defect, even when mom doesn't take a drug of any kind. If you are pregnant or planning a pregnancy, always let your doctor know before taking any drug, prescription or non-prescription, or herbal remedy.

. . . .

CYCLIZINE

Brand Names: Marezine, Marzine

Drug Use: This antihistamine is used to prevent nausea and vomiting associated with motion sickness.

Pregnancy Risk Category: **B**

Category B rating: The FDA assigns a drug to Category **B** for one of two reasons: (1) Studies show no evidence of fetal harm when using the drug in pregnant animals, but no controlled studies have been done using the drug in pregnant women, or (2) Studies show evidence of fetal harm when using the drug in pregnant animals, but controlled studies using the drug in pregnant women do not show evidence of fetal harm. Approximately 21% of prescription drugs fall in this category.

Animal Studies: Studies in pregnant animals treated with doses of this drug many times the usual human dose have been shown to cause birth defects such as cleft palate.

Human Studies: Cyclizine has not been shown to cause birth defects in pregnant women treated with this drug.

Remember: All pregnancies have a background risk of about 3% for a major birth defect, even when mom doesn't take a drug of any kind. If you are pregnant or planning a pregnancy, always let your doctor know before taking any drug, prescription or non-prescription, or herbal remedy.

. . . .

CYCLOBENZAPRINE

Brand Name: Flexeril

Drug Uses: This drug is approved by the FDA to relax skeletal muscles. It is also used to treat fibromyalgia.

Pregnancy Risk Category: **B**

Category B rating: The FDA assigns a drug to Category **B** for one of two reasons: (1) Studies show no evidence of fetal harm when using the drug in pregnant animals, but no controlled studies have been done using the drug in pregnant women, or (2) Studies show evidence of fetal harm when using the drug in pregnant animals, but controlled studies using the drug in pregnant women do not show evidence of fetal harm. Approximately 21% of prescription drugs fall in this category.

Animal Studies: Studies of pregnant mice, rats, and rabbits using this drug have shown no evidence of birth defects in their offspring.

Human Studies: Controlled studies using this drug in pregnant women have not been done.

Remember: All pregnancies have a background risk of about 3% for a major birth defect, even when mom doesn't take a drug of any kind. If you are pregnant or planning a pregnancy, always let your doctor know before taking any drug, prescription or non-prescription, or herbal remedy.

CYCLOPHOSPHAMIDE

Brand Names: Cytoxan, Neosar

Drug Use: This drug is approved by the FDA for the treatment of several types of cancer.

Pregnancy Risk Category: D

> **Category D rating:** The FDA assigns a drug to Category **D** when studies of pregnant women using the drug show evidence of fetal harm. Rarely, however, the potential benefit of using the drug in some life-threatening situations for mom may outweigh the potential risk of fetal harm. For example, when mom requires cancer treatment or when she has a serious disease for which safer drugs cannot be used or are less effective. Approximately 11% of prescription drugs fall in this category.

Animal Studies: Studies in pregnant mice, rats, and rabbits treated with this drug have shown birth defects in their offspring.

Human Studies: Infants with major birth defects as well as normal infants have been born to mothers taking this drug during pregnancy. This drug should not be used in the first trimester of pregnancy. Otherwise, the drug should only be used at other times in the case of serious or life-threatening illnesses where a safer drug will not work or cannot be used.

Remember: All pregnancies have a background risk of about 3% for a major birth defect, even when mom doesn't take a drug of any kind. If you are pregnant or planning a pregnancy, always let your doctor know before taking any drug, prescription or non-prescription, or herbal remedy.

. . . .

CYCLOSPORINE

Brand Names: Gengraf, Neoral, Sandimmune

Drug Use: This drug is approved by the FDA for use in suppressing the body's immunity to prevent the rejection of organ transplants.

Pregnancy Risk Category: C

> **Category C rating:** The FDA assigns a drug to Category C for one of two reasons: (1) Studies show evidence of fetal harm when using the drug in pregnant animals, but no controlled studies have been done using the drug in pregnant women, or (2) Studies using the drug in pregnant animals have not been done, and studies of pregnant women using the drug are insufficient to reach a conclusion. Thus, the drug should only be used if the potential benefit for mom is greater than the potential risk of fetal harm, which, in many cases, is unknown. Approximately 50% of prescription drugs fall in this category.

Animal Studies: In studies of pregnant rats and rabbits treated with toxic doses of this drug, fetal weight was reduced and fetal mortality was increased. However, no birth defects were found.

Human Studies: Based on limited experience treating pregnant women with this drug, it has not been shown to cause birth defects in humans.

Helpful Hints: This drug weakly interacts with grapefruit and grapefruit juice, which can cause harmful, and even life-threatening, side effects. Before taking this drug with grapefruit juice, or before consuming grapefruit or grapefruit juice during the day while taking this drug, first read the section "Grapefruit Juice–Drug Interactions Can Make You Sick" in the appendix of this book. Then discuss this with your pharmacist or the healthcare provider who prescribed this drug.

Remember: All pregnancies have a background risk of about 3% for a major birth defect, even when mom doesn't take a drug of any kind. If you are pregnant or planning a pregnancy, always let your doctor know before taking any drug, prescription or non-prescription, or herbal remedy.

• •

CYPROHEPTADINE

Brand Name: Periactin

Drug Use: This antihistamine has been approved by the FDA for the treatment of common seasonal and year-round allergies.

Pregnancy Risk Category: B

> **Category B rating:** The FDA assigns a drug to Category **B** for one of two reasons: (1) Studies show no evidence of fetal harm when using the drug in pregnant animals, but no controlled studies have been done using the drug in pregnant women, or (2) Studies show evidence of fetal harm when using the drug in pregnant animals, but controlled studies using the drug in pregnant women do not show evidence of fetal harm. Approximately 21% of prescription drugs fall in this category.

Animal Studies: Studies in pregnant mice, rats, and rabbits treated with up to 32 times the maximum recommended human dose of this drug revealed no evidence of fetal harm.

Human Studies: No controlled studies of this drug in pregnant women are available.

Remember: All pregnancies have a background risk of about 3% for a major birth defect, even when mom doesn't take a drug of any kind. If you are pregnant or planning a pregnancy, always let your doctor know before taking any drug, prescription or non-prescription, or herbal remedy.

. . . .

CYTARABINE

Brand Name: Depocyt

Drug Use: This drug is used to treat several types of leukemia.

Pregnancy Risk Category: D

> **Category D rating:** The FDA assigns a drug to Category **D** when studies of pregnant women using the drug show evidence of fetal harm. Rarely, however, the potential benefit of using the drug in some life-threatening situations for mom may outweigh the potential risk of fetal harm. For example, when mom requires cancer treatment or when she has a serious disease for which safer drugs cannot be used or are less effective. Approximately 11% of prescription drugs fall in this category.

Animal Studies: Cytarabine has caused major birth defects in pregnant mice and rats.

Human Studies: There are no controlled studies using this drug in pregnant women.

Remember: All pregnancies have a background risk of about 3% for a major birth defect, even when mom doesn't take a drug of any kind. If you are pregnant or planning a pregnancy, always let your doctor know before taking any drug, prescription or non-prescription, or herbal remedy.

. . . .

ADDITIONAL DRUGS AND THEIR FDA PREGNANCY RISK CATEGORIES

Since these additional drugs are uncommonly used in pregnancy, they are listed by generic name along with their FDA Pregnancy Risk Category without more detail:

Calcipotriene - C

Carbenicillin - B

Carboplatin - D

Carmustine - D

Cefaclor - B

Cefadroxil - B

Cefazolin - B

Cefdinir - B

Cefditoren - B

Cefepime - B

Cefixime - B

Cefprozil - B

Ceftazidime - B

Ceftibuten - B

Cefuroxime - B

Cetuximab - C

Cevimeline - C

Chlorhexidine - B

Chlorpheniramine - B

Chlorthalidone - B (D if used in gestational hypertension)

Chlorzoxazone - C

Cholestyramine - B

Ciclesonide - C

Ciclopirox - B

Cidofovir - C

Cinacalcet - C

Clobetasol - C

Clofarabine - D

Clomipramine - C

D

DESIPRAMINE

Brand Name: Norpramin

Drug Use: This drug is approved by the FDA for the treatment of depression.

Pregnancy Risk Category: C

> **Category C rating:** The FDA assigns a drug to Category C for one of two reasons: (1) Studies show evidence of fetal harm when using the drug in pregnant animals, but no controlled studies have been done using the drug in pregnant women, or (2) Studies using the drug in pregnant animals have not been done, and studies of pregnant women using the drug are insufficient to reach a conclusion. Thus, the drug should only be used if the potential benefit for mom is greater than the potential risk of fetal harm, which, in many cases, is unknown. Approximately 50% of prescription drugs fall in this category.

Animal Studies: No studies using this drug in pregnant animals have been reported.

Human Studies: Controlled studies using this drug in pregnant women have not been done. However, there are reports of women taking this drug during pregnancy, and no increased risk of birth defects was seen. When women do take desipramine throughout their entire pregnancies, their babies have an increased risk of experiencing withdrawal symptoms, such as fast heart rate and weight loss after birth.

Helpful Hints:

1. Studies show that antidepressants increase the risk of suicidal thinking and behavior in children,

adolescents, and young adults. Anyone considering the use of this drug or any other antidepressant in these patients must balance that risk with
the clinical need.

2. Almost all antidepressants carry some risk to the
developing fetus. However, we also know depression in a pregnant woman carries potential
risk for her health and for her unborn baby; for
example, low birth weight and prematurity. The
risks and benefits of medications and untreated
depression must be weighed carefully. If you are
pregnant and think you may have depression, or
if you already know you do, talk with your doctor so the two of you can create the right plan
for you and your unborn baby. (See "Antidepressants in Pregnancy" in the appendix of this book
for further information.)

Remember: All pregnancies have a background risk of
about 3% for a major birth defect, even when mom doesn't
take a drug of any kind. If you are pregnant or planning a
pregnancy, always let your doctor know before taking any
drug, prescription or non-prescription, or herbal remedy.

DEXAMETHASONE

Brand Name: Decadron. This drug is a member of the
corticosteroid family of drugs.

Drug Uses: This drug is approved by the FDA for the treatment of arthritis, severe allergies, asthma, certain types of
cancer, and other disorders.

Pregnancy Risk Categories: This drug has been assigned two pregnancy risk categories: **C** when used in

the second and third trimesters, and **D** when used in the first trimester. Approximately 12% of prescription drugs are assigned two pregnancy risk categories, depending on which trimester of pregnancy the drug is used.

> **Category C rating:** The FDA assigns a drug to Category **C** for one of two reasons: (1) Studies show evidence of fetal harm when using the drug in pregnant animals, but no controlled studies have been done using the drug in pregnant women, or (2) Studies using the drug in pregnant animals have not been done, and studies of pregnant women using the drug are insufficient to reach a conclusion. Thus, the drug should only be used if the potential benefit for mom is greater than the potential risk of fetal harm, which, in many cases, is unknown. Approximately 50% of prescription drugs fall in this category.

> **Category D rating:** The FDA assigns a drug to Category **D** when studies of pregnant women using the drug show evidence of fetal harm. Rarely, however, the potential benefit of using the drug in some life-threatening situations for mom may outweigh the potential risk of fetal harm. For example, when mom requires cancer treatment or when she has a serious disease for which safer drugs cannot be used or are less effective. Approximately 11% of prescription drugs fall in this category.

Animal Studies: The offspring of pregnant animals treated with this drug have shown a variety of toxic effects, such as decreased head size, decreased adrenal and placental weight, and increased liver weight.

Human Studies: Studies have linked this family of drugs to certain birth defects when pregnant women have taken the drug one month before to three months after conception. That is why this drug has a **D** risk rating if used in the first trimester of pregnancy.

Remember: All pregnancies have a background risk of about 3% for a major birth defect, even when mom doesn't take a drug of any kind. If you are pregnant or planning a pregnancy, always let your doctor know before taking any drug, prescription or non-prescription, or herbal remedy.

. . . .
DEXMETHYLPHENIDATE

Brand Name: Focalin

Drug Use: The FDA has approved this drug for the treatment of attention deficit hyperactivity disorder (ADHD).

Pregnancy Risk Category: C

> **Category C rating:** The FDA assigns a drug to Category **C** for one of two reasons: (1) Studies show evidence of fetal harm when using the drug in pregnant animals, but no controlled studies have been done using the drug in pregnant women, or (2) Studies using the drug in pregnant animals have not been done, and studies of pregnant women using the drug are insufficient to reach a conclusion. Thus, the drug should only be used if the potential benefit for mom is greater than the potential risk of fetal harm, which, in many cases, is unknown. Approximately 50% of prescription drugs fall in this category.

Animal Studies: When pregnant rats were treated with this drug, there was no increased risk of birth defects. However, at the highest doses tested, some of the developing fetuses showed delayed bone formation.

Human Studies: There are no reported human studies using this drug in pregnant women.

Remember: All pregnancies have a background risk of about 3% for a major birth defect, even when mom doesn't take a drug of any kind. If you are pregnant or planning a pregnancy, always let your doctor know before taking any drug, prescription or non-prescription, or herbal remedy.
. . . .
DEXTROMETHORPHAN

Brand Name: Dextromethorphan is an active ingredient in several cough syrups. These brands include Robitussin, Delsym, and Silphen.

Drug Use: The FDA has approved this drug for use as a cough suppressant.

Pregnancy Risk Category: C

> **Category C rating:** The FDA assigns a drug to Category C for one of two reasons: (1) Studies show evidence of fetal harm when using the drug in pregnant animals, but no controlled studies have been done using the drug in pregnant women, or (2) Studies using the drug in pregnant animals have not been done, and studies of pregnant women using the drug are insufficient to reach a conclusion. Thus, the drug should only be used if the potential benefit for mom is greater than the potential risk of fetal harm, which, in many cases, is unknown. Approximately 50% of prescription drugs fall in this category.

Animal Studies: One study conducted on chick embryos showed an increase of birth defects. There are no other reports, however, using dextromethorphan in pregnant animals.

Human Studies: Studies involving pregnant women treated with this drug have shown no link between this drug and birth defects.

Helpful Hints:

1. Some cough syrups contain ethanol (alcohol). Be sure to check the label on the bottle to see if ethanol is listed as an ingredient. Alcohol is known to cause birth defects in developing fetuses.

2. This drug weakly interacts with grapefruit and grapefruit juice, which can cause harmful, and even life-threatening, side effects. Before taking this drug with grapefruit juice, or before consuming grapefruit or grapefruit juice during the day while taking this drug, first read the section "Grapefruit Juice–Drug Interactions Can Make You Sick" in the appendix of this book. Then

discuss this with your pharmacist or the health-care provider who prescribed this drug.

Remember: All pregnancies have a background risk of about 3% for a major birth defect, even when mom doesn't take a drug of any kind. If you are pregnant or planning a pregnancy, always let your doctor know before taking any drug, prescription or non-prescription, or herbal remedy.

DIAZEPAM

Brand Name: Valium. This drug is a member of the benzodiazepine family of drugs.

Drug Uses: The FDA has approved diazepam for the treatment of anxiety, alcohol withdrawal symptoms, muscle spasms, and certain seizure disorders.

Pregnancy Risk Category: D

Category D rating: The FDA assigns a drug to Category **D** when studies of pregnant women using the drug show evidence of fetal harm. Rarely, however, the potential benefit of using the drug in some life-threatening situations for mom may outweigh the potential risk of fetal harm. For example, when mom requires cancer treatment or when she has a serious disease for which safer drugs cannot be used or are less effective. Approximately 11% of prescription drugs fall in this category.

Animal Studies: When pregnant mice were treated with diazepam, there was an increased risk of cleft palate, a hole in the roof of their mouth, in their offspring. Offspring of pregnant rats given this drug showed an increased risk of delayed behavioral development and cancers.

Human Studies: Studies on pregnant women taking this drug have shown that it crosses the placenta and enters the fetal circulation very easily. It probably accumulates in the fetus since concentrations of diazepam in the newborn baby's blood can be one to three times as high as the concentration of the drug in the mother's blood. There is conflict in the studies on pregnant women about whether or not this drug is associated with increased risk of birth defects. Withdrawal from this drug has been seen in newborn babies whose mothers took diazepam close to the time of delivery. Symptoms included shaking, irritability, diarrhea, and vomiting.

Helpful Hints: This drug strongly interacts with grapefruit and grapefruit juice, which can cause harmful, and even life-threatening, side effects. Before taking this drug with grapefruit juice, or before consuming grapefruit or grapefruit juice during the day while taking this drug, first read the section "Grapefruit Juice–Drug Interactions Can Make You Sick" in the appendix of this book. Then discuss this with your pharmacist or the healthcare provider who prescribed this drug.

Remember: All pregnancies have a background risk of about 3% for a major birth defect, even when mom doesn't take a drug of any kind. If you are pregnant or planning a pregnancy, always let your doctor know before taking any drug, prescription or non-prescription, or herbal remedy.

DIAZOXIDE

Brand Names: Hyperstat, Proglycem

Drug Use: The FDA has approved this drug for the treatment of severe high blood pressure.

Pregnancy Risk Category: C

Category C rating: The FDA assigns a drug to Category **C** for one of two reasons: (1) Studies show evidence of fetal harm when using the drug in pregnant animals, but no controlled studies have been done using the drug in pregnant women, or (2) Studies using the drug in pregnant animals have not been done, and studies of pregnant women using the drug are insufficient to reach a conclusion. Thus, the drug should only be used if the potential benefit for mom is greater than the potential risk of fetal harm, which, in many cases, is unknown. Approximately 50% of prescription drugs fall in this category.

Animal Studies: When pregnant rats, cats, and dogs were treated with this drug, their offspring showed decreased fetal and newborn survival as well as decreased fetal growth.

Human Studies: When given to pregnant women to lower blood pressure, this drug has been shown to lower the blood pressure too much, which then can decrease the blood flow to the fetus. This, in turn, may result in decreased oxygen delivery to the fetus. In addition, an increase in blood sugar in both mom and her baby has been also seen.

Helpful Hints: High blood pressure in pregnant women can be very serious. When it needs to be treated with medication, there are many options available. Those options include drugs which have less risk for mom and for her unborn baby than this medication does. It is important that you review these risks and benefits with your doctor and decide which option is best for you.

Remember: All pregnancies have a background risk of about 3% for a major birth defect, even when mom doesn't take a drug of any kind. If you are pregnant or planning a pregnancy, always let your doctor know before taking any drug, prescription or non-prescription, or herbal remedy.

DICUMAROL

Brand Name: Dicumarol

Drug Use: The FDA has approved dicumarol for use as a blood thinner to treat a variety of conditions. Dicumarol belongs to the coumarin family of drugs.

Pregnancy Risk Category: D

> **Category D rating:** The FDA assigns a drug to Category **D** when studies of pregnant women using the drug show evidence of fetal harm. Rarely, however, the potential benefit of using the drug in some life-threatening situations for mom may outweigh the potential risk of fetal harm. For example, when mom requires cancer treatment or when she has a serious disease for which safer drugs cannot be used or are less effective. Approximately 11% of prescription drugs fall in this category.

Animal Studies: No relevant data is available about using this drug in pregnant animals.

Human Studies: Several potential problems may occur when this drug is used in pregnancy. For example, human fetuses have shown brain defects, there has been an increased risk of miscarriage and stillbirth, prematurity, severe bleeding, seizures, deafness, and heart defects in these babies. The occurrence of these complications depends largely on the time in pregnancy the fetus is exposed to this drug. Exposure during the first trimester seems to have the most potential for these kinds of problems to occur.

Helpful Hints: There are many conditions that require a woman to be treated with a blood thinner during pregnancy. There are other medications, such as heparin, that pose much less risk to mom and her fetus than coumarin-type drugs.

Remember: All pregnancies have a background risk of about 3% for a major birth defect, even when mom doesn't take a drug of any kind. If you are pregnant or planning a pregnancy, always let your doctor know before taking any drug, prescription or non-prescription, or herbal remedy.

· ·

DIDANOSINE

Brand Name: Bidex

Drug Use: The FDA has approved this drug for the treatment of HIV infection.

Pregnancy Risk Category: B

> **Category B rating:** The FDA assigns a drug to Category **B** for one of two reasons: (1) Studies show no evidence of fetal harm when using the drug in pregnant animals, but no controlled studies have been done using the drug in pregnant women, or (2) Studies show evidence of fetal harm when using the drug in pregnant animals, but controlled studies using the drug in pregnant women do not show evidence of fetal harm. Approximately 21% of prescription drugs fall in this category.

Animal Studies: Studies using this drug in pregnant rats, rabbits, and mice have shown no increased risk of birth defects when given this drug.

Human Studies: Studies on pregnant women using this drug are limited. So far, no firm conclusions have been reached about the safety of this drug. However, results so far suggest that didanosine poses a low risk to the fetus.

Helpful Hints: The Centers for Disease Control recommends that women who have HIV continue their medication throughout pregnancy. The benefit of treating the mother likely outweighs any risk of medication to her unborn baby.

Remember: All pregnancies have a background risk of about 3% for a major birth defect, even when mom doesn't take a drug of any kind. If you are pregnant or planning a pregnancy, always let your doctor know before taking any drug, prescription or non-prescription, or herbal remedy.

. . . .

DIGOXIN

Brand Name: Lanoxin

Drug Uses: The FDA has approved digoxin for the treatment of congestive heart failure, atrial fibrillation, paroxysmal atrial tachycardia, and certain irregular heart rhythms.

Pregnancy Risk Category: C

> **Category C rating:** The FDA assigns a drug to Category **C** for one of two reasons: (1) Studies show evidence of fetal harm when using the drug in pregnant animals, but no controlled studies have been done using the drug in pregnant women, or (2) Studies using the drug in pregnant animals have not been done, and studies of pregnant women using the drug are insufficient to reach a conclusion. Thus, the drug should only be used if the potential benefit for mom is greater than the potential risk of fetal harm, which, in many cases, is unknown. Approximately 50% of prescription drugs fall in this category.

Animal Studies: When pregnant animals were treated with this drug, no increased risk of birth defects was seen.

Human Studies: The use of digitalis in pregnant women has not been linked with birth defects.

Helpful Hints: This drug weakly interacts with grapefruit and grapefruit juice, which can cause harmful, and even life-threatening, side effects. Before taking this drug with grapefruit juice, or before consuming grapefruit or grapefruit juice during the day while taking this drug, first read the section "Grapefruit Juice–Drug Interactions Can Make You Sick" in the appendix of this book. Then discuss this with your pharmacist or the healthcare provider who prescribed this drug.

Remember: All pregnancies have a background risk of about 3% for a major birth defect, even when mom doesn't take a drug of any kind. If you are pregnant or planning a pregnancy, always let your doctor know before taking any drug, prescription or non-prescription, or herbal remedy.

· ·

DIHYDROERGOTAMINE

Brand Name: D.H.E. 45

Drug Use: Dihydroergotamine is approved by the FDA for the treatment of migraine and cluster headaches.

Pregnancy Risk Category: X

> **Category X rating:** The FDA assigns a drug to Category **X** when studies have shown the risk of fetal harm clearly outweighs any potential maternal benefit from the drug. **Drugs in this category should not be used by pregnant women.** Approximately 5% of prescription drugs fall in this category.

Animal Studies: When pregnant rats were treated with this drug, their offspring showed decreased fetal weight and delayed bone formation. Studies in pregnant rabbits showed decreased fetal weight. In pregnant guinea pigs, this drug greatly reduced blood flow to the placenta, thereby decreasing blood flow and oxygen delivery to the fetus.

Human Studies: In studies performed more than 50 years ago, pregnant women were treated with this drug to induce labor.

Although the drug induced labor in many of those women, this use was associated with an increased risk of stillbirth, neonatal death, and newborn seizures. Investigators concluded the drug should not be used to induce labor.

Helpful Hints: Other medications are available to treat migraine and cluster headaches in pregnant women. If there is any chance you may be pregnant, avoid taking this medication.

Remember: All pregnancies have a background risk of about 3% for a major birth defect, even when mom doesn't take a drug of any kind. If you are pregnant or planning a pregnancy, always let your doctor know before taking any drug, prescription or non-prescription, or herbal remedy.

· ·

DILTIAZEM

Brand Names: Cardizem, Cartia, Dilacor, Tiazac

Drug Uses: The FDA has approved this drug for the treatment of angina, which is chest pain, high blood pressure, and irregular heart rhythms.

Pregnancy Risk Category: C

> **Category C rating:** The FDA assigns a drug to Category C for one of two reasons: (1) Studies show evidence of fetal harm when using the drug in pregnant animals, but no controlled studies have been done using the drug in pregnant women, or (2) Studies using the drug in pregnant animals have not been done, and studies of pregnant women using the drug are insufficient to reach a conclusion. Thus, the drug should only be used if the potential benefit for mom is greater than the potential risk of fetal harm, which, in many cases, is unknown. Approximately 50% of prescription drugs fall in this category.

Animal Studies: Studies conducted on pregnant rats, mice, and rabbits using this drug have shown an increase in fetal death and abnormal bone formation.

Human Studies: One report suggested a possible link between this drug and fetal heart defects when pregnant women have taken this drug. However, the report that suggested this link had a very small number of pregnant women in the study. Thus, no conclusive results were obtained.

Helpful Hints: This drug weakly interacts with grapefruit and grapefruit juice, which can cause harmful, and even life-threatening, side effects. Before taking this drug with grapefruit juice, or before consuming grapefruit or grapefruit juice during the day while taking this drug, first read the section "Grapefruit Juice–Drug Interactions Can Make You Sick" in the appendix of this book. Then discuss this with your pharmacist or the healthcare provider who prescribed this drug.

Remember: All pregnancies have a background risk of about 3% for a major birth defect, even when mom doesn't take a drug of any kind. If you are pregnant or planning a pregnancy, always let your doctor know before taking any drug, prescription or non-prescription, or herbal remedy.

DIPHENHYDRAMINE

Brand Name: Benadryl

Drug Uses: The FDA has approved this antihistamine for use in allergic reactions, insomnia, motion sickness, and cough.

Pregnancy Risk Category: B

> **Category B rating:** The FDA assigns a drug to Category **B** for one of two reasons: (1) Studies show no evidence of fetal harm when using the drug in pregnant animals, but no controlled studies have been done using the drug in pregnant women, or (2) Studies show evidence of fetal harm when using the drug in pregnant animals, but controlled studies using the drug in pregnant women do not show evidence of fetal harm. Approximately 21% of prescription drugs fall in this category.

Animal Studies: Studies on pregnant animals exposed to this drug have shown no evidence of fetal harm.

Human Studies: Most of the study results from pregnant women taking this drug have suggested that it is safe in pregnancy. However, one study did suggest a link between this drug and cleft palate, which is an opening in the roof of the mouth, but this association has not been demonstrated in other studies.

Helpful Hints: Some cough syrups contain ethanol (alcohol). Be sure to check the label on the bottle to see if ethanol is listed as an ingredient. Alcohol is known to cause birth defects in developing fetuses.

Remember: All pregnancies have a background risk of about 3% for a major birth defect, even when mom doesn't take a drug of any kind. If you are pregnant or planning a pregnancy, always let your doctor know before taking any drug, prescription or non-prescription, or herbal remedy.

DIPYRIDAMOLE

Brand Name: Persantine

Drug Uses: The FDA has approved this drug to help prevent blood clots. It is also used during cardiac stress testing.

Pregnancy Risk Category: B

> **Category B rating:** The FDA assigns a drug to Category **B** for one of two reasons: (1) Studies show no evidence of fetal harm when using the drug in pregnant animals, but no controlled studies have been done using the drug in pregnant women, or (2) Studies show evidence of fetal harm when using the drug in pregnant animals, but controlled studies using the drug in pregnant women do not show evidence of fetal harm. Approximately 21% of prescription drugs fall in this category.

Animal Studies: When pregnant mice, rats, and rabbits were treated with this drug, no fetal harm was demonstrated.

Human Studies: This drug is not associated with an increased risk of birth defects when taken by pregnant women.

Remember: All pregnancies have a background risk of about 3% for a major birth defect, even when mom doesn't take a drug of any kind. If you are pregnant or planning a pregnancy, always let your doctor know before taking any drug, prescription or non-prescription, or herbal remedy.

DISOPYRAMIDE

Brand Name: Norpace

Drug Use: The FDA has approved this drug for the treatment of a variety of irregular heart rhythms.

Pregnancy Risk Category: C

> **Category C rating:** The FDA assigns a drug to Category **C** for one of two reasons: (1) Studies show evidence of fetal harm when using the drug in pregnant animals, but no controlled studies have been done using the drug in pregnant women, or (2) Studies using the drug in pregnant animals have not been done, and studies of pregnant women using the drug are insufficient to reach a conclusion. Thus, the drug should only be used if the potential benefit for mom is greater than the potential risk of fetal harm, which, in many cases, is unknown. Approximately 50% of prescription drugs fall in this category.

Animal Studies: When pregnant animals have been treated with this drug, no fetal harm has been demonstrated.

Human Studies: This drug is not associated with an increased risk of birth defects in pregnant women.

Remember: All pregnancies have a background risk of about 3% for a major birth defect, even when mom doesn't take a drug of any kind. If you are pregnant or planning a pregnancy, always let your doctor know before taking any drug, prescription or non-prescription, or herbal remedy.

• •

DISULFIRAM

Brand Name: Antabuse

Drug Use: The FDA has approved this drug for the treatment of alcohol dependence.

Pregnancy Risk Category: C

> **Category C rating:** The FDA assigns a drug to Category C for one of two reasons: (1) Studies show evidence of fetal harm when using the drug in pregnant animals, but no controlled studies have been done using the drug in pregnant women, or (2) Studies using the drug in pregnant animals have not been done, and studies of pregnant women using the drug are insufficient to reach a conclusion. Thus, the drug should only be used if the potential benefit for mom is greater than the potential risk of fetal harm, which, in many cases, is unknown. Approximately 50% of prescription drugs fall in this category.

Animal Studies: When pregnant animals were treated with this drug, disulfiram has been shown to interfere with the very early development of the fetus. However, it has not been associated with definitive birth defects.

Human Studies: Pregnant women taking this drug have given birth to an occasional baby with a birth defect. However, the defects have not occurred in sufficient numbers to suggest a definite association between disulfiram and the resulting birth defects.

Helpful Hints: When alcohol is consumed, it is broken down in several steps as the body processes it. Disulfiram interferes with these, so that breakdown products build up, causing very unpleasant symptoms. This is how disulfiram discourages alcohol consumption.

Many of the birth defects seen in babies whose mothers took disulfiram during pregnancy are often associated with alcohol exposure in the womb. This finding suggests that some people taking disulfiram may continue to consume alcohol despite the unpleasant symptoms associated with the drug.

Remember: All pregnancies have a background risk of about 3% for a major birth defect, even when mom doesn't take a drug of any kind. If you are pregnant or planning a pregnancy, always let your doctor know before taking any drug, prescription or non-prescription, or herbal remedy.

DOCUSATE

Brand Name: Colace

Drug Use: The FDA has approved docusate for the treatment of constipation.

Pregnancy Risk Category: C

> **Category C rating:** The FDA assigns a drug to Category **C** for one of two reasons: (1) Studies show evidence of fetal harm when using the drug in pregnant animals, but no controlled studies have been done using the drug in pregnant women, or (2) Studies using the drug in pregnant animals have not been done, and studies of pregnant women using the drug are insufficient to reach a conclusion. Thus, the drug should only be used if the potential benefit for mom is greater than the potential risk of fetal harm, which, in many cases, is unknown. Approximately 50% of prescription drugs fall in this category.

Animal Studies: No studies have been done in pregnant animals using this drug.

Human Studies: When used by pregnant women, no fetal harm has been seen after exposure to this drug.

Remember: All pregnancies have a background risk of about 3% for a major birth defect, even when mom doesn't take a drug of any kind. If you are pregnant or planning a pregnancy, always let your doctor know before taking any drug, prescription or non-prescription, or herbal remedy.

• •

DONEPEZIL

Brand Name: Aricept

Drug Use: The FDA has approved this drug for the treatment of Alzheimer's dementia.

Pregnancy Risk Category: C

Category C rating: The FDA assigns a drug to Category C for one of two reasons: (1) Studies show evidence of fetal harm when using the drug in pregnant animals, but no controlled studies have been done using the drug in pregnant women, or (2) Studies using the drug in pregnant animals have not been done, and studies of pregnant women using the drug are insufficient to reach a conclusion. Thus, the drug should only be used if the potential benefit for mom is greater than the potential risk of fetal harm, which, in many cases, is unknown. Approximately 50% of prescription drugs fall in this category.

Animal Studies: Pregnant rats treated with this drug did not show an increased risk of birth defects. However, it was associated with a slight increase in the number of miscarriages.

Human Studies: There are no reports in which this drug was used to treat pregnant women.

Remember: All pregnancies have a background risk of about 3% for a major birth defect, even when mom doesn't take a drug of any kind. If you are pregnant or planning a pregnancy, always let your doctor know before taking any drug, prescription or non-prescription, or herbal remedy.

. . . .

DOXAZOSIN

Brand Name: Cardura

Drug Uses: The FDA has approved this drug for the treatment of high blood pressure. In men, it is also used to treat an enlarged prostate.

Pregnancy Risk Category: C

> **Category C rating:** The FDA assigns a drug to Category C for one of two reasons: (1) Studies show evidence of fetal harm when using the drug in pregnant animals, but no controlled studies have been done using the drug in pregnant women, or (2) Studies using the drug in pregnant animals have not been done, and studies of pregnant women using the drug are insufficient to reach a conclusion. Thus, the drug should only be used if the potential benefit for mom is greater than the potential risk of fetal harm, which, in many cases, is unknown. (Yes, it is confusing!) Approximately 50% of prescription drugs fall in this category.

Animal Studies: When given to pregnant rats, this drug was associated with delayed development of the offspring. Decreased fetal survival also occurred when this drug was given to pregnant rabbits. However, all of these effects were only seen at very high doses.

Human Studies: There are no reports of this drug being used in pregnant women.

Remember: All pregnancies have a background risk of about 3% for a major birth defect, even when mom doesn't take a drug of any kind. If you are pregnant or planning a pregnancy, always let your doctor know before taking any drug, prescription or non-prescription, or herbal remedy.

. . . .

DOXEPIN

Brand Name: Sinequan

Drug Use: The FDA has approved doxepin for the treatment of depression and anxiety.

Pregnancy Risk Category: C

Category C rating: The FDA assigns a drug to Category C for one of two reasons: (1) Studies show evidence of fetal harm when using the drug in pregnant animals, but no controlled studies have been done using the drug in pregnant women, or (2) Studies using the drug in pregnant animals have not been done, and studies of pregnant women using the drug are insufficient to reach a conclusion. Thus, the drug should only be used if the potential benefit for mom is greater than the potential risk of fetal harm, which, in many cases, is unknown. Approximately 50% of prescription drugs fall in this category.

Animal Studies: When this drug was administered to pregnant rats, rabbits, monkeys, and dogs, there was no increased risk of birth defects in the offspring. At very high doses, however, there was an association with increased newborn death in rats and rabbits.

Human Studies: Pregnant women taking this drug have not shown any evidence of fetal harm.

Helpful Hints:

1. Studies show that antidepressants increase the risk of suicidal thinking and behavior in children, adolescents, and young adults. Anyone considering the use of this drug or any other antidepressant in these patients must balance that risk with the clinical need.

2. Almost all antidepressants carry some risk to the developing fetus. However, we also know depression in a pregnant woman carries potential risk for her health and for her unborn baby; for example, low birth weight and prematurity. The risks and benefits of medications and untreated depression must be weighed carefully. If you are pregnant and think you may have depression, or if you already know you do, talk with your doctor so the two of you can create the right plan

for you and your unborn baby. (See "Antidepressants in Pregnancy" in the appendix of this book
for more detail.)

Remember: All pregnancies have a background risk
of about 3% for a major birth defect, even when mom
doesn't take a drug of any kind. If you are pregnant or
planning a pregnancy, always let your doctor know before taking any drug, prescription or non-prescription,
or herbal remedy.

DOXORUBICIN

Brand Name: Adriamycin

Drug Use: This drug is approved by the FDA for the
treatment of certain cancers.

Pregnancy Risk Category: D

> **Category D rating:** The FDA assigns a drug to Category **D** when
> studies of pregnant women using the drug show evidence of fetal
> harm. Rarely, however, the potential benefit of using the drug in
> some life-threatening situations for mom may outweigh the poten-
> tial risk of fetal harm. For example, when mom requires cancer
> treatment or when she has a serious disease for which safer drugs
> cannot be used or are less effective. Approximately 11% of pre-
> scription drugs fall in this category.

Animal Studies: When pregnant rats were treated with
this drug, a variety of birth defects were noted in the offspring. The drug was also associated with an increased
risk of miscarriage in pregnant rabbits.

Human Studies: When pregnant women have been
treated with this drug, their newborns have shown evidence of an increased risk of birth defects. However, in
most of these studies, the women taking the drug were
also taking other cancer-fighting medications. Some of

them were also exposed to radiation therapy. It is, therefore, difficult to distinguish which defects were caused by which treatments.

Helpful Hints: The National Study Commission on Cytotoxic Exposure has issued a statement regarding occupational exposure to this and other cancer-fighting drugs. The statement says that there is a possible association of exposure to these drugs, particularly during the first trimester, with birth defects and death of the fetus. The commission advises that caution be used when pregnant women handle these cancer-fighting drugs.

Remember: All pregnancies have a background risk of about 3% for a major birth defect, even when mom doesn't take a drug of any kind. If you are pregnant or planning a pregnancy, always let your doctor know before taking any drug, prescription or non-prescription, or herbal remedy.

DOXYCYCLINE

Brand Names: Dibramycin, Adoxa, Doryx, Periostat

Drug Uses: This antibiotic belongs to the tetracycline family of drugs. The FDA has approved this drug for the treatment of various bacterial infections. It is also used to prevent malaria.

Pregnancy Risk Category: **D**

Category D rating: The FDA assigns a drug to Category **D** when studies of pregnant women using the drug show evidence of fetal harm. Rarely, however, the potential benefit of using the drug in some life-threatening situations for mom may outweigh the potential risk of fetal harm. For example, when mom requires cancer treatment or when she has a serious disease for which safer drugs cannot be used or are less effective. Approximately 11% of prescription drugs fall in this category.

Animal Studies: No animal studies are available.

Human Studies: In the 1950s, this family of drugs was widely used to treat various infections in pregnant women. Only later did investigators realize that the tetracyclines were strongly associated with birth defects, especially involving the exposed baby's teeth. Also, it was shown to rarely cause severe liver problems in the pregnant woman taking the drug.

Helpful Hints: Members of this family of drugs can be useful, but they should be avoided in pregnancy, especially since safer and equally effective antibiotic options are available.

Remember: All pregnancies have a background risk of about 3% for a major birth defect, even when mom doesn't take a drug of any kind. If you are pregnant or planning a pregnancy, always let your doctor know before taking any drug, prescription or non-prescription, or herbal remedy.

• •

DOXYLAMINE

Brand Names: Unisom, Aldex

Drug Use: This antihistamine is approved by the FDA for use as a sedative and for use with other active ingredients in cough and cold preparations.

Pregnancy Risk Category: A

> **Category A rating:** The FDA assigns a drug to Category **A** when controlled studies using the drug in pregnant women do not show harmful fetal effects throughout pregnancy. Approximately 1% of prescription drugs fall in this category.

Animal Studies: Pregnant animals treated with this drug alone have shown no evidence of fetal harm.

Human Studies: There is no evidence of increased fetal risk when pregnant women have taken this drug.

However, this antihistamine was a component of the medical product Bendectin, which contained equal amounts of doxylamine, pyridoxine (which is vitamin B6), and dicyclomine. Bendectin was marketed in 1956 for the prevention and treatment of nausea and vomiting during pregnancy. The product was reformulated in 1976 to eliminate dicyclomine because that component was not found to contribute to the anti-nausea and vomiting effectiveness. Subsequently, more than 30 million women took this product during pregnancy, making it one of the most heavily prescribed drugs for nausea and vomiting in pregnancy. The United States manufacturer, however, stopped producing the drug combination in 1983 because of litigation and adverse media coverage over its alleged association with congenital limb defects. Thus, the two-drug combination is no longer available in the United States, but continues to be produced in Canada.

Helpful Hints: Some cough syrups contain ethanol (alcohol). Be sure to check the label on the bottle to see if ethanol is listed as an ingredient. Alcohol is known to cause birth defects in developing fetuses.

Remember: All pregnancies have a background risk of about 3% for a major birth defect, even when mom doesn't take a drug of any kind. If you are pregnant or planning a pregnancy, always let your doctor know before taking any drug, prescription or non-prescription, or herbal remedy.

DROPERIDOL

Brand Name: Inapsine

Drug Use: This drug is approved by the FDA for the treatment of nausea and vomiting.

Pregnancy Risk Category: C

Category C rating: The FDA assigns a drug to Category C for one of two reasons: (1) Studies show evidence of fetal harm when using the drug in pregnant animals, but no controlled studies have been done using the drug in pregnant women, or (2) Studies using the drug in pregnant animals have not been done, and studies of pregnant women using the drug are insufficient to reach a conclusion. Thus, the drug should only be used if the potential benefit for mom is greater than the potential risk of fetal harm, which, in many cases, is unknown. Approximately 50% of prescription drugs fall in this category.

Animal Studies: Pregnant animals treated with this drug have shown no increased risk of birth defects in their offspring. However, there was a slightly higher death rate than normal in newborn rats.

Human Studies: Studies involving pregnant women treated with this drug are limited. The information available suggests no increased risk of harm to the fetus.

Remember: All pregnancies have a background risk of about 3% for a major birth defect, even when mom doesn't take a drug of any kind. If you are pregnant or planning a pregnancy, always let your doctor know before taking any drug, prescription or non-prescription, or herbal remedy.

. . . .

ADDITIONAL DRUGS AND THEIR FDA PREGNANCY RISK CATEGORIES

Since these additional drugs are uncommonly used in pregnancy, they are listed by generic name along with

their FDA Pregnancy Risk Category without more detail:

Dacarbazine - C

Daclizumab - C

Dactinomycin - C

Danazol - X

Dantrolene - C

Daptomycin - B

Darbepoetin Alfa - C

Darifenacin - C

Daunorubicin - D

Decitabine - D

Deferasirox - B

Delavirdine - C

Demeclocycline - D

Denileukin - C

Dexrazoxane - C

Dextroamphetamine - C

Diclofenac - B (D if used in third trimester or near delivery)

Dicloxacillin - B

Dicyclomine - B

Diflunisal - C (D if used in third trimester or near delivery)

Diphenoxylate - C

Dipivefrin - B

Dobutamine - B

Docetaxel - D

Dofetilide - C

Dolasetron - B

Dopamine - C

Dornase Alfa - B

Dorzolamide - C

Dronabinol - C

Drotrecogin Alfa - C

Duloxetine - C (D if taken in second half of pregnancy)

Dutasteride - X

E

ENALAPRIL

Brand Name: Vasotec

Drug Use: This drug is approved by the FDA for the treatment of high blood pressure. The drug is also a member of the ACE inhibitor family of drugs. (See Helpful Hint on next page.)

Pregnancy Risk Categories: This drug has been assigned two pregnancy risk categories: **C** when used in the first trimester, and **D** when used in the second and third trimesters. Approximately 12% of prescription drugs are assigned two pregnancy risk categories, depending on which trimester of pregnancy the drug is used.

Category C rating: The FDA assigns a drug to Category **C** for one of two reasons: (1) Studies show evidence of fetal harm when using the drug in pregnant animals, but no controlled studies have been done using the drug in pregnant women, or (2) Studies using the drug in pregnant animals have not been done, and studies of pregnant women using the drug are insufficient to reach a conclusion. Thus, the drug should only be used if the potential benefit for mom is greater than the potential risk of fetal harm, which, in many cases, is unknown. Approximately 50% of prescription drugs fall in this category.

Category D rating: The FDA assigns a drug to Category **D** when studies of pregnant women using the drug show evidence of fetal harm. Rarely, however, the potential benefit of using the drug in some life-threatening situations for mom may outweigh the potential risk of fetal harm. For example, when mom requires cancer treatment or when she has a serious disease for which safer drugs cannot be used or are less effective. Approximately 11% of prescription drugs fall in this category.

Animal Studies: There are limited animal studies in which this drug has been used in pregnant animals. The main focus is on the studies in pregnant women.

Human Studies: The FDA has issued a Black Box Warning for this particular member of the ACE inhibitor family of drugs and for all drugs in this family. Members of the ACE inhibitor family of drugs can cause fetal harm and even death in the newborn baby. When pregnancy is detected, this drug should be discontinued as soon as possible.

This is the FDA's warning: Do not take enalapril if you are pregnant or breast feeding. If you become pregnant while taking enalapril, call your doctor immediately.

A Black Box Warning is the most serious prescription drug warning the FDA can require a drug company to issue.

A recent study reported in The New England Journal of Medicine found that pregnant women taking an ACE inhibitor during the first trimester had a 2.7 times greater risk of giving birth to a baby with a major birth defect than pregnant women taking non-ACE-inhibitor medications for high blood pressure, or those women who were not taking any medication for high blood pressure at all. The researchers concluded that first trimester exposure to ACE inhibitors is not safe and should be avoided. This study also suggests that assigning ACE inhibitors to Category **C** for the first trimester may in fact not be appropriate. (See "ACE Inhibitor Drugs in Pregnancy" in the appendix for more detail.)

Helpful Hints: This drug weakly interacts with grapefruit and grapefruit juice, which can cause harmful, and even life-threatening, side effects. Before taking this drug with grapefruit juice, or before consuming grapefruit or grapefruit juice during the day while taking this drug, first read the section "Grapefruit Juice–Drug Interactions Can Make You Sick" in the appendix of this book. Then discuss this with your pharmacist or the healthcare provider who prescribed this drug.

Remember: All pregnancies have a background risk of about 3% for a major birth defect, even when mom doesn't take a drug of any kind. If you are pregnant or planning a pregnancy, always let your doctor know before taking any drug, prescription or non-prescription, or herbal remedy.

ENOXAPARIN

Brand Name: Lobenox

Drug Use: This drug is approved by the FDA for the use as a heparin anticoagulant, or blood thinner.

Pregnancy Risk Category: B

> **Category B rating:** The FDA assigns a drug to Category **B** for one of two reasons: (1) Studies show no evidence of fetal harm when using the drug in pregnant animals, but no controlled studies have been done using the drug in pregnant women, or (2) Studies show evidence of fetal harm when using the drug in pregnant animals, but controlled studies using the drug in pregnant women do not show evidence of fetal harm. Approximately 21% of prescription drugs fall in this category.

Animal Studies: Studies using this drug in pregnant rats and rabbits have shown no evidence of an increased risk of birth defects in their offspring.

Human Studies: Controlled studies using this drug in pregnant women have not been done. One retrospective study, however, showed no increase in the risk of birth defects.

Remember: All pregnancies have a background risk of about 3% for a major birth defect, even when mom

doesn't take a drug of any kind. If you are pregnant or planning a pregnancy, always let your doctor know before taking any drug, prescription or non-prescription, or herbal remedy.

. . . .

EPINEPHRINE

Brand Name: Adrenalin

Drug Uses: This drug is approved by the FDA to relieve acute attacks of asthma, and for the treatment of select medical emergencies.

Pregnancy Risk Category: C

> **Category C rating:** The FDA assigns a drug to Category C for one of two reasons: (1) Studies show evidence of fetal harm when using the drug in pregnant animals, but no controlled studies have been done using the drug in pregnant women, or (2) Studies using the drug in pregnant animals have not been done, and studies of pregnant women using the drug are insufficient to reach a conclusion. Thus, the drug should only be used if the potential benefit for mom is greater than the potential risk of fetal harm, which, in many cases, is unknown. Approximately 50% of prescription drugs fall in this category.

Animal Studies: This drug readily crosses the placenta and has been shown to cause birth defects in the offspring of pregnant rats treated with epinephrine.

Human Studies: No controlled studies of epinephrine in pregnant women have been done. This drug can significantly reduce the oxygen supply to the developing fetus. One expert recommends avoiding the drug during the first trimester and during labor and delivery.

Remember: All pregnancies have a background risk of about 3% for a major birth defect, even when mom doesn't take a drug of any kind. If you are pregnant or planning a pregnancy, always let your doctor know

before taking any drug, prescription or non-prescription, or herbal remedy.

· ·

EPOETIN ALFA

Brand Names: Epogen, Procrit

Drug Uses: This drug is approved by the FDA for use in stimulating the production of red blood cells in the treatment of anemia and certain specific medical conditions.

Pregnancy Risk Category: C

> **Category C rating:** The FDA assigns a drug to Category **C** for one of two reasons: (1) Studies show evidence of fetal harm when using the drug in pregnant animals, but no controlled studies have been done using the drug in pregnant women, or (2) Studies using the drug in pregnant animals have not been done, and studies of pregnant women using the drug are insufficient to reach a conclusion. Thus, the drug should only be used if the potential benefit for mom is greater than the potential risk of fetal harm, which, in many cases, is unknown. Approximately 50% of prescription drugs fall in this category.

Animal Studies: In studies using this drug in pregnant rats, fetal toxicity was observed when mothers were treated with five times the equivalent human dose. No harmful effects were seen in the offspring of pregnant rabbits treated with this drug.

Human Studies: This drug does not cross the placenta when used in pregnant women. Because chronic anemia may pose a risk to mom and her unborn baby, it appears that the benefits of using this drug may outweigh the known risks of the drug in some instances.

Remember: All pregnancies have a background risk of about 3% for a major birth defect, even when mom doesn't take a drug of any kind. If you are pregnant or planning a pregnancy, always let your doctor know before taking any drug, prescription or non-prescription, or herbal remedy.

. . . .

ERGOTAMINE

Brand Name: Cafergot

Drug Use: This drug is approved by the FDA for the treatment of migraine headaches.

Pregnancy Risk Category: X

> **Category X rating:** The FDA assigns a drug to Category **X** when studies have shown the risk of fetal harm clearly outweighs any potential maternal benefit from the drug. **Drugs in this category should not be used by pregnant women.** Approximately 5% of prescription drugs fall in this category.

Animal Studies: Studies using this drug in pregnant mice, rats, and rabbits caused an increased mortality in the offspring, and delayed fetal growth.

Human Studies: Most experts consider ergotamine to be contraindicated in pregnancy, or to be used sparingly and with caution. Because the risks have not been adequately defined, ergotamine, in general, should not be used in pregnancy.

Remember: All pregnancies have a background risk of about 3% for a major birth defect, even when mom doesn't take a drug of any kind. If you are pregnant or planning a pregnancy, always let your doctor know before taking any drug, prescription or non-prescription, or herbal remedy.

. . . .

ERYTHROMYCIN

Brand Names: Zithromax, Biaxin, Ilosone

Drug Use: This antibiotic is approved by the FDA for the treatment of a variety of bacterial infections.

Pregnancy Risk Category: **B**

Category B rating: The FDA assigns a drug to Category **B** for one of two reasons: (1) Studies show no evidence of fetal harm when using the drug in pregnant animals, but no controlled studies have been done using the drug in pregnant women, or (2) Studies show evidence of fetal harm when using the drug in pregnant animals, but controlled studies using the drug in pregnant women do not show evidence of fetal harm. Approximately 21% of prescription drugs fall in this category.

Animal Studies: Studies in pregnant rats treated with this drug showed no evidence of birth defects in their offspring.

Human Studies: There are no controlled studies of pregnant women treated with this drug.

Helpful Hints:

1. In general, erythromycin is considered safe during pregnancy, except for erythromycin estolate, which can cause toxic liver reactions during pregnancy and should be avoided.

2. This drug weakly interacts with grapefruit and grapefruit juice, which can cause harmful, and even life-threatening, side effects. Before taking this drug with grapefruit juice, or before consuming grapefruit or grapefruit juice during the day while taking this drug, first read the section "Grapefruit Juice–Drug Interactions Can Make You Sick" in the appendix of this book. Then discuss this with your pharmacist or the healthcare provider who prescribed this drug.

Remember: All pregnancies have a background risk of about 3% for a major birth defect, even when mom doesn't take a drug of any kind. If you are pregnant or planning a pregnancy, always let your doctor know

before taking any drug, prescription or non-prescription, or herbal remedy.
. . . .

ESCITALOPRAM

Brand Name: Lexapro

Drug Use: This drug is approved by the FDA for the treatment of depression. It belongs to the family of selective serotonin reuptake inhibitors (SSRIs).

Pregnancy Risk Categories: This drug has been assigned two pregnancy risk categories: **C** when used in the first half of pregnancy, **D** when used in the second half, particularly near term and around the time of birth. Approximately 12% of prescription drugs are assigned two pregnancy risk categories, depending on which trimester of pregnancy the drug is used.

> **Category C rating:** The FDA assigns a drug to Category **C** for one of two reasons: (1) Studies show evidence of fetal harm when using the drug in pregnant animals, but no controlled studies have been done using the drug in pregnant women, or (2) Studies using the drug in pregnant animals have not been done, and studies of pregnant women using the drug are insufficient to reach a conclusion. Thus, the drug should only be used if the potential benefit for mom is greater than the potential risk of fetal harm, which, in many cases, is unknown. Approximately 50% of prescription drugs fall in this category.

> **Category D rating:** The FDA assigns a drug to Category **D** when studies of pregnant women using the drug show evidence of fetal harm. Rarely, however, the potential benefit of using the drug in some life-threatening situations for mom may outweigh the potential risk of fetal harm. For example, when mom requires cancer treatment or when she has a serious disease for which safer drugs cannot be used or are less effective. Approximately 11% of prescription drugs fall in this category.

Animal Studies: In pregnant rats treated with this drug, toxic effects on the offspring have been found when they were exposed to doses of the drug greater than human therapeutic doses.

Human Studies: There are no controlled studies using this drug in pregnant women. However, there are numerous case reports which have led to the **D** pregnancy risk category for the second half of pregnancy.

Newborns exposed to this drug and other members of the SSRI family of drugs in the second half of pregnancy have developed complications immediately after birth. These complications have required hospitalization, respiratory support, and tube feeding. These features are consistent with either a direct toxic effect of the drug or, possibly, abrupt withdrawal from the drug which occurs at birth, once the umbilical cord is cut. When treating a woman with a SSRI during the last half of pregnancy, the physician should carefully weigh these potential risks to the baby and the benefits of treatment to the mother.

Helpful Hints:

1. Studies show that antidepressants increase the risk of suicidal thinking and behavior in children, adolescents, and young adults. Anyone considering the use of this drug or any other antidepressant in these patients must balance that risk with the clinical need.

2. Almost all antidepressants carry some risk to the developing fetus. However, we also know depression in a pregnant woman carries potential risk for her health and for her unborn baby; for example, low birth weight and prematurity. The risks and benefits of medications and untreated depression must be weighed carefully. If you are pregnant and think you may have depression, or if you already know you do, talk with your doctor so the two of you can create the right plan for

you and your unborn baby. (See "Antidepressants in Pregnancy" in the appendix for more detail.)

Remember: All pregnancies have a background risk of about 3% for a major birth defect, even when mom doesn't take a drug of any kind. If you are pregnant or planning a pregnancy, always let your doctor know before taking any drug, prescription or non-prescription, or herbal remedy.

· ·

ETHAMBUTOL

Brand Name: Myambutol

Drug Use: This drug is approved by the FDA for the treatment of tuberculosis in combination with other anti-tuberculosis drugs.

Pregnancy Risk Category: B

> **Category B rating:** The FDA assigns a drug to Category **B** for one of two reasons: (1) Studies show no evidence of fetal harm when using the drug in pregnant animals, but no controlled studies have been done using the drug in pregnant women, or (2) Studies show evidence of fetal harm when using the drug in pregnant animals, but controlled studies using the drug in pregnant women do not show evidence of fetal harm. Approximately 21% of prescription drugs fall in this category.

Animal Studies: Studies of pregnant rats and rabbits treated with high doses of this drug showed higher risk of fetal mortality, but a low risk of birth defects.

Human Studies: There are no controlled studies of pregnant women using this drug. However, there are published reports of five women who were treated with this drug during pregnancy with no harmful birth defects.

Most experts consider this drug, along with isoniazid and rifampin, to be the safest therapy for tuberculosis.

Remember: All pregnancies have a background risk of about 3% for a major birth defect, even when mom doesn't take a drug of any kind. If you are pregnant or planning a pregnancy, always let your doctor know before taking any drug, prescription or non-prescription, or herbal remedy.

• •

ETHOSUXIMIDE

Brand Name: Zarontin

Drug Use: This drug is approved by the FDA for the treatment of certain seizure disorders.

Pregnancy Risk Category: C

> **Category C rating:** The FDA assigns a drug to Category **C** for one of two reasons: (1) Studies show evidence of fetal harm when using the drug in pregnant animals, but no controlled studies have been done using the drug in pregnant women, or (2) Studies using the drug in pregnant animals have not been done, and studies of pregnant women using the drug are insufficient to reach a conclusion. Thus, the drug should only be used if the potential benefit for mom is greater than the potential risk of fetal harm, which, in many cases, is unknown. Approximately 50% of prescription drugs fall in this category.

Animal Studies: Pregnant rodents treated with this drug showed an increased risk of bone formation defects.

Human Studies: No controlled studies using this drug in pregnant women are available. A limited number of case reports in pregnant women using this drug suggests the drug poses a low risk for fetal harm in humans.

Helpful Hint: In pregnant women with epilepsy, the first priority is to prevent seizures. This can be difficult because many seizure medications do not work quite as well during pregnancy. Sometimes the dose has to be increased or other medications added just to prevent seizures. Regardless, the healthiest situation for both mom and unborn baby is to have the fewest seizures possible.

Remember: All pregnancies have a background risk of about 3% for a major birth defect, even when mom doesn't take a drug of any kind. If you are pregnant or planning a pregnancy, always let your doctor know before taking any drug, prescription or non-prescription, or herbal remedy.

ADDITIONAL DRUGS AND THEIR FDA PREGNANCY RISK CATEGORIES

Since these additional drugs are uncommonly used in pregnancy, they are listed by generic name along with their FDA Pregnancy Risk Category without more detail:

Econazole - C
Efalizumab - C
Efavirenz - C
Eflornithine - C
Eletriptan - C
Emedastine - B
Emtricitabine - B
Enfuvirtide - B
Entecavir - C
Ephedrine - C
Epinastine - C
Epirubicin - D

Eplerenone - B
Eprosartan - C (D if taken in second or third trimester)
Eptifibatide - B
Erlotinib - D
Ertapenem - B
Esmolol - C
Esomeprazole - B
Estradiol - X
Estramustine - X
Estropipate - X

Eszopiclone - C

Etanercept - B

Etidronate - C

Etodolac - C (D if used in third trimester or near delivery)

Etoposide - D

Exemestane - D

Exenatide - C

Exetimibe - C

F

FAMOTIDINE

Brand Name: Pepcid

Drug Uses: This drug is approved by the FDA for the treatment of ulcers and/or gastroesophageal reflux disease (GERD) or "heartburn" and inflammation of the esophagus.

Pregnancy Risk Category: B

Category B rating: The FDA assigns a drug to Category **B** for one of two reasons: (1) Studies show no evidence of fetal harm when using the drug in pregnant animals, but no controlled studies have been done using the drug in pregnant women, or (2) Studies show evidence of fetal harm when using the drug in pregnant animals, but controlled studies using the drug in pregnant women do not show evidence of fetal harm. Approximately 21% of prescription drugs fall in this category.

Animal Studies: Pregnant rats and rabbits treated with this drug showed no evidence of fetal harm in the offspring.

Human Studies: A limited amount of information is available concerning pregnant women taking this drug. Due to the limited amount of information, no conclusions have been drawn about the overall safety of this drug.

Remember: All pregnancies have a background risk of about 3% for a major birth defect, even when mom doesn't take a drug of any kind. If you are pregnant or planning a pregnancy, always let your doctor know before taking any drug, prescription or non-prescription, or herbal remedy.

• •

FELODIPINE

Brand Name: Plendil

Drug Use: This drug is approved by the FDA for the treatment of high blood pressure. It belongs to the calcium channel blocker family of drugs.

Pregnancy Risk Category: C

> **Category C rating:** The FDA assigns a drug to Category C for one of two reasons: (1) Studies show evidence of fetal harm when using the drug in pregnant animals, but no controlled studies have been done using the drug in pregnant women, or (2) Studies using the drug in pregnant animals have not been done, and studies of pregnant women using the drug are insufficient to reach a conclusion. Thus, the drug should only be used if the potential benefit for mom is greater than the potential risk of fetal harm, which, in many cases, is unknown. Approximately 50% of prescription drugs fall in this category.

Animal Studies: In pregnant rabbits and monkeys treated with this drug, abnormalities of the fingers and toes were noted in the offspring. There was also an increased risk of stillbirth when the drug was administered to pregnant rats.

Human Studies: There have been no controlled studies of this drug in pregnant women. However, most experts feel there is no increased risk of fetal harm when using this drug in pregnancy.

Helpful Hints: This drug moderately interacts with grapefruit and grapefruit juice, which can cause harmful, and even life-threatening, side effects. Before taking this drug with grapefruit juice, or before consuming grapefruit or grapefruit juice during the day while taking this drug, first read the section "Grapefruit Juice–Drug Interactions Can Make You Sick" in the appendix of this book. Then discuss this with your pharmacist or the healthcare provider who prescribed this drug.

Remember: All pregnancies have a background risk of about 3% for a major birth defect, even when mom doesn't take a drug of any kind. If you are pregnant or planning a pregnancy, always let your doctor know before taking any drug, prescription or non-prescription, or herbal remedy.

FENTANYL

Brand Name: Sublimaze

Drug Use: This drug, which belongs to the narcotic family of drugs, is approved by the FDA for the treatment of pain in pregnant women.

Pregnancy Risk Categories: This drug has been assigned two pregnancy risk categories: **C** when used in the first two trimesters of pregnancy, and **D** when used near term or at the time of delivery. Approximately 12% of prescription drugs are assigned two pregnancy risk categories, depending on which trimester of pregnancy the drug is used.

Category C rating: The FDA assigns a drug to Category **C** for one of two reasons: (1) Studies show evidence of fetal harm when using the drug in pregnant animals, but no controlled studies have been done using the drug in pregnant women, or (2) Studies using the drug in pregnant animals have not been done, and studies of pregnant women using the drug are insufficient to reach a conclusion. Thus, the drug should only be used if the potential benefit for mom is greater than the potential risk of fetal harm, which, in many cases, is unknown. Approximately 50% of prescription drugs fall in this category.

Category D rating: The FDA assigns a drug to Category **D** when studies of pregnant women using the drug show evidence of fetal harm. Rarely, however, the potential benefit of using the drug in some life-threatening situations for mom may outweigh the potential risk of fetal harm. For example, when mom requires cancer treatment or when she has a serious disease for which safer drugs cannot be used or are less effective. Approximately 11% of prescription drugs fall in this category.

Animal Studies: When used in pregnant rats, fentanyl showed no increased risk of birth defects, but was associated with decreased fertility.

Human Studies: There are no controlled studies of this drug in pregnant women. However, there are case reports of newborn withdrawal symptoms when the drug has been used at the end of pregnancy or during labor. Thus, the drug received a Category **D** risk rating for this issue. These withdrawal symptoms consisted of jitteriness, irritability, and a high-pitched cry that often began within the first 24 hours after birth.

Helpful Hints: This drug weakly interacts with grapefruit and grapefruit juice, which can cause harmful, and even life-threatening, side effects. Before taking this drug with grapefruit juice, or before consuming grapefruit or grapefruit juice during the day while taking this drug, first read the section "Grapefruit Juice–Drug Interactions Can Make You Sick" in the appendix of this book. Then discuss this with your pharmacist or the healthcare provider who prescribed this drug.

Remember: All pregnancies have a background risk of about 3% for a major birth defect, even when mom doesn't take a drug of any kind. If you are pregnant or planning a pregnancy, always let your doctor know before taking any drug, prescription or non-prescription, or herbal remedy.

FILGRASTIM

Brand Name: Filgrastim

Drug Use: This drug is used to reduce the risk of infection in patients with cancer who are receiving certain types of chemotherapy.

Pregnancy Risk Category: C

Category C rating: The FDA assigns a drug to Category **C** for one of two reasons: (1) Studies show evidence of fetal harm when using the drug in pregnant animals, but no controlled studies have been done using the drug in pregnant women, or (2) Studies using the drug in pregnant animals have not been done, and studies of pregnant women using the drug are insufficient to reach a conclusion. Thus, the drug should only be used if the potential benefit for mom is greater than the potential risk of fetal harm, which, in many cases, is unknown. Approximately 50% of prescription drugs fall in this category.

Animal Studies: In pregnant rats treated with this drug, their offspring had a slightly decreased birth weight. There was also an increased risk of early fetal death when the drug was given to pregnant rabbits.

Human Studies: No controlled studies using this drug in pregnant women have been done. There have been no increased birth defects noted in case reports.

Remember: All pregnancies have a background risk of about 3% for a major birth defect, even when mom doesn't take a drug of any kind. If you are pregnant or planning a pregnancy, always let your doctor know before taking any drug, prescription or non-prescription, or herbal remedy.

FLUCONAZOLE

Brand Name: Diflucan

Drug Uses: This drug is approved by the FDA for the treatment of fungal infections, including yeast infections of the vagina, mouth, throat, esophagus, lungs, blood, and other organs. Fluconazole is also used to treat meningitis caused by various fungi.

Pregnancy Risk Category: C

Category C rating: The FDA assigns a drug to Category **C** for one of two reasons: (1) Studies show evidence of fetal harm when using the drug in pregnant animals, but no controlled studies have been done using the drug in pregnant women, or (2) Studies using the drug in pregnant animals have not been done, and studies of pregnant women using the drug are insufficient to reach a conclusion. Thus, the drug should only be used if the potential benefit for mom is greater than the potential risk of fetal harm, which, in many cases, is unknown. Approximately 50% of prescription drugs fall in this category.

Animal Studies: In studies with pregnant rats treated with this medication, spontaneous abortions were noted at a dose many times the recommended human dose. In pregnant rats, high doses produced increases in fetal birth defects. In addition, embryo deaths were observed at high doses as well.

Human Studies: Although the data is very limited, the use of fluconazole during the first trimester appears to potentially cause birth defects if continuous daily doses that exceed 400 mg per day are required. However, the published experience with the use of smaller doses, such as those prescribed for vaginal fungal infections, suggest that the risk for adverse outcomes is low, if it exists at all. In those instances in which continuous high-dose fluconazole is the only therapeutic choice during the first trimester, the patient should be informed of the potential risk to her unborn baby.

Remember: All pregnancies have a background risk of about 3% for a major birth defect, even when mom doesn't take a drug of any kind. If you are pregnant or planning a pregnancy, always let your doctor know before taking any drug, prescription or non-prescription, or herbal remedy.

FLUOXETINE

Brand Name: Prozac

Drug Use: This drug is approved by the FDA for the treatment of depression, obsessive-compulsive disorder, bulimia, and panic disorder. It belongs to the selective serotonin reuptake inhibitor (SSRI) family of medications.

Pregnancy Risk Categories: This drug has been assigned two pregnancy risk categories: **C** when used in the first half of pregnancy, **D** when used in the second half of pregnancy. Approximately 12% of prescription drugs are assigned two pregnancy risk categories, depending on which trimester of pregnancy the drug is used.

> **Category C rating:** The FDA assigns a drug to Category **C** for one of two reasons: (1) Studies show evidence of fetal harm when using the drug in pregnant animals, but no controlled studies have been done using the drug in pregnant women, or (2) Studies using the drug in pregnant animals have not been done, and studies of pregnant women using the drug are insufficient to reach a conclusion. Thus, the drug should only be used if the potential benefit for mom is greater than the potential risk of fetal harm, which, in many cases, is unknown. Approximately 50% of prescription drugs fall in this category.

> **Category D rating:** The FDA assigns a drug to Category **D** when studies of pregnant women using the drug show evidence of fetal harm. Rarely, however, the potential benefit of using the drug in some life-threatening situations for mom may outweigh the potential risk of fetal harm. For example, when mom requires cancer treatment or when she has a serious disease for which safer drugs cannot be used or are less effective. Approximately 11% of prescription drugs fall in this category.

Animal Studies: When this drug was given to pregnant rats and rabbits, there was no increase in birth defects. Pregnant rats, however, did have higher rates of stillbirth and decreased birth weights.

Human Studies: There are no controlled studies using this drug in pregnant women. However, there are numerous case reports involving SSRIs which have led to the **D** pregnancy risk category for this family of drugs when used in the second half of pregnancy.

Newborns exposed to members of the SSRI family of drugs in the second half of pregnancy have developed complications immediately after birth. These complications have required hospitalization, respiratory support, and tube feeding. These features are consistent with either a direct toxic effect of the drug or, possibly, abrupt withdrawal from the drug which occurs at birth, once the umbilical cord is cut. When treating a woman with a SSRI during the second half of pregnancy, the physician should carefully weigh these potential risks to the baby and the benefits of treatment to the mother.

Helpful Hints:

1. Studies show that antidepressants increase the risk of suicidal thinking and behavior in children, adolescents, and young adults. Anyone considering the use of this drug or any other antidepressant in these patients must balance that risk with the clinical need.

2. Almost all antidepressants carry some risk to the developing fetus. However, we also know depression in a pregnant woman carries potential risk for her health and for her unborn baby; for example, low birth weight and prematurity. The risks and benefits of medications and untreated depression must be weighed carefully. If you are pregnant and think you may have depression, or if you already know you do, talk with your doctor so the two of you can create the right plan for you and your unborn baby. (See "Antidepressants in Pregnancy" in the appendix for more details.)

Remember: All pregnancies have a background risk of about 3% for a major birth defect, even when mom

doesn't take a drug of any kind. If you are pregnant or planning a pregnancy, always let your doctor know before taking any drug, prescription or non-prescription, or herbal remedy.

∙∙∙∙∙∙∙∙∙∙∙∙∙∙∙∙∙∙∙∙∙∙∙∙∙∙∙∙∙∙∙∙∙∙∙∙

FLUPHENAZINE

Brand Names: Prolixin, Decanoate

Drug Use: This drug is an antipsychotic medication used to treat schizophrenia and psychotic symptoms such as hallucinations, delusions, and hostility.

Pregnancy Risk Category: C

> **Category C rating:** The FDA assigns a drug to Category **C** for one of two reasons: (1) Studies show evidence of fetal harm when using the drug in pregnant animals, but no controlled studies have been done using the drug in pregnant women, or (2) Studies using the drug in pregnant animals have not been done, and studies of pregnant women using the drug are insufficient to reach a conclusion. Thus, the drug should only be used if the potential benefit for mom is greater than the potential risk of fetal harm, which, in many cases, is unknown. Approximately 50% of prescription drugs fall in this category.

Animal Studies: When pregnant rats were treated with this drug, there were no adverse fetal effects. When given to pregnant mice, the only significant effect was that of reduced birth weight.

Human Studies: There are no controlled studies of this drug in pregnant women. However, anecdotal experience has raised concern on the part of some experts about an increased risk when this drug is used during the third trimester of pregnancy. The risk is related, primarily, to a few case reports in which the newborn of mothers who were taking this drug exhibited withdrawal symptoms for a period of time after birth.

Remember: All pregnancies have a background risk of about 3% for a major birth defect, even when mom doesn't take a drug of any kind. If you are pregnant or planning a pregnancy, always let your doctor know before taking any drug, prescription or non-prescription, or herbal remedy.

• •

FLUTICASONE

Brand Names: Flovent, which is the oral inhalation product; Flonase, which is the intranasal spray; and Cutivate, which is the topical form

Drug Uses: The FDA has approved this drug to help prevent asthma attacks, to treat season allergies, and to treat certain skin conditions.

Pregnancy Risk Category: C

> **Category C rating:** The FDA assigns a drug to Category C for one of two reasons: (1) Studies show evidence of fetal harm when using the drug in pregnant animals, but no controlled studies have been done using the drug in pregnant women, or (2) Studies using the drug in pregnant animals have not been done, and studies of pregnant women using the drug are insufficient to reach a conclusion. Thus, the drug should only be used if the potential benefit for mom is greater than the potential risk of fetal harm, which, in many cases, is unknown. Approximately 50% of prescription drugs fall in this category.

Animal Studies: When pregnant mice, rats, and rabbits were treated with this drug, they experienced embryonic growth retardation of their embryos and several types of birth defects.

Human Studies: There are no human studies in which pregnant women were treated with this drug. Because of the absence of human pregnancy experience, several experts have concluded that corticosteroids are better alternatives than this one. However, if a woman has shown a good response to fluticasone, it would be reasonable to continue her on this inhaled agent during pregnancy.

Remember: All pregnancies have a background risk of about 3% for a major birth defect, even when mom doesn't take a drug of any kind. If you are pregnant or planning a pregnancy, always let your doctor know before taking any drug, prescription or non-prescription, or herbal remedy.

- -

FLUVASTATIN

Brand Name: Lescol

Drug Use: The FDA has approved fluvastatin for the treatment of high cholesterol. This drug belongs to the "statin" family of drugs.

Pregnancy Risk Category: X

> **Category X rating:** The FDA assigns a drug to Category **X** when studies have shown the risk of fetal harm clearly outweighs any potential maternal benefit from the drug. **Drugs in this category should not be used by pregnant women.** Approximately 5% of prescription drugs fall in this category.

Animal Studies: Pregnant rats treated with this drug showed increased rates of stillbirth, illness in the offspring, and sickness of the pregnant rats, themselves, when given this drug. There was no increased risk of birth defects when fluvastatin was given to pregnant rats or rabbits.

Human Studies: There are no controlled studies using fluvastatin in pregnant women. All of the drugs in the statin family of drugs, including fluvastatin, have a pregnancy risk rating of **X**. The main reason is that

cholesterol and other products that are made from cholesterol are necessary for normal fetal development. Fluvastatin and the other drugs in the statin family lower
levels of cholesterol and, therefore, may interfere with
fetal development. Treating mom's high cholesterol is
important. However, stopping this treatment for the duration of pregnancy should have no significant effect on
her long-term cholesterol levels. Continuing the treatment, however, would put the fetus at unnecessary risk.
This is the primary reason why this family of drugs is
not indicated during pregnancy and is assigned to risk
Category **X**.

Helpful Hints:

1. Drugs that belong to the statin family of drugs,
    such as this one, should only be prescribed for
    women of childbearing age when they are highly
    unlikely to conceive and have been informed
    of the potential hazards, according to the FDA.
    Why? Because cholesterol is essential for nor-
    mal fetal development, and anything that lowers
    the serum level of cholesterol—which is what
    statins do—might adversely affect fetal develop-
    ment. If a woman becomes pregnant while tak-
    ing this drug, or any member of the statin family
    of drugs, it should be discontinued immediately
    and she should be told of the potential hazard to
    her unborn baby.

2. This drug weakly interacts with grapefruit and
    grapefruit juice, which can cause harmful, and
    even life-threatening, side effects. Before tak-
    ing this drug with grapefruit juice, or before
    consuming grapefruit or grapefruit juice dur-
    ing the day while taking this drug, first read

the section "Grapefruit Juice–Drug Interactions Can Make You Sick" in the appendix of this book. Then discuss this with your pharmacist or the healthcare provider who prescribed this drug.

Remember: All pregnancies have a background risk of about 3% for a major birth defect, even when mom doesn't take a drug of any kind. If you are pregnant or planning a pregnancy, always let your doctor know before taking any drug, prescription or non-prescription, or herbal remedy.

. . . .

FLUVOXAMINE

Brand Name: Luvox

Drug Uses: This drug is approved by the FDA for the treatment of depression and obsessive-compulsive disorder. It belongs to the selective serotonin reuptake inhibitor (SSRI) family of drugs.

Pregnancy Risk Categories: This drug has been assigned two pregnancy risk categories: **C** when used in the first half of pregnancy, **D** when used in the second half of pregnancy. Approximately 12% of prescription drugs are assigned two pregnancy risk categories, depending on which trimester of pregnancy the drug is used.

> **Category C rating:** The FDA assigns a drug to Category **C** for one of two reasons: (1) Studies show evidence of fetal harm when using the drug in pregnant animals, but no controlled studies have been done using the drug in pregnant women, or (2) Studies using the drug in pregnant animals have not been done, and studies of pregnant women using the drug are insufficient to reach a conclusion. Thus, the drug should only be used if the potential benefit for mom is greater than the potential risk of fetal harm, which, in many cases, is unknown. Approximately 50% of prescription drugs fall in this category.

Category D rating: The FDA assigns a drug to Category **D** when studies of pregnant women using the drug show evidence of fetal harm. Rarely, however, the potential benefit of using the drug in some life-threatening situations for mom may outweigh the potential risk of fetal harm. For example, when mom requires cancer treatment or when she has a serious disease for which safer drugs cannot be used or are less effective. Approximately 11% of prescription drugs fall in this category.

Animal Studies: In pregnant rats, this drug was associated with increased death rates in the offspring, as well as lower birth weights.

Human Studies: There are no controlled studies using this drug in pregnant women. However, there are numerous case reports involving SSRIs which have led to the **D** pregnancy risk category for this family of drugs when used in the second half of pregnancy.

Newborns exposed to members of the SSRI family of drugs in the second half of pregnancy have developed complications immediately after birth. These complications have required hospitalization, respiratory support, and tube feeding. These features are consistent with either a direct toxic effect of the drug or, possibly, abrupt withdrawal from the drug which occurs at birth, once the umbilical cord is cut. When treating a woman with a SSRI during the second half of pregnancy, the physician should carefully weigh these potential risks to the baby and the benefits of treatment to the mother.

Helpful Hints:

1. Almost all antidepressant medications carry some risk to the developing fetus. However, we know that depression in a pregnant woman also carries potential risk for her health and for her unborn baby. For example, low birth weight and prematurity are potential problems. The risks

and benefits of medications and untreated depression must be weighed carefully. If you are pregnant and think you may have depression, or if you already know you do, talk with your doctor so that the two of you can create the right plan for you.

In 2005, the FDA announced new labeling for antidepressants about the need to closely monitor patients for worsening of depression and the potential of increased suicidal thinking or suicidal behavior during treatment.

2. This drug weakly interacts with grapefruit and grapefruit juice, which can cause harmful, and even life-threatening, side effects. Before taking this drug with grapefruit juice, or before consuming grapefruit or grapefruit juice during the day while taking this drug, first read the section "Grapefruit Juice–Drug Interactions Can Make You Sick" in the appendix of this book. Then discuss this with your pharmacist or the healthcare provider who prescribed this drug.

Remember: All pregnancies have a background risk of about 3% for a major birth defect, even when mom doesn't take a drug of any kind. If you are pregnant or planning a pregnancy, always let your doctor know before taking any drug, prescription or non-prescription, or herbal remedy.

FOLIC ACID

Brand Name: Folic Acid

Drug Uses: The FDA has approved folic acid for the prevention of neural tube defects (open spine), to treat certain types of anemia, and as a nutritional supplement.

Pregnancy Risk Category: A

> **Category A rating:** The FDA assigns a drug to Category **A** when controlled studies using the drug in pregnant women do not show harmful fetal effects throughout pregnancy. Approximately 1% of prescription drugs fall in this category.

Animal Studies: No relevant information is available about the use of folic acid in pregnant animals.

Human Studies: The use of folic acid in pregnant women is well-studied. Supplementation with a multivitamin containing .4 mg of folic acid daily has been shown to lower the risk of a neural tube defect by two-thirds during pregnancy. However, it is important not to wait until one discovers one is pregnant before starting this supplementation. Rather, all women of childbearing age should take a multivitamin containing .4 mg of folic acid routinely.

Helpful Hints: Women who have a history of giving birth to a child with a neural tube defect, such as an open spine, should take ten times as much folic acid daily as the .4 mg daily recommended above. This amounts to 4 mg daily and requires a prescription from mom's obstetrician.

Women who take medications for seizures may also need extra folic acid daily during their pregnancy since many of these medications interfere with the absorption and metabolism of folic acid in the body. Ideally, this should be discussed with your obstetrician before you become pregnant.

Remember: All pregnancies have a background risk of about 3% for a major birth defect, even when mom doesn't take a drug of any kind. If you are pregnant or planning a pregnancy, always let your doctor know

before taking any drug, prescription or non-prescription, or herbal remedy.
. . . .

FOSINOPRIL

Brand Name: Monopril

Drug Uses: The FDA has approved fosinopril for the treatment of high blood pressure and congestive heart failure. It is a member of the ACE inhibitor family of drugs. (See Helpful Hint on next page.)

Pregnancy Risk Categories: This drug has been assigned two pregnancy risk categories: **C** when used in the first trimester, and **D** when used in the second and third trimesters. Approximately 12% of prescription drugs are assigned two pregnancy risk categories, depending on which trimester of pregnancy the drug is used.

> **Category C rating:** The FDA assigns a drug to Category **C** for one of two reasons: (1) Studies show evidence of fetal harm when using the drug in pregnant animals, but no controlled studies have been done using the drug in pregnant women, or (2) Studies using the drug in pregnant animals have not been done, and studies of pregnant women using the drug are insufficient to reach a conclusion. Thus, the drug should only be used if the potential benefit for mom is greater than the potential risk of fetal harm, which, in many cases, is unknown. Approximately 50% of prescription drugs fall in this category.

> **Category D rating:** The FDA assigns a drug to Category **D** when studies of pregnant women using the drug show evidence of fetal harm. Rarely, however, the potential benefit of using the drug in some life-threatening situations for mom may outweigh the potential risk of fetal harm. For example, when mom requires cancer treatment or when she has a serious disease for which safer drugs cannot be used or are less effective. Approximately 11% of prescription drugs fall in this category.

Animal Studies: In pregnant rats, this drug has been associated with an increased risk of defects involving the face and mouth in the offspring. No adverse fetal effects were seen when the drug was given to pregnant rabbits.

Human Studies: There are no controlled studies of pregnant women taking this drug. However, exposure of pregnant women to some drugs in this ACE inhibitor family of drugs has been associated with birth defects and even death of the fetus when taken in the second and third trimesters.

Helpful Hints: The FDA has issued the following Black Box Warning for this drug: "When used in pregnancy during the second and third trimesters, ACE inhibitors can cause injury and even death to the developing fetus. When pregnancy is detected, this drug should be discontinued as soon as possible." (See "ACE Inhibitor Drugs in Pregnancy" in the appendix for more details.)

A Black Box Warning is the most serious prescription drug warning the FDA can require a drug company to issue.

Remember: All pregnancies have a background risk of about 3% for a major birth defect, even when mom doesn't take a drug of any kind. If you are pregnant or planning a pregnancy, always let your doctor know before taking any drug, prescription or non-prescription, or herbal remedy.

FUROSEMIDE

Brand Name: Lasix

Drug Uses: This drug is approved by the FDA for the treatment of swelling and high blood pressure.

Pregnancy Risk Categories: This drug has been assigned two pregnancy risk categories: **C** throughout the pregnancy, and **D** if the drug is used to treat gestational hypertension, which is high blood pressure that develops during pregnancy. Approximately 12% of prescription drugs are assigned two pregnancy risk categories, depending on which trimester of pregnancy the drug is used.

> **Category C rating:** The FDA assigns a drug to Category C for one of two reasons: (1) Studies show evidence of fetal harm when using the drug in pregnant animals, but no controlled studies have been done using the drug in pregnant women, or (2) Studies using the drug in pregnant animals have not been done, and studies of pregnant women using the drug are insufficient to reach a conclusion. Thus, the drug should only be used if the potential benefit for mom is greater than the potential risk of fetal harm, which, in many cases, is unknown. Approximately 50% of prescription drugs fall in this category.

> **Category D rating:** The FDA assigns a drug to Category D when studies of pregnant women using the drug show evidence of fetal harm. Rarely, however, the potential benefit of using the drug in some life-threatening situations for mom may outweigh the potential risk of fetal harm. For example, when mom requires cancer treatment or when she has a serious disease for which safer drugs cannot be used or are less effective. Approximately 11% of prescription drugs fall in this category.

Animal Studies: In pregnant rats, furosemide was associated with bone defects in the offspring. This drug was also associated with enlargement of the kidneys in the offspring of pregnant rats and mice.

Human Studies: When taken by pregnant women, this drug has been associated with birth defects, but in no clear pattern, making a definitive relationship between the drug and the birth defects uncertain.

When hypertension develops during pregnancy, this event is associated with low blood volume in mom. In cases of low blood volume, the use of a diuretic (water pill) like furosemide can be dangerous. Thus, the drug has a **D** rating in pregnancy when used to treat hypertension that develops during pregnancy.

Remember: All pregnancies have a background risk of about 3% for a major birth defect, even when mom doesn't take a drug of any kind. If you are pregnant or planning a pregnancy, always let your doctor know before taking any drug, prescription or non-prescription, or herbal remedy.

ADDITIONAL DRUGS AND THEIR FDA PREGNANCY RISK CATEGORIES

Since these additional drugs are uncommonly used in pregnancy, they are listed by generic name along with their FDA Pregnancy Risk Category without more detail:

Famciclovir - B

Felbamate - C

Fenofibrate - C

Fexofenadine - C

Fenoprofen - B (D if used in third trimester or near delivery)

Flecainide - C

Flucytosine - C

Flumazenil - C

Flunisolide - C

Fluocinolone - C

Fluorouracil - D

Flurbiprofen - B (D if used in third trimester or near delivery)

Fondaparinux - B

Formoterol - C

Fosamprenavir - C

Foscarnet - C

Frovatriptan - C

G

GABAPENTIN

Brand Name: Neurontin

Drug Use: This drug is approved by the FDA for the treatment of seizures.

Pregnancy Risk Category: C

Category C rating: The FDA assigns a drug to Category **C** for one of two reasons: (1) Studies show evidence of fetal harm when using the drug in pregnant animals, but no controlled studies have been done using the drug in pregnant women, or (2) Studies using the drug in pregnant animals have not been done, and studies of pregnant women using the drug are insufficient to reach a conclusion. Thus, the drug should only be used if the potential benefit for mom is greater than the potential risk of fetal harm, which, in many cases, is unknown. Approximately 50% of prescription drugs fall in this category.

Animal Studies: Pregnant mice and rats treated with this drug showed delayed ossification of bones in the offspring.

Human Studies: Controlled studies using this drug in pregnant women have not been reported.

Helpful Hints:
1. In pregnant women with epilepsy, the first priority is to prevent seizures. This can be difficult because many seizure medications do not work quite as well during pregnancy. Sometimes the dose has to be increased or other medications added just to prevent seizures. Regardless, the healthiest situation for both mom and unborn baby is to have the fewest seizures possible.

2. Do not discontinue this drug abruptly because you may precipitate a seizure. Instead, discuss gradually tapering off this drug's use with your doctor.

Remember: All pregnancies have a background risk of about 3% for a major birth defect, even when mom doesn't take a drug of any kind. If you are pregnant or planning a pregnancy, always let your doctor know before taking any drug, prescription or non-prescription, or herbal remedy.

∙ ∙

GEMFIBROZIL

Brand Names: Gemcor, Lopid

Drug Use: This drug is approved by the FDA for the treatment of high blood cholesterol

Pregnancy Risk Category: C

> **Category C rating:** The FDA assigns a drug to Category **C** for one of two reasons: (1) Studies show evidence of fetal harm when using the drug in pregnant animals, but no controlled studies have been done using the drug in pregnant women, or (2) Studies using the drug in pregnant animals have not been done, and studies of pregnant women using the drug are insufficient to reach a conclusion. Thus, the drug should only be used if the potential benefit for mom is greater than the potential risk of fetal harm, which, in many cases, is unknown. Approximately 50% of prescription drugs fall in this category.

Animal Studies: Studies using this drug in pregnant rats and rabbits have shown harmful effects, including liver cancer in the rat offspring and a decrease in litter size in rabbits. However, two additional studies have shown no harmful effects in rats or rabbits.

Human Studies: Controlled studies using this drug in pregnant women have not been done. One case report involving a pregnant woman who started taking this drug at twenty weeks of pregnancy showed no harmful effects to her baby.

Remember: All pregnancies have a background risk of about 3% for a major birth defect, even when mom doesn't take a drug of any kind. If you are pregnant or planning a pregnancy, always let your doctor know before taking any drug, prescription or non-prescription, or herbal remedy.

GENTAMICIN

Brand Names: Garamycin, Genoptic, Gentacidin, Gentak

Drug Use: This antibiotic is approved by the FDA for the treatment of various bacterial infections. The drug belongs to the aminoglycoside family of drugs.

Pregnancy Risk Category: C

> **Category C rating:** The FDA assigns a drug to Category C for one of two reasons: (1) Studies show evidence of fetal harm when using the drug in pregnant animals, but no controlled studies have been done using the drug in pregnant women, or (2) Studies using the drug in pregnant animals have not been done, and studies of pregnant women using the drug are insufficient to reach a conclusion. Thus, the drug should only be used if the potential benefit for mom is greater than the potential risk of fetal harm, which, in many cases, is unknown. (Yes, it is confusing!) Approximately 50% of prescription drugs fall in this category.

Animal Studies: Studies using this drug in pregnant rats have shown kidney toxicity and high blood pressure in their offspring.

Human Studies: No controlled studies of pregnant women using this drug are available. Unlike other drugs in this family of drugs, hearing toxicity in the newborn has not been reported as an effect of exposure to this drug during pregnancy.

The FDA has issued the following Black Box Warning concerning this family of drugs:

"Injectable drugs in this family of drugs have been associated with significant kidney or hearing toxicity. Although kidney damage may be reversible, hearing toxicity may not. Monitoring of blood levels of this drug and kidney function are required."

A Black Box Warning is the most serious prescription drug warning the FDA can require a drug company to issue.

Remember: All pregnancies have a background risk of about 3% for a major birth defect, even when mom doesn't take a drug of any kind. If you are pregnant or planning a pregnancy, always let your doctor know before taking any drug, prescription or non-prescription, or herbal remedy.

GLIMEPIRIDE

Brand Name: Amaryl

Drug Use: This drug is approved by the FDA for use as an adjunct to diet and exercise in the treatment of Type 2 diabetes.

Pregnancy Risk Category: C

Category C rating: The FDA assigns a drug to Category **C** for one of two reasons: (1) Studies show evidence of fetal harm when using the drug in pregnant animals, but no controlled studies have been done using the drug in pregnant women, or (2) Studies using the drug in pregnant animals have not been done, and studies of pregnant women using the drug are insufficient to reach a conclusion. Thus, the drug should only be used if the potential benefit for mom is greater than the potential risk of fetal harm, which, in many cases, is unknown. Approximately 50% of prescription drugs fall in this category.

Animal Studies: Studies of pregnant rats and rabbits treated with extremely high doses of this drug have not found an increase in birth defects in their offspring.

Human Studies: Controlled studies of this drug in pregnant women have not been done. Most experts, including the American College of Obstetricians and Gynecologists (ACOG), recommend that insulin be used for Type 1 and Type 2 diabetes in pregnancy.

Remember: All pregnancies have a background risk of about 3% for a major birth defect, even when mom doesn't take a drug of any kind. If you are pregnant or planning a pregnancy, always let your doctor know before taking any drug, prescription or non-prescription, or herbal remedy.

GLIPIZIDE

Brand Name: Glucotrol

Drug Use: This drug is approved by the FDA for use as an oral drug to treat Type 2 diabetes. It is not approved for use in treating Type 1 diabetes.

Pregnancy Risk Category: C

> **Category C rating:** The FDA assigns a drug to Category C for one of two reasons: (1) Studies show evidence of fetal harm when using the drug in pregnant animals, but no controlled studies have been done using the drug in pregnant women, or (2) Studies using the drug in pregnant animals have not been done, and studies of pregnant women using the drug are insufficient to reach a conclusion. Thus, the drug should only be used if the potential benefit for mom is greater than the potential risk of fetal harm, which, in many cases, is unknown. Approximately 50% of prescription drugs fall in this category.

Animal Studies: There are no studies showing an increased risk of birth defects in the offspring of animals treated with this drug.

Human Studies: Controlled studies in pregnant women have not been done. This drug is not the drug of choice to treat pregnant diabetics. Most experts, including the American College of Obstetricians and Gynecologists (ACOG), recommend that insulin be used for Type 1 and Type 2 diabetes occurring during pregnancy.

Remember: All pregnancies have a background risk of about 3% for a major birth defect, even when mom doesn't take a drug of any kind. If you are pregnant or planning a pregnancy, always let your doctor know before taking any drug, prescription or non-prescription, or herbal remedy.

· ·

GLYBURIDE

Brand Names: Diabeta, Glynase, Micronase

Drug Use: This drug is approved by the FDA for the treatment of Type 2 diabetes.

Pregnancy Risk Category: C

> **Category C rating:** The FDA assigns a drug to Category **C** for one of two reasons: (1) Studies show evidence of fetal harm when using the drug in pregnant animals, but no controlled studies have been done using the drug in pregnant women, or (2) Studies using the drug in pregnant animals have not been done, and studies of pregnant women using the drug are insufficient to reach a conclusion. Thus, the drug should only be used if the potential benefit for mom is greater than the potential risk of fetal harm, which, in many cases, is unknown. Approximately 50% of prescription drugs fall in this category.

Animal Studies: No birth defects were found in the off-spring of pregnant mice, rats, and rabbits treated with this drug.

Human Studies: There are no controlled studies in which this drug was used to treat pregnant women. Insulin remains the treatment of choice for treating diabetes in pregnancy, according to most experts, including the American College of Obstetricians and Gynecologists (ACOG).

Remember: All pregnancies have a background risk of about 3% for a major birth defect, even when mom doesn't take a drug of any kind. If you are pregnant or planning a pregnancy, always let your doctor know before taking any drug, prescription or non-prescription, or herbal remedy.

GUAIFENESIN

Brand Names: This drug is an active ingredient in dozens of medications including Robitussin, Sudafed Multi-Symptom Cough & Cold, and Vicks Formula 44D Decongestant.

Drug Use: This drug is approved by the FDA for use as an expectorant.

Pregnancy Category: C

> **Category C rating:** The FDA assigns a drug to Category C for one of two reasons: (1) Studies show evidence of fetal harm when using the drug in pregnant animals, but no controlled studies have been done using the drug in pregnant women, or (2) Studies using the drug in pregnant animals have not been done, and studies of pregnant women using the drug are insufficient to reach a conclusion. Thus, the drug should only be used if the potential benefit for mom is greater than the potential risk of fetal harm, which, in many cases, is unknown. Approximately 50% of prescription drugs fall in this category.

Animal Studies: No animal studies using this drug are available.

Human Studies: A variety of non-controlled studies of pregnant women using this drug have shown no relationship of this drug with birth defects.

Remember: All pregnancies have a background risk of about 3% for a major birth defect, even when mom doesn't take a drug of any kind. If you are pregnant or planning a pregnancy, always let your doctor know before taking any drug, prescription or non-prescription, or herbal remedy.

• •

GUANETHIDINE

Brand Name: Ismelin

Drug Use: This drug is approved by the FDA for the treatment of high blood pressure.

Pregnancy Risk Category: C

> **Category C rating:** The FDA assigns a drug to Category C for one of two reasons: (1) Studies show evidence of fetal harm when using the drug in pregnant animals, but no controlled studies have been done using the drug in pregnant women, or (2) Studies using the drug in pregnant animals have not been done, and studies of pregnant women using the drug are insufficient to reach a conclusion. Thus, the drug should only be used if the potential benefit for mom is greater than the potential risk of fetal harm, which, in many cases, is unknown. Approximately 50% of prescription drugs fall in this category.

Animal Studies: Studies in pregnant animals have shown no increased risk for fetal harm when using this drug.

Human Studies: There are no controlled studies using this drug in pregnant women. This drug is the last choice for treating increased blood pressure in pregnancy. It has been replaced by safer, more effective drugs.

Remember: All pregnancies have a background risk of about 3% for a major birth defect, even when mom doesn't take a drug of any kind. If you are pregnant or planning a pregnancy, always let your doctor know before taking any drug, prescription or non-prescription, or herbal remedy.

. . . .

GUANFACINE

Brand Name: Intuniv, Tenex

Drug Use: This drug is approved by the FDA for the treatment of high blood pressure.

Pregnancy Risk Category: B

> **Category B rating:** The FDA assigns a drug to Category **B** for one of two reasons: (1) Studies show no evidence of fetal harm when using the drug in pregnant animals, but no controlled studies have been done using the drug in pregnant women, or (2) Studies show evidence of fetal harm when using the drug in pregnant animals, but controlled studies using the drug in pregnant women do not show evidence of fetal harm. Approximately 21% of prescription drugs fall in this category.

Animal Studies: No adverse fetal effects were seen in pregnant rats and rabbits treated with this drug.

Human Studies: There are no controlled studies using this drug in pregnant women. Thus, the data available is very limited.

Remember: All pregnancies have a background risk of about 3% for a major birth defect, even when mom doesn't take a drug of any kind. If you are pregnant or planning a pregnancy, always let your doctor know before taking any drug, prescription or non-prescription, or herbal remedy.

. . . .

ADDITIONAL DRUGS AND THEIR FDA PREGNANCY RISK CATEGORIES

Since these additional drugs are uncommonly used in pregnancy, they are listed by generic name along with

their FDA Pregnancy Risk Category without more detail:

Galantamine - B

Ganciclovir - C

Gatifloxacin - C

Gefitinib - D

Gemifloxacin - C

Gemtuzumab - D

Glatiramer - B

Glycopyrrolate - B

Granisetron - B

Griseofluvin - C

H

HALOPERIDOL

Brand Name: Haldol

Drug Uses: This drug is approved by the FDA for the treatment of psychosis and Tourette's syndrome.

Pregnancy Risk Category: C

> **Category C rating:** The FDA assigns a drug to Category C for one of two reasons: (1) Studies show evidence of fetal harm when using the drug in pregnant animals, but no controlled studies have been done using the drug in pregnant women, or (2) Studies using the drug in pregnant animals have not been done, and studies of pregnant women using the drug are insufficient to reach a conclusion. Thus, the drug should only be used if the potential benefit for mom is greater than the potential risk of fetal harm, which, in many cases, is unknown. Approximately 50% of prescription drugs fall in this category.

Animal Studies: When given to pregnant rodents, haloperidol was not associated with an increased risk of birth defects. However, the animals did show decreased fertility and a higher rate of newborn death.

Human Studies: There are no controlled studies using haloperidol in pregnant women, and there is actually very little information about using the drug in pregnant women. Some reports have shown that babies whose mothers were taking haloperidol close to the time of delivery showed signs of withdrawal from the drug after birth.

Remember: All pregnancies have a background risk of about 3% for a major birth defect, even when mom doesn't

take a drug of any kind. If you are pregnant or planning a pregnancy, always let your doctor know before taking any drug, prescription or non-prescription, or herbal remedy.

HALOTHANE

Brand Name: Halothane

Drug Use: This drug is approved by the FDA for use as a general anesthetic.

Pregnancy Risk Category: B

> **Category B rating:** The FDA assigns a drug to Category **B** for one of two reasons: (1) Studies show no evidence of fetal harm when using the drug in pregnant animals, but no controlled studies have been done using the drug in pregnant women, or (2) Studies show evidence of fetal harm when using the drug in pregnant animals, but controlled studies using the drug in pregnant women do not show evidence of fetal harm. Approximately 21% of prescription drugs fall in this category.

Animal Studies: When pregnant animals have been exposed to halothane, there has been an association in some animals with a variety of birth defects. However, the cause and effect was not always clear.

Human Studies: There is a limited amount of data concerning the use of halothane in pregnant women. There are no controlled studies. Overall, the various case reports suggest that it poses a low risk to the fetus and the newborn.

Helpful Hints: All drugs used for anesthesia, including halothane, can cause some difficulty breathing for the newborn immediately after birth. These breathing difficulties, however, are usually temporary, requiring little more than close observation for the first day or two of life.

Remember: All pregnancies have a background risk of about 3% for a major birth defect, even when mom doesn't take a drug of any kind. If you are pregnant or planning a pregnancy, always let your doctor know before taking any drug, prescription or non-prescription, or herbal remedy.

HEPARIN

Brand Name: Heparin

Drug Uses: Heparin is one of several kinds of "blood thinners" that helps prevent blood clots from forming. It is approved by the FDA for treating deep venous thrombosis, which means clots in the deep veins. It is also used to treat pulmonary embolism, which are clots in the deep veins that have broken loose and traveled to veins in the lungs.

Pregnancy Risk Category: C

> **Category C rating:** The FDA assigns a drug to Category C for one of two reasons: (1) Studies show evidence of fetal harm when using the drug in pregnant animals, but no controlled studies have been done using the drug in pregnant women, or (2) Studies using the drug in pregnant animals have not been done, and studies of pregnant women using the drug are insufficient to reach a conclusion. Thus, the drug should only be used if the potential benefit for mom is greater than the potential risk of fetal harm, which, in many cases, is unknown. Approximately 50% of prescription drugs fall in this category.

Animal Studies: Apparently, studies in pregnant animals have not been done using heparin.

Human Studies: Controlled studies using heparin in pregnant women have not been done.

Helpful Hints: Heparin does not cross the placental barrier. Even though heparin does not cross the placenta, and should not cause birth defects, it still should only be given to pregnant women if clearly needed.

Remember: All pregnancies have a background risk of about 3% for a major birth defect, even when mom doesn't take a drug of any kind. If you are pregnant or planning a pregnancy, always let your doctor know before taking any drug, prescription or non-prescription, or herbal remedy.

HEPATITIS B VACCINE

Brand Names: Engerix-B, Recombivax HB

Drug Use: Hepatitis B vaccine is used to prevent hepatitis B infection.

Pregnancy Risk Category: C

> **Category C rating:** The FDA assigns a drug to Category C for one of two reasons: (1) Studies show evidence of fetal harm when using the drug in pregnant animals, but no controlled studies have been done using the drug in pregnant women, or (2) Studies using the drug in pregnant animals have not been done, and studies of pregnant women using the drug are insufficient to reach a conclusion. Thus, the drug should only be used if the potential benefit for mom is greater than the potential risk of fetal harm, which, in many cases, is unknown. Approximately 50% of prescription drugs fall in this category.

Animal Studies: No animal studies have been done with this vaccine.

Human Studies: No adverse effect on the developing fetus has been observed when pregnant women have been immunized using this vaccine.

Helpful Hints: The Centers for Disease Control and Prevention (CDC) states that pregnancy is not a contraindication to hepatitis B vaccination. The CDC also advises that pregnant women at risk for hepatitis B viral infection should be vaccinated.

Remember: All pregnancies have a background risk of about 3% for a major birth defect, even when mom doesn't take a drug of any kind. If you are pregnant or planning a pregnancy, always let your doctor know before taking any drug, prescription or non-prescription, or herbal remedy.

· ·

HYDRALAZINE

Brand Name: Apresoline

Drug Use: This drug is approved by the FDA for the treatment of hypertension, which is high blood pressure.

Pregnancy Risk Category: C

> **Category C rating:** The FDA assigns a drug to Category C for one of two reasons: (1) Studies show evidence of fetal harm when using the drug in pregnant animals, but no controlled studies have been done using the drug in pregnant women, or (2) Studies using the drug in pregnant animals have not been done, and studies of pregnant women using the drug are insufficient to reach a conclusion. Thus, the drug should only be used if the potential benefit for mom is greater than the potential risk of fetal harm, which, in many cases, is unknown. Approximately 50% of prescription drugs fall in this category.

Animal Studies: This drug has caused birth defects in mice when 20 to 30 times the maximum daily human dose was used, and possibly in rabbits when 10 to 15 times the maximum daily human dose was used.

Human Studies: There are no controlled studies which have used this drug in pregnant women. Clinical experience does not include any evidence of adverse effects on the unborn baby. Still, this drug should be used during pregnancy only if the expected benefit exceeds the potential risk to the fetus.

Remember: All pregnancies have a background risk of about 3% for a major birth defect, even when mom doesn't

take a drug of any kind. If you are pregnant or planning a pregnancy, always let your doctor know before taking any drug, prescription or non-prescription, or herbal remedy.

· ·

HYDROCODONE

Brand Name: Vicodin (combination of hydrocodone and acetaminophen)

Drug Use: Hydrocodone is a narcotic agent related to codeine. It is combined with other drugs for moderate to severe pain relief.

Pregnancy Risk Categories: This drug has been assigned two pregnancy risk categories: **C** and **D** if used for prolonged periods or in high doses near term. Approximately 12% of prescription drugs are assigned two pregnancy risk categories, depending on which trimester of pregnancy the drug is used.

> **Category C rating:** The FDA assigns a drug to Category **C** for one of two reasons: (1) Studies show evidence of fetal harm when using the drug in pregnant animals, but no controlled studies have been done using the drug in pregnant women, or (2) Studies using the drug in pregnant animals have not been done, and studies of pregnant women using the drug are insufficient to reach a conclusion. Thus, the drug should only be used if the potential benefit for mom is greater than the potential risk of fetal harm, which, in many cases, is unknown. Approximately 50% of prescription drugs fall in this category.

> **Category D rating:** The FDA assigns a drug to Category **D** when studies of pregnant women using the drug show evidence of fetal harm. Rarely, however, the potential benefit of using the drug in some life-threatening situations for mom may outweigh the potential risk of fetal harm. For example, when mom requires cancer treatment or when she has a serious disease for which safer drugs cannot be used or are less effective. Approximately 11% of prescription drugs fall in this category.

Animal Studies: When given to pregnant hamsters, a single dose of hydrocodone (the narcotic ingredient in

Vicodin) increased the risk of birth defects, including cranial defects.

Human Studies: Limited studies in pregnant women showed that using Vicodin for a prolonged time during the end of pregnancy may cause narcotic withdrawal symptoms after delivery in the baby. These symptoms include irritability and excessive crying, tremors, overactive reflexes, fast breathing, increased stooling, sneezing, yawning, vomiting, and fever. For this reason, this drug is assigned to pregnancy risk category **D** if used for prolonged periods or in high doses at term.

Remember: All pregnancies have a background risk of about 3% for a major birth defect even when mom doesn't take a drug of any kind. If you are pregnant or planning a pregnancy, always let your doctor know before taking any drug, prescription or non-prescription, or herbal remedy.

. . . .

HYDROCORTISONE

Brand Name: Cortef

Drug Uses: This drug is approved by the FDA for a variety of uses, including the treatment of endocrine disorders, rheumatic disorders, collagen diseases including lupus, dermatologic diseases involving the skin, allergy difficulties, various disorders of the eye, breathing problems, blood disorders, various cancers, and a variety of other disorders.

Pregnancy Risk Categories: This drug has been assigned two pregnancy risk categories: **C** when used in the second and third trimesters, and **D** when used in the first trimester. Approximately 12% of prescription drugs are assigned two pregnancy risk categories, depending on which trimester of pregnancy the drug is used.

> **Category C rating:** The FDA assigns a drug to Category **C** for one of two reasons: (1) Studies show evidence of fetal harm when using the drug in pregnant animals, but no controlled studies have been done using the drug in pregnant women, or (2) Studies using the drug in pregnant animals have not been done, and studies of pregnant women using the drug are insufficient to reach a conclusion. Thus, the drug should only be used if the potential benefit for mom is greater than the potential risk of fetal harm, which, in many cases, is unknown. Approximately 50% of prescription drugs fall in this category.

> **Category D rating:** The FDA assigns a drug to Category **D** when studies of pregnant women using the drug show evidence of fetal harm. Rarely, however, the potential benefit of using the drug in some life-threatening situations for mom may outweigh the potential risk of fetal harm. For example, when mom requires cancer treatment or when she has a serious disease for which safer drugs cannot be used or are less effective. Approximately 11% of prescription drugs fall in this category.

Animal Studies: This drug, when given to pregnant animals, has been associated with a variety of birth defects.

Human Studies: However, when given to pregnant women, the same effects have not been found. But concern about birth defects is high enough that the pregnancy risk factor is **D** if this drug is used in the first trimester of pregnancy.

Helpful Hints: Infants born of mothers who have received substantial doses of this drug during pregnancy should be carefully observed for signs of decreased adrenal gland function.

Remember: All pregnancies have a background risk of about 3% for a major birth defect, even when mom doesn't take a drug of any kind. If you are pregnant or planning a pregnancy, always let your doctor know

before taking any drug, prescription or non-prescription, or herbal remedy.

· ·

HYDROMORPHONE

Brand Names: Dilaudid, Palladone

Drug Use: This drug is approved by the FDA for the management of pain in patients where a narcotic analgesic is appropriate.

Pregnancy Risk Categories: This drug has been assigned two pregnancy risk categories: **C** when used routinely during pregnancy and **D** when used for a prolonged period of time or just prior to delivery, placing the unborn baby at risk for depressed respirations after birth. Approximately 12% of prescription drugs are assigned two pregnancy risk categories, depending on which trimester of pregnancy the drug is used.

> **Category C rating:** The FDA assigns a drug to Category **C** for one of two reasons: (1) Studies show evidence of fetal harm when using the drug in pregnant animals, but no controlled studies have been done using the drug in pregnant women, or (2) Studies using the drug in pregnant animals have not been done, and studies of pregnant women using the drug are insufficient to reach a conclusion. Thus, the drug should only be used if the potential benefit for mom is greater than the potential risk of fetal harm, which, in many cases, is unknown. Approximately 50% of prescription drugs fall in this category.

> **Category D rating:** The FDA assigns a drug to Category **D** when studies of pregnant women using the drug show evidence of fetal harm. Rarely, however, the potential benefit of using the drug in some life-threatening situations for mom may outweigh the potential risk of fetal harm. For example, when mom requires cancer treatment or when she has a serious disease for which safer drugs cannot be used or are less effective. Approximately 11% of prescription drugs fall in this category.

Animal Studies: When pregnant rats were treated with this drug, no evidence was found of birth defects in their offspring. However, the drug did produce skull defects in hamsters when given during pregnancy.

Human Studies: This drug crosses the placenta and should be used in pregnant women only if the potential benefit justifies the potential risk to the unborn baby. Infants born to mothers who become physically dependant on this medication may also be physically dependant and have breathing difficulties, along with withdrawal symptoms.

Remember: All pregnancies have a background risk of about 3% for a major birth defect, even when mom doesn't take a drug of any kind. If you are pregnant or planning a pregnancy, always let your doctor know before taking any drug, prescription or non-prescription, or herbal remedy.

HYDROXYCHLOROQUINE

Brand Name: Plaquenil

Drug Uses: This drug is approved by the FDA for the treatment of malaria. It is also used to treat lupus and rheumatoid arthritis.

Pregnancy Risk Category: C

> **Category C rating:** The FDA assigns a drug to Category C for one of two reasons: (1) Studies show evidence of fetal harm when using the drug in pregnant animals, but no controlled studies have been done using the drug in pregnant women, or (2) Studies using the drug in pregnant animals have not been done, and studies of pregnant women using the drug are insufficient to reach a conclusion. Thus, the drug should only be used if the potential benefit for mom is greater than the potential risk of fetal harm, which, in many cases, is unknown. Approximately 50% of prescription drugs fall in this category.

Animal Studies: Studies in pregnant mice showed this drug crosses the placenta rapidly. It accumulates selectively in the structure of the fetal eyes and is retained in the eye tissue for up to five months after the drug has been eliminated from the rest of the body.

Human Studies: This drug does not seem to pose a significant risk to the fetus, especially when lower doses are used. No reports of eye or ear abnormalities after exposure during pregnancy have been located. The CDC states that the drug may be used during pregnancy for the treatment of malaria.

Remember: All pregnancies have a background risk of about 3% for a major birth defect, even when mom doesn't take a drug of any kind. If you are pregnant or planning a pregnancy, always let your doctor know before taking any drug, prescription or non-prescription, or herbal remedy.

HYDROXYUREA

Brand Names: Droxia, Hydrea

Drug Uses: This drug is approved by the FDA for the reduction of painful crises and to reduce the need for blood transfusions in adult patients with sickle cell anemia.

Pregnancy Risk Category: D

> **Category D rating:** The FDA assigns a drug to Category **D** when studies of pregnant women using the drug show evidence of fetal harm. Rarely, however, the potential benefit of using the drug in some life-threatening situations for mom may outweigh the potential risk of fetal harm. For example, when mom requires cancer treatment or when she has a serious disease for which safer drugs cannot be used or are less effective. Approximately 11% of prescription drugs fall in this category.

Animal Studies: This drug has been shown to cause a variety of birth defects in a variety of pregnant animals, including mice, hamsters, cats, swine, dogs, and monkeys.

Human Studies: There are no controlled studies using this drug in pregnant women. If this drug is used during pregnancy, or if the patient becomes pregnant while taking this drug, the patient should be advised of the potential harm to her unborn baby. Women of childbearing age should be advised to avoid becoming pregnant while taking this medication.

Remember: All pregnancies have a background risk of about 3% for a major birth defect, even when mom doesn't take a drug of any kind. If you are pregnant or planning a pregnancy, always let your doctor know before taking any drug, prescription or non-prescription, or herbal remedy.

∙ ∙

HYDROXYZINE

Brand Names: Atarax, Vistaril

Drug Uses: This drug is approved by the FDA for the treatment of anxiety, as well as itching due to allergic conditions, and as a sedative when used as premedication and following general anesthesia.

Pregnancy Risk Category: C

> **Category C rating:** The FDA assigns a drug to Category **C** for one of two reasons: (1) Studies show evidence of fetal harm when using the drug in pregnant animals, but no controlled studies have been done using the drug in pregnant women, or (2) Studies using the drug in pregnant animals have not been done, and studies of pregnant women using the drug are insufficient to reach a conclusion. Thus, the drug should only be used if the potential benefit for mom is greater than the potential risk of fetal harm, which, in many cases, is unknown. Approximately 50% of prescription drugs fall in this category.

Animal Studies: When this drug was given to pregnant mice, rats, and rabbits, it induced fetal birth defects in the rat and mouse in doses substantially higher than the human therapeutic range.

Human Studies: Unlike studies in pregnant animals, this drug, when used in pregnant women, has not shown evidence of causing birth defects. Thus, the human data suggests low risk. On the other hand, drug withdrawal has been reported in two newborns exposed near the time of delivery.

Remember: All pregnancies have a background risk of about 3% for a major birth defect, even when mom doesn't take a drug of any kind. If you are pregnant or planning a pregnancy, always let your doctor know before taking any drug, prescription or non-prescription, or herbal remedy.

ADDITIONAL DRUGS AND THEIR FDA PREGNANCY RISK CATEGORIES

Since these additional drugs are uncommonly used in pregnancy, they are listed by generic name along with their FDA Pregnancy Risk Category without more detail:

Hetastarch - C

Histrelin - X

Human Papillomavirus (HPV) Vaccine - B

Hydrochlorothiazide - B

I

IBUPROFEN

Brand Names: This drug is an active ingredient in more than 80 drug products, including Motrin and Advil.

Drug Use: This drug is approved by the FDA for the relief of pain, tenderness, swelling, and stiffness caused by osteoarthritis and rheumatoid arthritis. This drug belongs to the non-steroidal, anti-inflammatory (NSAID) family of drugs. (See Helpful Hint on next page.)

Pregnancy Risk Categories: This drug has been assigned two pregnancy risk categories: a **B** rating when used in the first two trimesters of pregnancy, and a **D** rating when used in the third trimester or near delivery. Approximately 12% of prescription drugs are assigned two pregnancy risk categories, depending on which trimester of pregnancy the drug is used.

> **Category B rating:** The FDA assigns a drug to Category **B** for one of two reasons: (1) Studies show no evidence of fetal harm when using the drug in pregnant animals, but no controlled studies have been done using the drug in pregnant women, or (2) Studies show evidence of fetal harm when using the drug in pregnant animals, but controlled studies using the drug in pregnant women do not show evidence of fetal harm. Approximately 21% of prescription drugs fall in this category.

> **Category D rating:** The FDA assigns a drug to Category **D** when studies of pregnant women using the drug show evidence of fetal harm. Rarely, however, the potential benefit of using the drug in some life-threatening situations for mom may outweigh the potential risk of fetal harm. For example, when mom requires cancer treatment or when she has a serious disease for which safer drugs cannot be used or are less effective. Approximately 11% of prescription drugs fall in this category.

Animal Studies: Studies in pregnant rats and rabbits using ibuprofen found no increase of birth defects in the offspring.

Human Studies: Controlled studies using this drug in pregnant women are not available.

Helpful Hints: Ibuprofen should be avoided during the third trimester of pregnancy, especially near the time of delivery. Why? Because NSAIDs have seriously harmed the fetus, leading to life-threatening illness after birth and even death. These potential effects apply to all NSAIDs, whether purchased by prescription or over-the-counter without a prescription. They also explain why NSAIDs have been assigned a **D** pregnancy risk category when used in the third trimester of pregnancy. (See "Non-Steroidal, Anti-Inflammatory Drugs (NSAIDs) in Pregnancy" in the appendix for more details.)

Remember: All pregnancies have a background risk of about 3% for a major birth defect, even when mom doesn't take a drug of any kind. If you are pregnant or planning a pregnancy, always let your doctor know before taking any drug, prescription or non-prescription, or herbal remedy.

IMIPRAMINE

Brand Names: Antipress, Tofranil

Drug Uses: This drug is approved by the FDA for the treatment of depression. It is also used to treat bed wetting.

Pregnancy Risk Category: C

Category C rating: The FDA assigns a drug to Category **C** for one of two reasons: (1) Studies show evidence of fetal harm when using the drug in pregnant animals, but no controlled studies have

been done using the drug in pregnant women, or (2) Studies using the drug in pregnant animals have not been done, and studies of pregnant women using the drug are insufficient to reach a conclusion. Thus, the drug should only be used if the potential benefit for mom is greater than the potential risk of fetal harm, which, in many cases, is unknown. Approximately 50% of prescription drugs fall in this category.

Animal Studies: Studies using this drug in pregnant mice, rats, rabbits, and monkeys have shown no evidence of birth defects in their offspring.

Human Studies: No controlled prospective studies in pregnant women are available. Uncontrolled, retrospective studies involving pregnant women have shown no increase in the incidence of birth defects. However, withdrawal symptoms have been reported in infants born to mothers taking this drug during pregnancy.

Helpful Hints:

1. Studies show that antidepressants increase the risk of suicidal thinking and behavior in children, adolescents, and young adults. Anyone considering the use of this drug or any other antidepressant in these patients must balance that risk with the clinical need.

2. Almost all antidepressants carry some risk to the developing fetus. However, we also know depression in a pregnant woman carries potential risk for her health and for her unborn baby; for example, low birth weight and prematurity. The risks and benefits of medications and untreated depression must be weighed carefully. If you are pregnant and think you may have depression, or if you already know you do, talk with your doctor so the two of you can create the right

plan for you and your unborn baby. (See "Anti-depressants in Pregnancy" in the appendix for more details.)

Remember: All pregnancies have a background risk of about 3% for a major birth defect, even when mom doesn't take a drug of any kind. If you are pregnant or planning a pregnancy, always let your doctor know before taking any drug, prescription or non-prescription, or herbal remedy.

INDOMETHACIN

Brand Name: Indocin

Drug Use: This drug is approved by the FDA for the treatment of pain and inflammation of osteoarthritis, rheumatoid arthritis, ankylosing spondylitis, tendonitis, and bursitis. This drug belongs to the non-steroidal, anti-inflammatory (NSAID) family of drugs. (See Helpful Hint on next page.)

Pregnancy Risk Categories: This drug has been assigned two pregnancy risk categories: **B** during the first two trimesters of pregnancy, and **D** if used for longer than 48 hours, or after 34 weeks of pregnancy, or close to the time of delivery. Approximately 12% of prescription drugs are assigned two pregnancy risk categories, depending on which trimester of pregnancy the drug is used.

> **Category B rating:** The FDA assigns a drug to Category **B** for one of two reasons: (1) Studies show no evidence of fetal harm when using the drug in pregnant animals, but no controlled studies have been done using the drug in pregnant women, or (2) Studies show evidence of fetal harm when using the drug in pregnant animals, but controlled studies using the drug in pregnant women do not show evidence of fetal harm. Approximately 21% of prescription drugs fall in this category.

Category D rating: The FDA assigns a drug to Category **D** when studies of pregnant women using the drug show evidence of fetal harm. Rarely, however, the potential benefit of using the drug in some life-threatening situations for mom may outweigh the potential risk of fetal harm. For example, when mom requires cancer treatment or when she has a serious disease for which safer drugs cannot be used or are less effective. Approximately 11% of prescription drugs fall in this category.

Animal Studies: Studies in pregnant mice and rats treated with this drug have shown various abnormalities of the skeleton in the offspring of mice, but not in rats.

Human Studies: Controlled studies using this drug in pregnant women are not available.

Helpful Hints: When taken in the third trimester of pregnancy, NSAIDs have seriously harmed the fetus, leading to life-threatening illness after birth and even death. These potential effects apply to all NSAIDs, whether purchased by prescription or over-the-counter without a prescription. They also explain why NSAIDs have been assigned a **D** pregnancy risk category. (See "Non-Steroidal, Anti-Inflammatory Drugs (NSAIDs) in Pregnancy" in the Appendix for more details.)

Remember: All pregnancies have a background risk of about 3% for a major birth defect, even when mom doesn't take a drug of any kind. If you are pregnant or planning a pregnancy, always let your doctor know before taking any drug, prescription or non-prescription, or herbal remedy.

• •

INFLUENZA VACCINE

Brand Names: 2010–2011 Seasonal Influenza Vaccine

Drug Use: This vaccine is used to prevent or modify seasonal influenza infection.

Pregnancy Risk Category: C

Category C rating: The FDA assigns a drug to Category C for one of two reasons: (1) Studies show evidence of fetal harm when using the drug in pregnant animals, but no controlled studies have been done using the drug in pregnant women, or (2) Studies using the drug in pregnant animals have not been done, and studies of pregnant women using the drug are insufficient to reach a conclusion. Thus, the drug should only be used if the potential benefit for mom is greater than the potential risk of fetal harm, which, in many cases, is unknown. Approximately 50% of prescription drugs fall in this category.

Animal Studies: No animal studies have been done with this vaccine.

Human Studies: No adverse effect on the developing fetus has been observed when pregnant women have been immunized using the seasonal influenza vaccine.

Helpful Hints:

1. When this book went to press, a key FDA advisory committee had already recommended that protection against the 2009 H1N1 virus (formerly known as the "swine flu" virus) be included in the 2010–2011 seasonal influenza vaccine starting in the fall of 2010. This means that most Americans will be able to return to the traditional routine of having one flu vaccine to protect them against the major circulating flu viruses. The World Health Organization has also made the same recommendation. Consult your doctor, local health department, or the CDC web site (www.CDC.gov) as the 2010–2011 influenza season draws closer.

2. Annual influenza vaccination is considered safe and benefits all age groups, including pregnant women who are at increased risk for influenza complications.

Remember: All pregnancies have a background risk of about 3% for a major birth defect, even when mom doesn't take a drug of any kind. If you are pregnant or planning a pregnancy, always let your doctor know before taking any drug, prescription or non-prescription, or herbal remedy.

• •

INSULIN

Brand Names: Humulin, Iletin, Novolin, Velosulin

Drug Use: This drug is approved by the FDA for the control of blood sugar in diabetes.

Pregnancy Risk Category: B

> **Category B rating:** The FDA assigns a drug to Category **B** for one of two reasons: (1) Studies show no evidence of fetal harm when using the drug in pregnant animals, but no controlled studies have been done using the drug in pregnant women, or (2) Studies show evidence of fetal harm when using the drug in pregnant animals, but controlled studies using the drug in pregnant women do not show evidence of fetal harm. Approximately 21% of prescription drugs fall in this category.

Animal Studies: Studies of pregnant animals treated with insulin have yielded inconclusive results regarding any association of this drug with birth defects in the offspring.

Human Studies: Controlled studies of pregnant women taking insulin are not available. However, insulin is the drug of choice for managing diabetes during pregnancy. Non-pregnant diabetic women should make every effort to establish the best dose of insulin for good control of their blood sugar before becoming pregnant. This is because infants of diabetic mothers are at risk for an increased incidence of birth defects, three to five times that of non-diabetic women, if their blood sugars are not controlled when they become pregnant. Insulin does not cross the placenta into the fetal circulation.

Helpful Hints: It is extremely important for diabetic women of childbearing age to have their diabetes well controlled before becoming pregnant. This statement bears repeating because if a woman has controlled diabetes prior to becoming pregnant, her risk of having a baby with a major birth defect is no greater than the risk of women who do not have diabetes.

Remember: All pregnancies have a background risk of about 3% for a major birth defect, even when mom doesn't take a drug of any kind. If you are pregnant or planning a pregnancy, always let your doctor know before taking any drug, prescription or non-prescription, or herbal remedy.

· ·

INTERFERON, ALFA

Brand Name: Roferon-A

Drug Uses: This drug is approved by the FDA for the treatment of chronic hepatitis C and hairy cell leukemia.

Pregnancy Risk Category: C

>   **Category C rating:** The FDA assigns a drug to Category **C** for one of two reasons: (1) Studies show evidence of fetal harm when using the drug in pregnant animals, but no controlled studies have been done using the drug in pregnant women, or (2) Studies using the drug in pregnant animals have not been done, and studies of pregnant women using the drug are insufficient to reach a conclusion. Thus, the drug should only be used if the potential benefit for mom is greater than the potential risk of fetal harm, which, in many cases, is unknown. Approximately 50% of prescription drugs fall in this category.

Animal Studies: Several studies of pregnant rats and rabbits treated with this drug found no increase in birth defects or adverse developmental changes in the offspring. However, this drug was associated with a significant increase in spontaneous abortions in monkeys treated with 20–500 times the human dose.

Human Studies: There are no controlled studies of pregnant women taking this drug. However, based on a limited number of human cases, interferon, alfa does not seem to pose a risk to the developing embryo and fetus.

Remember: All pregnancies have a background risk of about 3% for a major birth defect, even when mom doesn't take a drug of any kind. If you are pregnant or planning a pregnancy, always let your doctor know before taking any drug, prescription or non-prescription, or herbal remedy.
• •

INTERFERON, BETA

Brand Names: Betaseron, Avonex

Drug Uses: This drug is approved by the FDA for the treatment of multiple sclerosis. It is also an investigational drug for the treatment of AIDS, some cancers, and acute hepatitis.

Pregnancy Risk Category: C

> **Category C rating:** The FDA assigns a drug to Category C for one of two reasons: (1) Studies show evidence of fetal harm when using the drug in pregnant animals, but no controlled studies have been done using the drug in pregnant women, or (2) Studies using the drug in pregnant animals have not been done, and studies of pregnant women using the drug are insufficient to reach a conclusion. Thus, the drug should only be used if the potential benefit for mom is greater than the potential risk of fetal harm, which, in many cases, is unknown. Approximately 50% of prescription drugs fall in this category.

Animal Studies: Studies in pregnant monkeys using this drug found no increase in birth defects.

Human Studies: No controlled studies have been done in pregnant women using this drug and no published case reports are available.

Helpful Hints: A pregnancy registry has been established to monitor pregnancy outcomes of women exposed to Betaseron while pregnant. Providers or their patients can obtain additional information online at www.beta seronpregnancyregistry.com. Patients can be registered by calling 1-800-478-7049.

Remember: All pregnancies have a background risk of about 3% for a major birth defect, even when mom doesn't take a drug of any kind. If you are pregnant or planning a pregnancy, always let your doctor know before taking any drug, prescription or non-prescription, or herbal remedy.

INTERFERON, GAMMA

Brand Name: Actimmune

Drug Use: This drug is approved by the FDA for the reduction of the frequency and severity of serious infections in patients with chronic granulomatous disease. Its use in pregnancy is rare.

Pregnancy Risk Category: C

Category C rating: The FDA assigns a drug to Category **C** for one of two reasons: (1) Studies show evidence of fetal harm when using the drug in pregnant animals, but no controlled studies have been done using the drug in pregnant women, or (2) Studies using the drug in pregnant animals have not been done, and studies of pregnant women using the drug are insufficient to reach a conclusion. Thus, the drug should only be used if the potential benefit for mom is greater than the potential risk of fetal harm, which, in many cases, is unknown. Approximately 50% of prescription drugs fall in this category.

Animal Studies: In studies of pregnant monkeys and mice treated with 100 times the human dose of Interferon, Gamma there was an increase of fetal death.

Human Studies: No reports describing the use of this drug in pregnant women have been found.

Remember: All pregnancies have a background risk of about 3% for a major birth defect, even when mom doesn't take a drug of any kind. If you are pregnant or planning a pregnancy, always let your doctor know before taking any drug, prescription or non-prescription, or herbal remedy.

• •

IPRATROPIUM

Brand Name: Atrovent

Drug Use: This drug is approved by the FDA for the treatment of airway spasm associated with chronic lung disease, bronchitis, and emphysema.

Pregnancy Risk Category: B

> **Category B rating:** The FDA assigns a drug to Category **B** for one of two reasons: (1) Studies show no evidence of fetal harm when using the drug in pregnant animals, but no controlled studies have been done using the drug in pregnant women, or (2) Studies show evidence of fetal harm when using the drug in pregnant animals, but controlled studies using the drug in pregnant women do not show evidence of fetal harm. Approximately 21% of prescription drugs fall in this category.

Animal Studies: Studies of pregnant mice, rats, and rabbits treated with this drug have shown no increase in the incidence of birth defects in their offspring.

Human Studies: Controlled studies of pregnant women taking this drug are unavailable.

Although little data is available concerning this drug's use in pregnant women, the consensus appears to be there is no evidence that this drug causes fetal harm.

Remember: All pregnancies have a background risk of about 3% for a major birth defect, even when mom doesn't take a drug of any kind. If you are pregnant or planning a pregnancy, always let your doctor know before taking any drug, prescription or non-prescription, or herbal remedy.

IRBESARTAN

Brand Name: Avapro

Drug Use: This drug is approved by the FDA for the treatment of hypertension, which is high blood pressure. This drug belongs to the family of drugs called angiotensin II inhibitors.

Pregnancy Risk Categories: This drug has been assigned two pregnancy risk categories: **C** if used in the first trimester, and **D** if used in the second or third trimesters. Approximately 12% of prescription drugs are assigned two pregnancy risk categories, depending on which trimester of pregnancy the drug is used.

Category C rating: The FDA assigns a drug to Category **C** for one of two reasons: (1) Studies show evidence of fetal harm when using the drug in pregnant animals, but no controlled studies have been done using the drug in pregnant women, or (2) Studies using the drug in pregnant animals have not been done, and studies of pregnant women using the drug are insufficient to reach a conclusion. Thus, the drug should only be used if the potential benefit for mom is greater than the potential risk of fetal harm, which, in many cases, is unknown. Approximately 50% of prescription drugs fall in this category.

Category D rating: The FDA assigns a drug to Category **D** when studies of pregnant women using the drug show evidence of fetal harm. Rarely, however, the potential benefit of using the drug in some life-threatening situations for mom may outweigh the potential risk of fetal harm. For example, when mom requires cancer treatment or when she has a serious disease for which safer drugs cannot be used or are less effective. Approximately 11% of prescription drugs fall in this category.

Animal Studies: Studies of pregnant rats treated with this drug have revealed malformations of the fetal kidneys. Moreover, studies in pregnant rabbits have shown increased maternal mortality and spontaneous abortions.

Human Studies: No controlled studies or case reports of pregnant women taking this drug are available. Since the manner in which this drug works is similar to the manner in which the family of so-called ACE inhibitors work, the use of this drug during the second and third trimesters may cause birth defects and fetal and newborn toxicity identical to that seen with the ACE inhibitor family of drugs. These defects include abnormalities of the fetal skull and kidney defects. They also include growth retardation, prematurity, and newborn hypotension, which is low blood pressure.

Helpful Hints: The potential problems with using this drug during the second and third trimesters of pregnancy make it imperative that you check with your doctor immediately if you are taking this drug and think you are pregnant.

Remember: All pregnancies have a background risk of about 3% for a major birth defect, even when mom doesn't take a drug of any kind. If you are pregnant or planning a pregnancy, always let your doctor know before taking any drug, prescription or non-prescription, or herbal remedy.

ISONIAZID

Brand Name: Isoniazid

Drug Use: This drug is approved by the FDA for the prevention and treatment of tuberculosis.

Pregnancy Risk Category: C

Category C rating: The FDA assigns a drug to Category C for one of two reasons: (1) Studies show evidence of fetal harm when using the drug in pregnant animals, but no controlled studies have been done using the drug in pregnant women, or (2) Studies using the drug in pregnant animals have not been done, and studies of pregnant women using the drug are insufficient to reach a conclusion. Thus, the drug should only be used if the potential benefit for mom is greater than the potential risk of fetal harm, which, in many cases, is unknown. Approximately 50% of prescription drugs fall in this category.

Animal Studies: Studies in pregnant mice, rats, and rabbits treated with this drug found no association between the drug and birth defects in the offspring.

Human Studies: Controlled studies in pregnant women using this drug are not available. However, several retrospective studies found no relationship between isoniazid and fetal birth defects.

Helpful Hints: The American Thoracic Society recommends using this drug to treat tuberculosis occurring during pregnancy because "untreated TB represents a far greater hazard to a pregnant woman and her fetus than does treatment of the disease."

Remember: All pregnancies have a background risk of about 3% for a major birth defect, even when mom doesn't take a drug of any kind. If you are pregnant or planning a pregnancy, always let your doctor know before taking any drug, prescription or non-prescription, or herbal remedy.

ISOPROTERENOL

Brand Name: Isuprel

Drug Use: This drug is approved by the FDA for the treatment of certain types of irregular heart rhythms.

Pregnancy Risk Category: C

Category C rating: The FDA assigns a drug to Category C for one of two reasons: (1) Studies show evidence of fetal harm when using the drug in pregnant animals, but no controlled studies have been done using the drug in pregnant women, or (2) Studies using the drug in pregnant animals have not been done, and studies of pregnant women using the drug are insufficient to reach a conclusion. Thus, the drug should only be used if the potential benefit for mom is greater than the potential risk of fetal harm, which, in many cases, is unknown. Approximately 50% of prescription drugs fall in this category.

Animal Studies: Studies in pregnant rats and rabbits treated with this drug found no increased incidence of birth defects. However, similar studies in hamsters did.

Human Studies: No controlled studies using this drug in pregnant women and no case reports linking the human use of this drug to birth defects have been found.

Remember: All pregnancies have a background risk of about 3% for a major birth defect, even when mom doesn't take a drug of any kind. If you are pregnant or planning a pregnancy, always let your doctor know before taking any drug, prescription or non-prescription, or herbal remedy.
. . . .

ISOSORBIDE MONONITRATE

Brand Names: Imdur, ISMO. This drug is the active ingredient in more than 20 different medical products.

Drug Use: This drug is approved by the FDA for the treatment and prevention of angina pectoris, which is chest pain.

Pregnancy Risk Category: C

Category C rating: The FDA assigns a drug to Category C for one of two reasons: (1) Studies show evidence of fetal harm when

using the drug in pregnant animals, but no controlled studies have been done using the drug in pregnant women, or (2) Studies using the drug in pregnant animals have not been done, and studies of pregnant women using the drug are insufficient to reach a conclusion. Thus, the drug should only be used if the potential benefit for mom is greater than the potential risk of fetal harm, which, in many cases, is unknown. Approximately 50% of prescription drugs fall in this category.

Animal Studies: No harmful fetal effects were found in pregnant rats and rabbits treated with moderate doses of this drug. However, in high doses, treatment in rats was associated with prolonged gestation, stillbirth, and newborn death.

Human Studies: No controlled studies or case reports of pregnant women taking this drug are available.

Remember: All pregnancies have a background risk of about 3% for a major birth defect, even when mom doesn't take a drug of any kind. If you are pregnant or planning a pregnancy, always let your doctor know before taking any drug, prescription or non-prescription, or herbal remedy.

ISOTRETINOIN

Brand Names: Accutane, Claravis

Drug Use: This drug is approved by the FDA for the treatment of severe acne unresponsive to conventional treatment.

Pregnancy Risk Category: X

Category X rating: The FDA assigns a drug to Category **X** when studies have shown the risk of fetal harm clearly outweighs any potential maternal benefit from the drug. **Drugs in this category should not be used by pregnant women.** Approximately 5% of prescription drugs fall in this category.

Animal Studies: The high probability for birth defects, especially those involving the brain, face, and limbs, in the offspring of pregnant animals treated with this drug was well-documented before it was approved for human use in 1982.

Human Studies: No controlled studies in pregnant women using this drug are available. However, the FDA and the CDC have received reports of more than 150 cases of isotretinoin-exposed pregnancies. Of 154 exposed pregnancies, 95 were electively aborted, 12 aborted spontaneously, 26 infants were born without major defects, and 21 had major defects. The pattern of major defects predominantly involved the brain, face, and heart. Thus, isotretinoin is a potent and well-known cause of birth defects.

Helpful Hints: In 2005, the FDA notified healthcare professionals and patients about a stronger isotretinoin management program called iPledge, which was designed to minimize pregnancy exposures to this drug.

Several years ago, the FDA issued the following Black Box Warning:

"Accutane must not be used by female patients who are or who may become pregnant. There is an extremely high risk that severe birth defects will result if pregnancy occurs while taking Accutane in any amount, even for short periods of time. Potentially, any fetus exposed during pregnancy can be affected. There are no accurate means of determining whether an exposed fetus has been affected."

"Birth defects which have been documented following Accutane exposure include abnormalities of the face, eyes, ears, skull, central nervous system, heart, thymus and parathyroid glands. Also, cases with IQ scores of less than 85 with or without other abnormalities have been reported. There is an increased risk of spontaneous abortion and premature birth."

"Because of Accutane's tendency to cause birth defects and to minimize fetal exposure, Accutane is approved for marketing only under a special restricted distribution program approved by the FDA. This program is also called iPledge. Accutane must only be prescribed by health-care providers who are registered and activated with the iPledge program. Accutane must only be dispensed by a pharmacy registered and activated with iPledge, and must only be dispensed to patients who are registered and meet all of the requirements of iPledge. For more specifics, please refer to the FDA website www.fda.gov."

A Black Box Warning is the most serious prescription drug warning the FDA can require a drug company to issue.

Remember: All pregnancies have a background risk of about 3% for a major birth defect, even when mom doesn't take a drug of any kind. If you are pregnant or planning a pregnancy, always let your doctor know before taking any drug, prescription or non-prescription, or herbal remedy.

ADDITIONAL DRUGS AND THEIR FDA PREGNANCY RISK CATEGORIES

Since these additional drugs are uncommonly used in pregnancy, they are listed by generic name along with

their FDA Pregnancy Risk Category without more detail:

Ibandronate - C

Ibutilide - C

Idarubicin - D

Ifosfamide - D

Iloprost - C

Imatinib - D

Imiquimod - C

Inamrinone - C

Indapamide - B (D if used in gestational hypertension)

Indinavir - C

Infliximab - B

Irinotecan - D

Isradipine - C

Itraconazole - C

Ivermectin - C

K

KANAMYCIN

Brand Name: Kantrex

Drug Use: This antibiotic is approved by the FDA for the treatment of a variety of bacterial infections. It belongs to the family of aminoglycoside antibiotics.

Pregnancy Risk Category: D

> **Category D rating:** The FDA assigns a drug to Category **D** when studies of pregnant women using the drug show evidence of fetal harm. Rarely, however, the potential benefit of using the drug in some life-threatening situations for mom may outweigh the potential risk of fetal harm. For example, when mom requires cancer treatment or when she has a serious disease for which safer drugs cannot be used or are less effective. Approximately 11% of prescription drugs fall in this category.

Animal Studies: Studies in pregnant rats and rabbits using low doses of this drug have revealed no evidence of impaired fertility or birth defects. However, studies in pregnant rats and guinea pigs using very large doses of the drug led to hearing impairment in the offspring.

Human Studies: There are no controlled studies in pregnant women taking this drug. Clinical experience has not shown any evidence of adverse effects of the drug on the human fetus. A retrospective study of 391 pregnant women who had received the drug for prolonged periods of time during their pregnancies found that nine children of those 391 mothers did develop a hearing loss. Except for this incidence of hearing loss, there are no reports of birth defects associated with the use of kanamycin in human pregnancy.

However, if the drug is used during pregnancy, or if the patient becomes pregnant while taking this drug, the patient should be made aware of the potential hazard for hearing loss in her unborn baby.

Helpful Hints: The concern about hearing loss in babies exposed to kanamycin before birth was raised when it was found that another member of the aminoglycoside family of antibiotics, namely streptomycin, has caused total, irreversible congenital deafness in children whose mothers received the drug during pregnancy. Since kanamycin is a member of the same family of antibiotics, concern over hearing loss extends to every member of this antibiotic family.

Remember: All pregnancies have a background risk of about 3% for a major birth defect, even when mom doesn't take a drug of any kind. If you are pregnant or planning a pregnancy, always let your doctor know before taking any drug, prescription or non-prescription, or herbal remedy.

• •

KETAMINE

Brand Name: Ketalar

Drug Use: This drug is approved by the FDA for use as a general anesthetic.

Pregnancy Risk Category: B

> **Category B rating:** The FDA assigns a drug to Category **B** for one of two reasons: (1) Studies show no evidence of fetal harm when using the drug in pregnant animals, but no controlled studies have been done using the drug in pregnant women, or (2) Studies show evidence of fetal harm when using the drug in

pregnant animals, but controlled studies using the drug in pregnant women do not show evidence of fetal harm. Approximately 21% of prescription drugs fall in this category.

Animal Studies: Studies of pregnant rats, mice, rabbits, and dogs exposed to this drug have found no increased risk of birth defects or other harmful fetal effects.

Human Studies: Ketamine anesthesia used close to the time of delivery of pregnant women may be associated with temporary newborn respiratory depression. These effects are usually avoided with the use of lower maternal doses. No reports of birth defects associated with ketamine anesthesia have been found.

Remember: All pregnancies have a background risk of about 3% for a major birth defect, even when mom doesn't take a drug of any kind. If you are pregnant or planning a pregnancy, always let your doctor know before taking any drug, prescription or non-prescription, or herbal remedy.

· ·

KETOROLAC

Brand Name: Toradol

Drug Use: This drug is approved by the FDA for short-term pain relief. This drug is a member of the non-steroidal anti-inflammatory family of drugs (NSAIDs). (See Helpful Hint on next page.)

Pregnancy Risk Categories: This drug has been assigned two pregnancy risk categories: **C** when used in the first and second trimesters of pregnancy, and **D** when used in the third trimester or near delivery. Approximately 12% of prescription drugs are assigned two pregnancy risk categories, depending on which trimester of pregnancy the drug is used.

Category C rating: The FDA assigns a drug to Category **C** for one of two reasons: (1) Studies show evidence of fetal harm when using the drug in pregnant animals, but no controlled studies have been done using the drug in pregnant women, or (2) Studies using the drug in pregnant animals have not been done, and studies of pregnant women using the drug are insufficient to reach a conclusion. Thus, the drug should only be used if the potential benefit for mom is greater than the potential risk of fetal harm, which, in many cases, is unknown. Approximately 50% of prescription drugs fall in this category.

Category D rating: The FDA assigns a drug to Category **D** when studies of pregnant women using the drug show evidence of fetal harm. Rarely, however, the potential benefit of using the drug in some life-threatening situations for mom may outweigh the potential risk of fetal harm. For example, when mom requires cancer treatment or when she has a serious disease for which safer drugs cannot be used or are less effective. Approximately 11% of prescription drugs fall in this category.

Animal Studies: Studies of pregnant rats and rabbits using this drug have revealed no evidence of birth defects in the offspring.

Human Studies: There are no controlled studies using this drug in pregnant women.

Helpful Hints: When taken in the third trimester of pregnancy, NSAIDs have seriously harmed the fetus, leading to life-threatening illness after birth and even death. These potential effects apply to all NSAIDs, whether purchased by prescription or over-the-counter without a prescription. They also explain why NSAIDs have been assigned a **D** pregnancy risk category. (See "Non-Steroidal, Anti-Inflammatory Drugs (NSAIDs) in Pregnancy" in the appendix for more details.)

Remember: All pregnancies have a background risk of about 3% for a major birth defect, even when mom doesn't take a drug of any kind. If you are pregnant or

planning a pregnancy, always let your doctor know before taking any drug, prescription or non-prescription, or herbal remedy.

. . . .

ADDITIONAL DRUGS AND THEIR FDA PREGNANCY RISK CATEGORIES

Since these additional drugs are uncommonly used in pregnancy, they are listed by generic name along with their FDA Pregnancy Risk Category without more detail:

Ketoconazole - C

Ketoprofen - B (D if used in third trimester or near delivery)

Ketotifen - C

L

LABETALOL

Brand Names: There are 13 branded drug products in which labetalol is an active ingredient, including Trandate and Normodyne.

Drug Uses: This drug is approved by the FDA for the treatment of hypertension (high blood pressure). The drug belongs to the beta-blocker family of drugs. It is also used to treat chest pain and patients with tetanus.

Pregnancy Risk Category: C

> **Category C rating:** The FDA assigns a drug to Category C for one of two reasons: (1) Studies show evidence of fetal harm when using the drug in pregnant animals, but no controlled studies have been done using the drug in pregnant women, or (2) Studies using the drug in pregnant animals have not been done, and studies of pregnant women using the drug are insufficient to reach a conclusion. Thus, the drug should only be used if the potential benefit for mom is greater than the potential risk of fetal harm, which, in many cases, is unknown. Approximately 50% of prescription drugs fall in this category.

Animal Studies: When pregnant rats and rabbits were treated with labetalol, there were no adverse effects on the offspring.

Human Studies: There are no controlled studies of this drug in pregnant women.

Helpful Hints: Labetalol given to pregnant women with hypertension does not appear to affect the usual course of labor and delivery.

Remember: All pregnancies have a background risk of about 3% for a major birth defect, even when mom doesn't take a drug of any kind. If you are pregnant or planning a pregnancy, always let your doctor know before taking any drug, prescription or non-prescription, or herbal remedy.

. . . .

LAMIVUDINE

Brand Name: Epivir

Drug Uses: This drug is approved by the FDA for the treatment of HIV infection and for the treatment of chronic hepatitis B.

Pregnancy Risk Category: C

> **Category C rating:** The FDA assigns a drug to Category C for one of two reasons: (1) Studies show evidence of fetal harm when using the drug in pregnant animals, but no controlled studies have been done using the drug in pregnant women, or (2) Studies using the drug in pregnant animals have not been done, and studies of pregnant women using the drug are insufficient to reach a conclusion. Thus, the drug should only be used if the potential benefit for mom is greater than the potential risk of fetal harm, which, in many cases, is unknown. Approximately 50% of prescription drugs fall in this category.

Animal Studies: Studies in pregnant rabbits treated with this drug showed an increased risk of fetal death when the drug was given in human doses.

Human Studies: There are no controlled studies of this drug in pregnant women and in case reports there has been no increase reported of birth defects in babies whose mothers took this drug during pregnancy.

Helpful Hints:

1. The clinical experience from using this drug in pregnant women suggests that lamivudine poses a low risk of birth defects to the fetus.

2. The CDC recommends that women who have HIV continue their medication throughout pregnancy. The benefit of treating the mother likely outweighs any risk of medication to her unborn baby.

Remember: All pregnancies have a background risk of about 3% for a major birth defect, even when mom doesn't take a drug of any kind. If you are pregnant or planning a pregnancy, always let your doctor know before taking any drug, prescription or non-prescription, or herbal remedy.

· ·

LAMOTRIGINE

Brand Name: Lamictal

Drug Uses: This drug is approved by the FDA for the treatment of bipolar disorder and certain types of seizures. Lamotrigine is a member of the folic acid antagonist family of drugs.

Pregnancy Risk Category: C

> **Category C rating:** The FDA assigns a drug to Category C for one of two reasons: (1) Studies show evidence of fetal harm when using the drug in pregnant animals, but no controlled studies have been done using the drug in pregnant women, or (2) Studies using the drug in pregnant animals have not been done, and studies of pregnant women using the drug are insufficient to reach a conclusion. Thus, the drug should only be used if the potential benefit for mom is greater than the potential risk of fetal harm, which, in many cases, is unknown. Approximately 50% of prescription drugs fall in this category.

Animal Studies: When pregnant rats and mice were treated with this drug, there was an increased risk of decreased fetal weight and delayed bone formation. At even higher doses, pregnant rats experienced an increased incidence of fetal death. In addition, this drug is associated with decreased folate levels in pregnant rats. Folate or folic acid is critical in the development of a normal spinal column.

Human Studies: There are no controlled studies using this drug in pregnant women.

Helpful Hints:

1. Many drugs taken to control seizures, including lamotrigine, can decrease the levels of folate or folic acid in the pregnant mom. Since folate is critical for the development of the spine and brain, it is crucial for pregnant women to have an adequate intake of folic acid at all times. Thus, it is very important for a woman who has a seizure disorder and is taking this or other medications for those seizures, to discuss the possible need for additional folic acid before becoming pregnant.

2. In pregnant women with a seizure disorder, the first priority is to prevent seizures. This can be difficult at times because many seizure medications do not work quite as well during pregnancy. Sometimes the dose has to be increased or an additional medication added just to prevent seizures. Whatever doses and medications are needed to minimize the risk of seizures seem to be the safest for mom and baby.

Remember: All pregnancies have a background risk of about 3% for a major birth defect, even when mom doesn't take a drug of any kind. If you are pregnant or planning a pregnancy, always let your doctor know before taking any drug, prescription or non-prescription, or herbal remedy.

. . . .

LANSOPRAZOLE

Brand Name: Prevacid

Drug Uses: This drug is approved by the FDA for the treatment of gastroesophageal reflux disease (GERD) or "heartburn," gastric ulcer, duodenal ulcer, the prevention of ulcers in the first place, and certain other conditions that involve increased stomach acid production.

Pregnancy Risk Category: B

> **Category B rating:** The FDA assigns a drug to Category **B** for one of two reasons: (1) Studies show no evidence of fetal harm when using the drug in pregnant animals, but no controlled studies have been done using the drug in pregnant women, or (2) Studies show evidence of fetal harm when using the drug in pregnant animals, but controlled studies using the drug in pregnant women do not show evidence of fetal harm. Approximately 21% of prescription drugs fall in this category.

Animal Studies: This drug has not been associated with an increased incidence of fetal birth defects when given to pregnant rabbits. It has, however, been shown to cause dose-related tumors in the offspring in pregnant mice and rats.

Human Studies: No controlled studies using this drug in pregnant women have been done. Overall, the clinical impression by experts is that it poses a low risk for the unborn baby.

Helpful Hints: This drug weakly interacts with grapefruit and grapefruit juice, which can cause harmful, and even life-threatening, side effects. Before taking this drug with grapefruit juice, or before consuming grapefruit or grapefruit juice during the day while taking this drug, first read the section "Grapefruit Juice–Drug Interactions Can Make You Sick" in the appendix of this book. Then discuss this with your pharmacist or the healthcare provider who prescribed this drug.

Remember: All pregnancies have a background risk of about 3% for a major birth defect, even when mom doesn't take a drug of any kind. If you are pregnant or planning a pregnancy, always let your doctor know before taking any drug, prescription or non-prescription, or herbal remedy.

- -

LATANOPROST

Brand Name: Xalatan

Drug Use: This topical eye preparation is approved by the FDA to reduce pressure within the eye.

Pregnancy Risk Category: C

> **Category C rating:** The FDA assigns a drug to Category **C** for one of two reasons: (1) Studies show evidence of fetal harm when using the drug in pregnant animals, but no controlled studies have been done using the drug in pregnant women, or (2) Studies using the drug in pregnant animals have not been done, and studies of pregnant women using the drug are insufficient to reach a conclusion. Thus, the drug should only be used if the potential benefit for mom is greater than the potential risk of fetal harm, which, in many cases, is unknown. Approximately 50% of prescription drugs fall in this category.

Animal Studies: In pregnant monkeys taking this drug, there was an increased amount of pigment noted in the iris of offspring.

Human Studies: There are no controlled studies using this drug in pregnant women.

Remember: All pregnancies have a background risk of about 3% for a major birth defect, even when mom doesn't take a drug of any kind. If you are pregnant or

planning a pregnancy, always let your doctor know before taking any drug, prescription or non-prescription, or herbal remedy.

· ·

LEFLUNOMIDE

Brand Name: Arava

Drug Use: This drug is approved by the FDA for the treatment of rheumatoid arthritis.

Pregnancy Risk Category: X

> **Category X rating:** The FDA assigns a drug to Category **X** when studies have shown the risk of fetal harm clearly outweighs any potential maternal benefit from the drug. **Drugs in this category should not be used by pregnant women.** Approximately 5% of prescription drugs fall in this category.

Animal Studies: This drug causes birth defects in pregnant animals exposed to the drug.

Human Studies: Very little information about the use of this drug in pregnant women is available. In light of the results of animal studies and this lack of information, the FDA has issued the following Black Box Warning:

"Pregnancy must be excluded before the start of treatment with Arava. Arava is contraindicated in pregnant women, or women of childbearing potential who are not using reliable contraception. Pregnancy must be avoided during Arava treatment or prior to the completion of the drug elimination procedure after Arava treatment."

A Black Box Warning is the most serious prescription drug warning the FDA can require a drug company to issue.

Helpful Hints: This drug stays in the body for a very long time. It may actually take up to two years for the body to completely clear it. It is critical that any woman of childbearing age use reliable birth control if she plans to take or is taking this drug. Furthermore, birth control must be continued for a prolonged period of time even after stopping the drug.

Remember: All pregnancies have a background risk of about 3% for a major birth defect, even when mom doesn't take a drug of any kind. If you are pregnant or planning a pregnancy, always let your doctor know before taking any drug, prescription or non-prescription, or herbal remedy.

. . . .

LEVETIRACETAM

Brand Name: Keppra

Drug Use: This drug is approved by the FDA for the treatment of seizures.

Pregnancy Risk Category: C

> **Category C rating:** The FDA assigns a drug to Category C for one of two reasons: (1) Studies show evidence of fetal harm when using the drug in pregnant animals, but no controlled studies have been done using the drug in pregnant women, or (2) Studies using the drug in pregnant animals have not been done, and studies of pregnant women using the drug are insufficient to reach a conclusion. Thus, the drug should only be used if the potential benefit for mom is greater than the potential risk of fetal harm, which, in many cases, is unknown. Approximately 50% of prescription drugs fall in this category.

Animal Studies: In pregnant rats treated with this drug, there has been an increased risk of bony abnormalities and slow growth of the fetus. With increasing doses, there was also increased risk of fetal death and altered behavior patterns in the offspring of these rats. Similar effects were seen when this drug was given to pregnant rabbits.

Human Studies: There is little known information about the use of this drug in pregnant women. One of the authors has had a personal experience with a pregnant patient treated with this drug during pregnancy. In addition to levetiracetam, the patient required two additional anti-seizure medications throughout her pregnancy. She did have approximately one seizure per month during her pregnancy, yet delivered a full-term, healthy male. No birth defects were noted in the newborn.

Helpful Hints:

1. In pregnant women with epilepsy, the first priority is to prevent seizures. This can be difficult because many seizure medications do not work quite as well during pregnancy. Sometimes the dose has to be increased or other medications added just to prevent seizures. Regardless, the healthiest situation for both mom and unborn baby is to have the fewest seizures possible.

2. Many anti-seizure medications can decrease the level of folate or folic acid in the pregnant woman. Since folate is critical for the normal development of the spinal column and brain, many women with epilepsy may need additional intake of folic acid throughout their pregnancy. It is not known if levetiracetam causes folic acid deficiency, but it will usually be combined with other anticonvulsants, some of which may cause folic acid deficiency.

Remember: All pregnancies have a background risk of about 3% for a major birth defect, even when mom doesn't take a drug of any kind. If you are pregnant or planning a pregnancy, always let your doctor know

before taking any drug, prescription or non-prescription, or herbal remedy.

· ·

LEVODOPA

Brand Name: Simemet

Drug Use: The FDA has approved Levodopa for the treatment and prevention of symptoms related to Parkinson's disease. This drug is often combined with a second drug called carbidopa, which enhances Levodopa's effectiveness.

Pregnancy Risk Category: C

> **Category C rating:** The FDA assigns a drug to Category C for one of two reasons: (1) Studies show evidence of fetal harm when using the drug in pregnant animals, but no controlled studies have been done using the drug in pregnant women, or (2) Studies using the drug in pregnant animals have not been done, and studies of pregnant women using the drug are insufficient to reach a conclusion. Thus, the drug should only be used if the potential benefit for mom is greater than the potential risk of fetal harm, which, in many cases, is unknown. Approximately 50% of prescription drugs fall in this category.

Animal Studies: This drug has been associated with an increased risk of birth defects when given to pregnant rabbits. At higher doses, the offspring of pregnant mice have shown a decrease in birth weight.

Human Studies: There is very little information available about the use of this drug in pregnant women. Clinically, no definitive adverse effects have been seen.

Remember: All pregnancies have a background risk of about 3% for a major birth defect, even when mom doesn't take a drug of any kind. If you are pregnant or planning a pregnancy, always let your doctor know before taking any drug, prescription or non-prescription, or herbal remedy.

· ·

LEVOFLOXACIN

Brand Name: Levaquin

Drug Use: This drug is approved by the FDA for treating a variety of bacterial infections, including pneumonia, prostatitis, kidney infection, sinusitis, and others.

Pregnancy Risk Category: C

> **Category C rating:** The FDA assigns a drug to Category C for one of two reasons: (1) Studies show evidence of fetal harm when using the drug in pregnant animals, but no controlled studies have been done using the drug in pregnant women, or (2) Studies using the drug in pregnant animals have not been done, and studies of pregnant women using the drug are insufficient to reach a conclusion. Thus, the drug should only be used if the potential benefit for mom is greater than the potential risk of fetal harm, which, in many cases, is unknown. Approximately 50% of prescription drugs fall in this category.

Animal Studies: In high doses, this drug is associated with a decrease in fetal weight and an increased risk of fetal death when given to pregnant rats.

Human Studies: There have been no controlled studies using this drug in pregnant women.

Remember: All pregnancies have a background risk of about 3% for a major birth defect, even when mom doesn't take a drug of any kind. If you are pregnant or planning a pregnancy, always let your doctor know before taking any drug, prescription or non-prescription, or herbal remedy.

· ·

LEVOTHYROXINE

Brand Names: Levothyroid, Levoxyl, Synthroid, Unithroid

Drug Use: This drug is approved by the FDA for the treatment of hypothyroidism, which means underactive thyroid.

Pregnancy Risk Category: **A**

> **Category A rating:** The FDA assigns a drug to Category **A** when controlled studies using the drug in pregnant women do not show harmful fetal effects throughout pregnancy. Approximately 1% of prescription drugs fall in this category.

Animal Studies: There are no studies available in which this drug was used to treat pregnant animals.

Human Studies: Clinical experience with this drug in pregnant women has shown that it is safe for use in pregnancy.

Helpful Hints: This drug weakly interacts with grapefruit and grapefruit juice, which can cause harmful, and even life-threatening, side effects. Before taking this drug with grapefruit juice, or before consuming grapefruit or grapefruit juice during the day while taking this drug, first read the section "Grapefruit Juice–Drug Interactions Can Make You Sick" in the appendix of this book. Then discuss this with your pharmacist or the healthcare provider who prescribed this drug.

Remember: All pregnancies have a background risk of about 3% for a major birth defect, even when mom doesn't take a drug of any kind. If you are pregnant or planning a pregnancy, always let your doctor know before taking any drug, prescription or non-prescription, or herbal remedy.

LIDOCAINE

Brand Names: More than 50 medical preparations containing this drug are on the market, including Xylocaine, Lidoderm, and Xylocaine Topical.

Drug Uses: The FDA has approved Lidocaine for use as a local anesthetic in a variety of forms, and also to treat life-threatening irregular heart rhythms.

Pregnancy Risk Category: **B**

> **Category B rating:** The FDA assigns a drug to Category **B** for one of two reasons: (1) Studies show no evidence of fetal harm when using the drug in pregnant animals, but no controlled studies have been done using the drug in pregnant women, or (2) Studies show evidence of fetal harm when using the drug in pregnant animals, but controlled studies using the drug in pregnant women do not show evidence of fetal harm. Approximately 21% of prescription drugs fall in this category.

Animal Studies: Limited studies performed on pregnant animals receiving this drug did not show any evidence of increased fetal harm.

Human Studies: There are no controlled studies using this drug in pregnant women. Various case reports indicate the drug is not associated with birth defects.

Remember: All pregnancies have a background risk of about 3% for a major birth defect, even when mom doesn't take a drug of any kind. If you are pregnant or planning a pregnancy, always let your doctor know before taking any drug, prescription or non-prescription, or herbal remedy.

• •

LISINOPRIL

Brand Names: Prinivil, Zestril

Drug Uses: This drug is approved by the FDA for the treatment of high blood pressure, congestive heart failure, and acute heart attack. Lisinopril belongs to the ACE inhibitor family of drugs. (See Helpful Hint on next page.)

Pregnancy Risk Categories: This drug has been assigned two pregnancy risk categories: **C** when used in the first trimester, and **D** when used in the second and third trimesters. Approximately 12% of prescription drugs are assigned two pregnancy risk categories, depending on which trimester of pregnancy the drug is used.

Category C rating: The FDA assigns a drug to Category **C** for one of two reasons: (1) Studies show evidence of fetal harm when using the drug in pregnant animals, but no controlled studies have been done using the drug in pregnant women, or (2) Studies using the drug in pregnant animals have not been done, and studies of pregnant women using the drug are insufficient to reach a conclusion. Thus, the drug should only be used if the potential benefit for mom is greater than the potential risk of fetal harm, which, in many cases, is unknown. Approximately 50% of prescription drugs fall in this category.

Category D rating: The FDA assigns a drug to Category **D** when studies of pregnant women using the drug show evidence of fetal harm. Rarely, however, the potential benefit of using the drug in some life-threatening situations for mom may outweigh the potential risk of fetal harm. For example, when mom requires cancer treatment or when she has a serious disease for which safer drugs cannot be used or are less effective. Approximately 11% of prescription drugs fall in this category.

Animal Studies: When pregnant mice, rats, and rabbits were treated with this medication, there were no adverse fetal effects.

Human Studies: When taken in the first trimester of pregnancy, lisinopril appears to have no adverse fetal effects. Thus, its pregnancy risk rating for the first trimester is **C**. However, the FDA has issued the following Black Box Warning for this drug and all ACE inhibitors:

"When used in pregnancy during the second and third trimesters, ACE inhibitors can cause injury and even death to the developing fetus. When pregnancy is detected, this drug should be discontinued as soon as possible."

A Black Box Warning is the most serious prescription drug warning the FDA can require a drug company to issue.

Helpful Hints: It is important to reemphasize the following: "When used in pregnancy during the second and third trimesters, ACE inhibitors can cause injury and even death to the developing fetus." (See "Ace Inhibitor Drugs in Pregnancy" in the appendix for more details.)

Remember: All pregnancies have a background risk of about 3% for a major birth defect, even when mom doesn't take a drug of any kind. If you are pregnant or planning a pregnancy, always let your doctor know before taking any drug, prescription or non-prescription, or herbal remedy.

LITHIUM

Brand Names: Eskalith, Lithobid

Drug Uses: This drug is approved by the FDA for treating bipolar disorder and mania.

Pregnancy Risk Category: D

> **Category D rating:** The FDA assigns a drug to Category **D** when studies of pregnant women using the drug show evidence of fetal harm. Rarely, however, the potential benefit of using the drug in some life-threatening situations for mom may outweigh the potential risk of fetal harm. For example, when mom requires cancer treatment or when she has a serious disease for which safer drugs cannot be used or are less effective. Approximately 11% of prescription drugs fall in this category.

Animal Studies: In pregnant rats, lithium has been associated with an increased risk of birth defects, especially those involving the heart.

Human Studies: Although there have not been any controlled studies of lithium use in pregnant women, a variety of case reports and retrospective studies reveal that lithium has been associated with birth defects, most often involving the heart. The risk is probably greatest in the first trimester of pregnancy, when these structures are formed.

Helpful Hints: Lithium is a very effective drug for controlling the symptoms of bipolar disorder. It also carries increased risk to the fetus. Thus, this drug should not be used in pregnancy except under exceptional circumstances when the benefit for mom's health outweighs the potential risk for her unborn baby.

Remember: All pregnancies have a background risk of about 3% for a major birth defect, even when mom doesn't take a drug of any kind. If you are pregnant or planning a pregnancy, always let your doctor know before taking any drug, prescription or non-prescription, or herbal remedy.

LORATADINE

Brand Names: Claritin, Alavert

Drug Uses: This drug is approved by the FDA for the treatment of allergic rhinitis (seasonal allergies) and hives.

Pregnancy Risk Category: B

> **Category B rating:** The FDA assigns a drug to Category **B** for one of two reasons: (1) Studies show no evidence of fetal harm when using the drug in pregnant animals, but no controlled studies have been done using the drug in pregnant women, or (2) Studies show evidence of fetal harm when using the drug in pregnant animals, but controlled studies using the drug in pregnant women do not show evidence of fetal harm. Approximately 21% of prescription drugs fall in this category.

Animal Studies: When loratadine was given to pregnant rats and rabbits, no adverse effects were noted in their offspring.

Human Studies: Although there are no controlled studies of pregnant women taking this drug, clinical experience suggests that it is not associated with an increased risk of birth defects.

Remember: All pregnancies have a background risk of about 3% for a major birth defect, even when mom doesn't take a drug of any kind. If you are pregnant or planning a pregnancy, always let your doctor know before taking any drug, prescription or non-prescription, or herbal remedy.

LORAZEPAM

Brand Name: Ativan

Drug Uses: This drug is approved by the FDA for the treatment of anxiety, insomnia, seizures, and nausea associated with chemotherapy. This drug is a member of the benzodiazepine family of drugs.

Pregnancy Risk Category: D

> **Category D rating:** The FDA assigns a drug to Category **D** when studies of pregnant women using the drug show evidence of fetal harm. Rarely, however, the potential benefit of using the drug in some life-threatening situations for mom may outweigh the potential risk of fetal harm. For example, when mom requires cancer treatment or when she has a serious disease for which safer drugs cannot be used or are less effective. Approximately 11% of prescription drugs fall in this category.

Animal Studies: When pregnant rats, mice, and rabbits were treated with this medication, there was an increased risk of birth defects in their offspring. It has also been associated with an increased risk of fetal death in pregnant rabbits.

Human Studies: There are no controlled studies in which this drug was used in pregnant women. However, a variety of case reports and retrospective studies have indicated that occasionally babies whose mothers have taken this medication suffer respiratory depression shortly after birth. In addition, unborn babies exposed to this benzodiazepine family of drugs have an increased risk of anal atresia, which is a failure of the anus to open during fetal development. Fortunately, this condition can be treated surgically after birth.

Helpful Hints: This drug should be avoided in pregnancy. However, it is possible that on rare occasions the potential benefit for mom may outweigh the potential risk for her unborn baby.

Remember: All pregnancies have a background risk of about 3% for a major birth defect, even when mom doesn't take a drug of any kind. If you are pregnant or planning a pregnancy, always let your doctor know before taking any drug, prescription or non prescription, or herbal remedy.

· ·

LOSARTAN

Brand Name: Cozaar

Drug Uses: This drug is approved by the FDA for the treatment of high blood pressure and diabetic kidney disease. It belongs to a family of drugs that is a cousin to the ACE inhibitor family of drugs. Thus, it may affect the fetus in a similar manner as the members of the ACE inhibitor family of drugs.

Pregnancy Risk Categories: This drug has been assigned two pregnancy risk categories: **C** when used in the first trimester and **D** when used in the second and third trimesters. Approximately 12% of prescription drugs are assigned two pregnancy risk categories, depending on which trimester of pregnancy the drug is used.

Category C rating: The FDA assigns a drug to Category **C** for one of two reasons: (1) Studies show evidence of fetal harm when

using the drug in pregnant animals, but no controlled studies have been done using the drug in pregnant women, or (2) Studies using the drug in pregnant animals have not been done, and studies of pregnant women using the drug are insufficient to reach a conclusion. Thus, the drug should only be used if the potential benefit for mom is greater than the potential risk of fetal harm, which, in many cases, is unknown. Approximately 50% of prescription drugs fall in this category.

Category D rating: The FDA assigns a drug to Category **D** when studies of pregnant women using the drug show evidence of fetal harm. Rarely, however, the potential benefit of using the drug in some life-threatening situations for mom may outweigh the potential risk of fetal harm. For example, when mom requires cancer treatment or when she has a serious disease for which safer drugs cannot be used or are less effective. Approximately 11% of prescription drugs fall in this category.

Animal Studies: When used in the treatment of pregnant rats, losartan has been associated with decreased fetal weight, kidney disease, and increased fetal death.

Human Studies: Although no controlled studies using losartan in pregnant women have been done, clinical experience shows that this drug is associated with several potentially severe problems for the fetus, particularly if taken in the second and third trimesters. These problems include birth defects, kidney failure, decreased amount of amniotic fluid, failure of the fetal lungs to mature appropriately prior to birth, decreased fetal growth, and even death. For these reasons, the drug is assigned to category **D** when used in the second and third trimesters.

Helpful Hints:

1. Losartan is an effective drug for lowering blood pressure. Unfortunately, in pregnancy, it is thought that it also lowers fetal blood pressure. This lowered fetal blood pressure leads to decreased blood flow to the kidney, which results in decreased urine

production, which, in turn, results in decreased amniotic fluid, which, in turn, adversely affects fetal lung development.

2. Ideally, women who are taking losartan and planning to become pregnant should discuss possibly discontinuing the drug and switching to a safer drug before becoming pregnant.

3. This drug weakly interacts with grapefruit and grapefruit juice, which can cause harmful, and even life-threatening, side effects. Before taking this drug with grapefruit juice, or before consuming grapefruit or grapefruit juice during the day while taking this drug, first read the section "Grapefruit Juice–Drug Interactions Can Make You Sick" in the appendix of this book. Then discuss this with your pharmacist or the healthcare provider who prescribed this drug.

4. The FDA has issued the following Black Box Warning:
"When used in pregnancy during the second and third trimesters, drugs that act directly on the renin-angiotensin system, which this drug does, can cause injury and even death to the developing fetus. When pregnancy is detected, this drug should be discontinued as soon as possible."

A Black Box Warning is the most serious prescription drug warning the FDA can require a drug company to issue.

Remember: All pregnancies have a background risk of about 3% for a major birth defect, even when mom doesn't take a drug of any kind. If you are pregnant or planning a pregnancy, always let your doctor know

before taking any drug, prescription or non-prescription, or herbal remedy.
· ·

LOVASTATIN

Brand Names: Mevacor, Altoprev

Drug Uses: This drug is approved by the FDA for the treatment of high cholesterol and to lower the risk of heart attack. It is a member of the "statin" family of drugs.

Pregnancy Risk Category: X

> **Category X rating:** The FDA assigns a drug to Category **X** when studies have shown the risk of fetal harm clearly outweighs any potential maternal benefit from the drug. **Drugs in this category should not be used by pregnant women.** Approximately 5% of prescription drugs fall in this category.

Animal Studies: When given to pregnant mice and rats, lovastatin has been associated with decreased fetal weight and increased risk of bony defects.

Human Studies: There are no controlled studies using this drug in pregnant women.

Cholesterol is essential for normal fetal development. But because lovastatin and the other members of the statin family of drugs lower serum cholesterol, they may inadvertently interfere with normal fetal development. According to experts, stopping treatment for the duration of pregnancy should have no significant effect on mom's long-term cholesterol level. Continuing treatment, however, may put the fetus at unnecessary risk. This explains why this family of drugs, including lovastatin, has been assigned a pregnancy risk category of **X**.

Helpful Hints:

1. Drugs that belong to the statin family of drugs, such as this one, should only be prescribed for women of childbearing age when they are highly unlikely to conceive and have been informed of the potential hazards, according to the FDA. Why? Because cholesterol is essential for normal fetal development, and anything that lowers the serum level of cholesterol—which is what statins do—might adversely affect fetal development. If a woman becomes pregnant while taking this drug, or any member of the statin family of drugs, it should be discontinued immediately and she should be told of the potential hazard to her unborn baby.

2. This drug strongly interacts with grapefruit and grapefruit juice, which can cause harmful, and even life-threatening, side effects. Before taking this drug with grapefruit juice, or before consuming grapefruit or grapefruit juice during the day while taking this drug, first read the section "Grapefruit Juice–Drug Interactions Can Make You Sick" in the appendix of this book. Then discuss this with your pharmacist or the healthcare provider who prescribed this drug.

Remember: All pregnancies have a background risk of about 3% for a major birth defect, even when mom doesn't take a drug of any kind. If you are pregnant or planning a pregnancy, always let your doctor know before taking any drug, prescription or non-prescription, or herbal remedy.

. . . .

ADDITIONAL DRUGS AND THEIR FDA PREGNANCY RISK CATEGORIES

Since these additional drugs are uncommonly used in pregnancy, they are listed by generic name along with their FDA Pregnancy Risk Category without more detail:

Lactulose - B

Laronidase - B

Lepirudin - B

Letrozole - D

Leucovorin - C

Leuprolide - X

Levalbuterol - C

Lindane - B

Linezolid - C

Lodoxamide - B

Lomustine - D

Loperamide - B

Lopinavir - C

Loracarbef - B

Loteprednol - C

Lubiprostone - C

Lutropin Alfa - X

M

MAGNESIUM SULFATE

Brand Name: Magnesium Sulfate

Drug Uses: This drug is approved by the FDA for the treatment of magnesium deficiency and to prevent or control seizures in severe toxemia in pregnancy.

Pregnancy Risk Category: B

> **Category B rating:** The FDA assigns a drug to Category **B** for one of two reasons: (1) Studies show no evidence of fetal harm when using the drug in pregnant animals, but no controlled studies have been done using the drug in pregnant women, or (2) Studies show evidence of fetal harm when using the drug in pregnant animals, but controlled studies using the drug in pregnant women do not show evidence of fetal harm. Approximately 21% of prescription drugs fall in this category.

Animal Studies: No studies in pregnant animals have been located.

Human Studies: There are no reports of fetal birth defects associated with treatment with magnesium sulfate in pregnancy. When given by continuous infusion, especially for more than 24 hours prior to delivery to control seizures in toxemic mothers, this drug may cause magnesium toxicity in the newborn, including respiratory depression which may require resuscitation and respirator support. Thus, it is important to have the necessary equipment and personnel available when a baby is born whose mother has been receiving magnesium sulfate during labor.

Remember: All pregnancies have a background risk of about 3% for a major birth defect, even when mom doesn't take a drug of any kind. If you are pregnant or planning a pregnancy, always let your doctor know before taking any drug, prescription or non-prescription, or herbal remedy.

MEBENDAZOLE

Brand Name: Mebendazole

Drug Use: This drug is approved by the FDA for the treatment of intestinal parasites, whipworms, pinworms, roundworms, and hookworms.

Pregnancy Risk Category: C

> **Category C rating:** The FDA assigns a drug to Category C for one of two reasons: (1) Studies show evidence of fetal harm when using the drug in pregnant animals, but no controlled studies have been done using the drug in pregnant women, or (2) Studies using the drug in pregnant animals have not been done, and studies of pregnant women using the drug are insufficient to reach a conclusion. Thus, the drug should only be used if the potential benefit for mom is greater than the potential risk of fetal harm, which, in many cases, is unknown. Approximately 50% of prescription drugs fall in this category.

Animal Studies: When pregnant rats were treated with this medication, an increased incidence of spontaneous abortion and birth defects resulted in the offspring.

Human Studies: There are no controlled studies using this drug in pregnant women. However, surveys of women who have taken the drug during the first trimester of pregnancy showed that the incidence of spontaneous abortion and birth defects did not exceed that found in the general population.

Remember: All pregnancies have a background risk of about 3% for a major birth defect, even when mom doesn't

take a drug of any kind. If you are pregnant or planning a pregnancy, always let your doctor know before taking any drug, prescription or non-prescription, or herbal remedy.

MECLIZINE

Brand Name: Antivert

Drug Use: This drug is approved by the FDA for the management of nausea, vomiting, and dizziness associated with motion sickness.

Pregnancy Risk Category: B

> **Category B rating:** The FDA assigns a drug to Category **B** for one of two reasons: (1) Studies show no evidence of fetal harm when using the drug in pregnant animals, but no controlled studies have been done using the drug in pregnant women, or (2) Studies show evidence of fetal harm when using the drug in pregnant animals, but controlled studies using the drug in pregnant women do not show evidence of fetal harm. Approximately 21% of prescription drugs fall in this category.

Animal Studies: When pregnant rats were treated with this drug at 25 to 50 times the human dose, there was an increased incidence of cleft palate, which is a hole in the roof of the mouth.

Human Studies: Studies in pregnant women have not shown an increase in birth defects in their babies. Despite the above-mentioned animal findings, it appears the possibility of fetal harm is remote.

Remember: All pregnancies have a background risk of about 3% for a major birth defect, even when mom doesn't take a drug of any kind. If you are pregnant or planning a pregnancy, always let your doctor know before taking any drug, prescription or non-prescription, or herbal remedy.

. . . .

MEDROXYPROGESTERONE

Brand Name: Depo-Provera

Drug Use: This drug is approved by the FDA for the prevention of pregnancy. It is a long-term, injectable contraceptive given at threemonth intervals.

Pregnancy Risk Category: X

> **Category X rating:** The FDA assigns a drug to Category **X** when studies have shown the risk of fetal harm clearly outweighs any potential maternal benefit from the drug. **Drugs in this category should not be used by pregnant women.** Approximately 5% of prescription drugs fall in this category.

Animal Studies: Studies in pregnant animals treated with this drug showed that it causes dose-related birth defects and toxicity in the offspring of pregnant animals.

Human Studies: In contrast to the above-mentioned animal studies, inadvertent exposure in human pregnancies does not result in a significant risk of birth defects.

Helpful Hints: The FDA has issued the following black box warning:

"Women who use Depo-Provera contraceptive injection may lose significant bone mineral density. Bone loss is greater with increasing duration of use and may not be completely reversible. Depo-Provera contraception injection should be used as a long-term birth control method (longer than two years) only if other birth control methods are inadequate."

A Black Box Warning is the most serious prescription drug warning the FDA can require a drug company to issue.

Remember: All pregnancies have a background risk of about 3% for a major birth defect, even when mom doesn't

take a drug of any kind. If you are pregnant or planning a pregnancy, always let your doctor know before taking any drug, prescription or non-prescription, or herbal remedy.

∙ ∙

MEFENAMIC ACID

Brand Name: Ponstel

Drug Use: This drug is approved by the FDA for the relief of mild to moderate pain in patients for no longer than a week. It belongs to the non-steroidal anti-inflammatory disease (NSAID) family of drugs. (See Helpful Hint on next page.)

Pregnancy Risk Categories: This drug has been assigned two pregnancy risk categories: **C** when used in the first and second trimesters, and **D** if used in the third trimester or near delivery. Approximately 12% of prescription drugs are assigned two pregnancy risk categories, depending on which trimester of pregnancy the drug is used.

> **Category C rating:** The FDA assigns a drug to Category **C** for one of two reasons: (1) Studies show evidence of fetal harm when using the drug in pregnant animals, but no controlled studies have been done using the drug in pregnant women, or (2) Studies using the drug in pregnant animals have not been done, and studies of pregnant women using the drug are insufficient to reach a conclusion. Thus, the drug should only be used if the potential benefit for mom is greater than the potential risk of fetal harm, which, in many cases, is unknown. Approximately 50% of prescription drugs fall in this category.

> **Category D rating:** The FDA assigns a drug to Category **D** when studies of pregnant women using the drug show evidence of fetal harm. Rarely, however, the potential benefit of using the drug in some life-threatening situations for mom may outweigh the potential risk of fetal harm. For example, when mom requires cancer treatment or when she has a serious disease for which safer drugs cannot be used or are less effective. Approximately 11% of prescription drugs fall in this category.

Animal Studies: When pregnant rats and rabbits were treated with this medication, there was no increase in risk for birth defects in the offspring.

Human Studies: There are no controlled studies in pregnant women using this drug.

Helpful Hints: When taken in the third trimester of pregnancy, NSAIDs have seriously harmed the fetus, leading to life-threatening illness after birth and even death. These potential effects apply to all NSAIDs, whether purchased by prescription or over-the-counter without a prescription. They also explain why NSAIDs have been assigned a **D** pregnancy risk category. (See "Non-Steroidal, Anti-Inflammatory Drugs (NSAIDs) in Pregnancy" in the appendix for more details.)

Remember: All pregnancies have a background risk of about 3% for a major birth defect, even when mom doesn't take a drug of any kind. If you are pregnant or planning a pregnancy, always let your doctor know before taking any drug, prescription or non-prescription, or herbal remedy.

· ·

MELOXICAM

Brand Name: Mobic

Drug Use: This drug is approved by the FDA for the relief of the pain from osteoarthritis. It is a member of the non-steroidal, anti-inflammatory family of drugs (NSAIDs). (See Helpful Hint on next page.)

Pregnancy Risk Categories: This drug has been assigned two pregnancy risk categories: **C** when used in the first and second trimesters of pregnancy, and **D** if used in the third trimester or near term. Approximately

12% of prescription drugs are assigned two pregnancy risk categories, depending on which trimester of pregnancy the drug is used.

Category C rating: The FDA assigns a drug to Category **C** for one of two reasons: (1) Studies show evidence of fetal harm when using the drug in pregnant animals, but no controlled studies have been done using the drug in pregnant women, or (2) Studies using the drug in pregnant animals have not been done, and studies of pregnant women using the drug are insufficient to reach a conclusion. Thus, the drug should only be used if the potential benefit for mom is greater than the potential risk of fetal harm, which, in many cases, is unknown. Approximately 50% of prescription drugs fall in this category.

Category D rating: The FDA assigns a drug to Category **D** when studies of pregnant women using the drug show evidence of fetal harm. Rarely, however, the potential benefit of using the drug in some life-threatening situations for mom may outweigh the potential risk of fetal harm. For example, when mom requires cancer treatment or when she has a serious disease for which safer drugs cannot be used or are less effective. Approximately 11% of prescription drugs fall in this category.

Animal Studies: When pregnant rabbits were treated with 65 times the dose normally used in humans, their offspring showed an increased incidence of heart defects. However, when pregnant rats were treated with only two times the human dose, there was no increase in birth defects noted.

Human Studies: There are no controlled studies of this drug in pregnant women.

Helpful Hints: When taken in the third trimester of pregnancy, NSAIDs have seriously harmed the fetus, leading to life-threatening illness after birth and even death. These potential effects apply to all NSAIDs, whether purchased by prescription or over-the-counter without a prescription. They also explain why NSAIDs have been assigned a **D** pregnancy risk category. (See

"Non-Steroidal, Anti-Inflammatory Drugs (NSAIDs) in Pregnancy" in the appendix for more details.)

Remember: All pregnancies have a background risk of about 3% for a major birth defect, even when mom doesn't take a drug of any kind. If you are pregnant or planning a pregnancy, always let your doctor know before taking any drug, prescription or non-prescription, or herbal remedy.

• •

MEPERIDINE

Brand Name: Demerol

Drug Use: This drug is approved by the FDA for the treatment of moderate to severe pain.

Pregnancy Risk Categories: This drug has been assigned two pregnancy risk categories: **B** for routine use throughout pregnancy, and **D** for prolonged periods of use during pregnancy or near term. Approximately 12% of prescription drugs are assigned two pregnancy risk categories, depending on which trimester of pregnancy the drug is used.

> **Category B rating:** The FDA assigns a drug to Category **B** for one of two reasons: (1) Studies show no evidence of fetal harm when using the drug in pregnant animals, but no controlled studies have been done using the drug in pregnant women, or (2) Studies show evidence of fetal harm when using the drug in pregnant animals, but controlled studies using the drug in pregnant women do not show evidence of fetal harm. Approximately 21% of prescription drugs fall in this category.

> **Category D rating:** The FDA assigns a drug to Category **D** when studies of pregnant women using the drug show evidence of fetal harm. Rarely, however, the potential benefit of using the drug in some life-threatening situations for mom may outweigh the potential risk of fetal harm. For example, when mom requires cancer treatment or when she has a serious disease for which safer drugs cannot be used or are less effective. Approximately 11% of prescription drugs fall in this category.

Animal Studies: Controlled studies in which meperidine was used to treat pregnant animals could not be found.

Human Studies: There are no controlled studies using meperidine in pregnant women. However, uncontrolled studies have shown no association of meperidine use in pregnancy with major birth defects.

Helpful Hints: This drug's primary use in pregnancy is during labor and delivery. Like all narcotics, maternal and neonatal addiction is possible if the drug is given for a prolonged period of time. Fatal respiratory depression in the newborn is the primary concern of using this drug during pregnancy. In order to minimize this possibility, adequate equipment and personnel should be available to immediately intervene if a baby is born whose mother has been taking meperidine during labor.

Remember: All pregnancies have a background risk of about 3% for a major birth defect, even when mom doesn't take a drug of any kind. If you are pregnant or planning a pregnancy, always let your doctor know before taking any drug, prescription or non-prescription, or herbal remedy.

MEPROBAMATE

Brand Name: Meprobamate

Drug Use: This drug is approved by the FDA for the use in treating anxiety disorders.

Pregnancy Risk Category: C

Category C rating: The FDA assigns a drug to Category **C** for one of two reasons: (1) Studies show evidence of fetal harm when using the drug in pregnant animals, but no controlled studies have been done using the drug in pregnant women, or (2) Studies using the drug in pregnant animals have not been done, and studies of pregnant women using the drug are insufficient to reach a conclusion.

Thus, the drug should only be used if the potential benefit for mom is greater than the potential risk of fetal harm, which, in many cases, is unknown. Approximately 50% of prescription drugs fall in this category.

Animal Studies: Several studies using this drug in pregnant animals have shown an association with birth defects in the offspring.

Human Studies: A number of reports have linked the use of this drug in pregnant women to an increase in birth defects. As a result, many experts recommend avoiding this drug, especially during the first trimester of pregnancy.

Remember: All pregnancies have a background risk of about 3% for a major birth defect, even when mom doesn't take a drug of any kind. If you are pregnant or planning a pregnancy, always let your doctor know before taking any drug, prescription or non-prescription, or herbal remedy.

. . . .

MERCAPTOPURINE

Brand Name: Purinethol

Drug Use: This drug is approved by the FDA for use in treating acute lymphatic leukemia in combination with other drugs.

Pregnancy Risk Category: D

Category D rating: The FDA assigns a drug to Category **D** when studies of pregnant women using the drug show evidence of fetal harm. Rarely, however, the potential benefit of using the drug in some life-threatening situations for mom may outweigh the potential risk of fetal harm. For example, when mom requires cancer treatment or when she has a serious disease for which safer drugs cannot be used or are less effective. Approximately 11% of prescription drugs fall in this category.

Animal Studies: Very little has been published about pregnant animals treated with this drug.

Human Studies: Since this drug is usually given in combination with other drugs, it is often difficult to isolate which drug, if any, might have caused a particular birth defect or fetal harm. Regardless, sufficient uncontrolled studies have linked the drug to various birth defects, which warrants a **D** category rating for this drug.

Remember: All pregnancies have a background risk of about 3% for a major birth defect, even when mom doesn't take a drug of any kind. If you are pregnant or planning a pregnancy, always let your doctor know before taking any drug, prescription or non-prescription, or herbal remedy.

MESALAMINE

Brand Names: Apriso, Asacol

Drug Use: This drug is approved by the FDA for the treatment of ulcerative colitis.

Pregnancy Risk Category: B

> **Category B rating:** The FDA assigns a drug to Category **B** for one of two reasons: (1) Studies show no evidence of fetal harm when using the drug in pregnant animals, but no controlled studies have been done using the drug in pregnant women, or (2) Studies show evidence of fetal harm when using the drug in pregnant animals, but controlled studies using the drug in pregnant women do not show evidence of fetal harm. Approximately 21% of prescription drugs fall in this category.

Animal Studies: Studies using this drug in pregnant rats and rabbits have shown no increase in risk of birth defects in the offspring.

Human Studies: No controlled studies using this drug have been done in pregnant women.

Remember: All pregnancies have a background risk of about 3% for a major birth defect, even when mom doesn't take a drug of any kind. If you are pregnant or planning a pregnancy, always let your doctor know before taking any drug, prescription or non-prescription, or herbal remedy.

. . . .

METFORMIN

Brand Names: Fortamet, Glucophage

Drug Use: This drug is approved by the FDA for the treatment of Type 2 diabetes.

Pregnancy Risk Category: B

> **Category B rating:** The FDA assigns a drug to Category **B** for one of two reasons: (1) Studies show no evidence of fetal harm when using the drug in pregnant animals, but no controlled studies have been done using the drug in pregnant women, or (2) Studies show evidence of fetal harm when using the drug in pregnant animals, but controlled studies using the drug in pregnant women do not show evidence of fetal harm. Approximately 21% of prescription drugs fall in this category.

Animal Studies: When this drug was used in pregnant rats and rabbits, studies showed no increase in birth defects in the offspring.

Human Studies: No controlled studies have been done in pregnant women.

Helpful Hints: Most experts, including the American College of Obstetricians and Gynecologists (ACOG), recommend insulin to treat Type 2 diabetes during pregnancy.

Remember: All pregnancies have a background risk of about 3% for a major birth defect, even when mom doesn't take a drug of any kind. If you are pregnant or planning a pregnancy, always let your doctor know before taking any drug, prescription or non-prescription, or herbal remedy.

METHADONE

Brand Name: Dolophine

Drug Use: This drug is approved by the FDA for use in pregnancy as part of a heroin treatment program.

Pregnancy Risk Categories: This drug has been assigned two pregnancy risk categories: **B** for routine use throughout pregnancy, and **D** if used for prolonged periods or in high doses near term. Approximately 12% of prescription drugs are assigned two pregnancy risk categories, depending on which trimester of pregnancy the drug is used.

Category B rating: The FDA assigns a drug to Category **B** for one of two reasons: (1) Studies show no evidence of fetal harm when using the drug in pregnant animals, but no controlled studies have been done using the drug in pregnant women, or (2) Studies show evidence of fetal harm when using the drug in pregnant animals, but controlled studies using the drug in pregnant women do not show evidence of fetal harm. Approximately 21% of prescription drugs fall in this category.

Category D rating: The FDA assigns a drug to Category **D** when studies of pregnant women using the drug show evidence of fetal harm. Rarely, however, the potential benefit of using the drug in some life-threatening situations for mom may outweigh the potential risk of fetal harm. For example, when mom requires cancer treatment or when she has a serious disease for which safer drugs cannot be used or are less effective. Approximately 11% of prescription drugs fall in this category.

Animal Studies: Studies in a variety of pregnant animals treated with this drug have shown mixed results with extremely high doses producing a variety of birth defects, while lower doses were not associated with birth defects in the offspring.

Human Studies: Studies of pregnant women treated with methadone have not found an increased risk of birth defects. Newborn drug withdrawal and low birth weight seem to be the main concerns.

Helpful Hints:

1. Babies born to mothers on a Methadone Maintenance Program may be physically dependant and suffer withdrawal symptoms after birth. Personnel responsible for such a baby's care after birth should be aware that the mom is participating in such a program and the potential implications for the baby. This might mean the need for resuscitation and treatment of withdrawal symptoms.

2. This drug weakly interacts with grapefruit and grapefruit juice, which can cause harmful, and even life-threatening, side effects. Before taking this drug with grapefruit juice, or before consuming grapefruit or grapefruit juice during the day while taking this drug, first read the section "Grapefruit Juice–Drug Interactions Can Make You Sick" in the appendix of this book. Then discuss this with your pharmacist or the healthcare provider who prescribed this drug.

Remember: All pregnancies have a background risk of about 3% for a major birth defect, even when mom doesn't take a drug of any kind. If you are pregnant or planning a pregnancy, always let your doctor know before taking any drug, prescription or non-prescription, or herbal remedy.

· ·

METHIMAZOLE

Brand Name: Tapazole

Drug Use: This drug is approved by the FDA for the medical treatment of hyperthyroidism, which is an overactive thyroid.

Pregnancy Risk Category: **D**

> **Category D rating:** The FDA assigns a drug to Category **D** when studies of pregnant women using the drug show evidence of fetal harm. Rarely, however, the potential benefit of using the drug in some life-threatening situations for mom may outweigh the potential risk of fetal harm. For example, when mom requires cancer treatment or when she has a serious disease for which safer drugs cannot be used or are less effective. Approximately 11% of prescription drugs fall in this category.

Animal Studies: The results of any studies that may have been done in pregnant animals are not available.

Human Studies: In the past, methimazole was an effective treatment for hyperthyroidism complicated by pregnancy. However, it has been associated with enough birth defects that it has been assigned a **D** pregnancy risk category. For instance, the drug rapidly crosses the placenta and may induce a thyroid goiter and even hypothyroidism, which means underactive thyroid, in the newborn. Thus, this drug is not necessarily the drug of choice for treating maternal hyperthyroidism complicated by pregnancy.

Remember: All pregnancies have a background risk of about 3% for a major birth defect, even when mom doesn't take a drug of any kind. If you are pregnant or planning a pregnancy, always let your doctor know before taking any drug, prescription or non-prescription, or herbal remedy.

METHOTREXATE

Brand Name: Methotrexate

Drug Uses: This drug is approved by the FDA for use to treat severe, disabling psoriasis; severe, active rheumatoid arthritis; and certain types of cancer. This drug is a member of the folic acid antagonist family of drugs.

Pregnancy Risk Category: **X**

Category X rating: The FDA assigns a drug to Category **X** when studies have shown the risk of fetal harm clearly outweighs any potential maternal benefit from the drug. **Drugs in this category should not be used by pregnant women.** Approximately 5% of prescription drugs fall in this category.

Animal Studies: When pregnant rats and rabbits were treated with methotrexate, a variety of birth defects were produced in their offspring, depending on the timing of methotrexate treatment during those pregnancies. For example, when pregnant rabbits were treated with methotrexate on the 12th day of pregnancy, 94% of the fetuses were malformed.

Human Studies: When used in pregnant women, the drug is toxic for the embryo, causes fetal birth defects, and places pregnant women at risk for spontaneous miscarriage.

According to the FDA's Black Box Warning:

"Methotrexate has been reported to cause fetal death and/or congenital anomalies (birth defects). Therefore it is not recommended for women of childbearing potential unless there is clear medical evidence that the benefits can be expected to outweigh the considerable risk. Pregnant women with psoriasis or rheumatoid arthritis should not receive methotrexate."

A Black Box Warning is the most serious prescription drug warning the FDA can require a drug company to issue.

Helpful Hints:

1. Women of childbearing potential should not be started on methotrexate until pregnancy is excluded and should be fully counseled on the

serious risk to the fetus should they become pregnant while undergoing treatment.

2. Pregnancy should be avoided if either partner is receiving methotrexate; during or for a minimum of three months after therapy for male patients, and during or for at least one ovulatory cycle after therapy for female patients.

Remember: All pregnancies have a background risk of about 3% for a major birth defect, even when mom doesn't take a drug of any kind. If you are pregnant or planning a pregnancy, always let your doctor know before taking any drug, prescription or non-prescription, or herbal remedy.

METHYLDOPA

Brand Name: Methyldopa

Drug Use: This drug is approved by the FDA for the treatment of hypertension, which is high blood pressure.

Pregnancy Risk Category: B

Category B rating: The FDA assigns a drug to Category **B** for one of two reasons: (1) Studies show no evidence of fetal harm when using the drug in pregnant animals, but no controlled studies have been done using the drug in pregnant women, or (2) Studies show evidence of fetal harm when using the drug in pregnant animals, but controlled studies using the drug in pregnant women do not show evidence of fetal harm. Approximately 21% of prescription drugs fall in this category.

Animal Studies: When pregnant mice, rabbits, and rats were treated with this drug, there was no evidence of harm to the offspring.

Human Studies: No controlled studies have been done in pregnant women. Published reports in which methyldopa was used throughout pregnancy indicate it is unlikely that this drug is harmful to the fetus. Follow-up studies have shown no significant differences in growth and development when treated and non-treated children were compared.

Remember: All pregnancies have a background risk of about 3% for a major birth defect, even when mom doesn't take a drug of any kind. If you are pregnant or planning a pregnancy, always let your doctor know before taking any drug, prescription or non-prescription, or herbal remedy.

METHYLPHENIDATE

Brand Names: Concerta, Methylin, Ritalin

Drug Use: This drug is approved by the FDA for the treatment of attention deficit hyperactivity disorder (ADHD).

Pregnancy Risk Category: C

> **Category C rating:** The FDA assigns a drug to Category C for one of two reasons: (1) Studies show evidence of fetal harm when using the drug in pregnant animals, but no controlled studies have been done using the drug in pregnant women, or (2) Studies using the drug in pregnant animals have not been done, and studies of pregnant women using the drug are insufficient to reach a conclusion. Thus, the drug should only be used if the potential benefit for mom is greater than the potential risk of fetal harm, which, in many cases, is unknown. Approximately 50% of prescription drugs fall in this category.

Animal Studies: Studies of pregnant rabbits treated with this drug showed no evidence of birth defects up to a dose of a drug that was 11 times the maximum recommended human dose. However, open spine defects of the fetus were observed at doses 40 times the maximum recommended human dose.

Human Studies: No controlled studies have been done using this drug in pregnant women.

Remember: All pregnancies have a background risk of about 3% for a major birth defect, even when mom doesn't take a drug of any kind. If you are pregnant or planning a pregnancy, always let your doctor know before taking any drug, prescription or non-prescription, or herbal remedy.

· ·

METHYLPREDNISOLONE

Brand Names: Solu-Medrol, Medrol, Depo-Medrol

Drug Uses: This drug is approved by the FDA for the treatment of a variety of endocrine disorders, rheumatic disorders, collagen diseases, skin disorders, and a long list of other medical problems.

Pregnancy Risk Category: C

> **Category C rating:** The FDA assigns a drug to Category C for one of two reasons: (1) Studies show evidence of fetal harm when using the drug in pregnant animals, but no controlled studies have been done using the drug in pregnant women, or (2) Studies using the drug in pregnant animals have not been done, and studies of pregnant women using the drug are insufficient to reach a conclusion. Thus, the drug should only be used if the potential benefit for mom is greater than the potential risk of fetal harm, which, in many cases, is unknown. Approximately 50% of prescription drugs fall in this category.

Animal Studies: Pregnant mice, rats, and rabbits treated with this drug have shown an increased incidence of birth defects.

Human Studies: Adequate studies in pregnant women are not available. Many experts recommend avoiding this medication during the first three months of pregnancy. They also recommend limiting its use in the remainder of pregnancy if possible. If used in pregnancy, it is important to observe those newborns for possible adrenal deficiency.

Helpful Hints: This drug weakly interacts with grapefruit and grapefruit juice, which can cause harmful, and even life-threatening, side effects. Before taking this drug with grapefruit juice, or before consuming grapefruit or grapefruit juice during the day while taking this drug, first read the section "Grapefruit Juice–Drug Interactions Can Make You Sick" in the appendix of this book. Then discuss this with your pharmacist or the healthcare provider who prescribed this drug.

Remember: All pregnancies have a background risk of about 3% for a major birth defect, even when mom doesn't take a drug of any kind. If you are pregnant or planning a pregnancy, always let your doctor know before taking any drug, prescription or non-prescription, or herbal remedy.

• •

METHYSERGIDE

Brand Name: Sansert

Drug Uses: This drug is approved by the FDA to prevent disabling vascular headaches, migraines, and cluster neuralgia.

Pregnancy Risk Category: X

> **Category X rating:** The FDA assigns a drug to Category **X** when studies have shown the risk of fetal harm clearly outweighs any potential maternal benefit from the drug. **Drugs in this category should not be used by pregnant women.** Approximately 5% of prescription drugs fall in this category.

Animal Studies: No information from animal studies is available.

Human Studies: Controlled studies using this drug in pregnant women are not available. This drug has been assigned to a pregnancy risk category of **X** primarily because of its tendency to stimulate the uterus to contract and bring on labor as well as its tendency to interfere with oxygen delivery to the fetus. Thus, this drug should not be taken in pregnancy.

Remember: All pregnancies have a background risk of about 3% for a major birth defect, even when mom doesn't take a drug of any kind. If you are pregnant or planning a pregnancy, always let your doctor know before taking any drug, prescription or non-prescription, or herbal remedy.

METOCLOPRAMIDE

Brand Name: Reglan

Drug Use: This drug is approved by the FDA for the treatment of gastro-esophageal reflux disease (GERD), which causes heartburn.

Pregnancy Risk Category: B

Category B rating: The FDA assigns a drug to Category **B** for one of two reasons: (1) Studies show no evidence of fetal harm when using the drug in pregnant animals, but no controlled studies have been done using the drug in pregnant women, or (2) Studies show evidence of fetal harm when using the drug in pregnant animals, but controlled studies using the drug in pregnant women do not show evidence of fetal harm. Approximately 21% of prescription drugs fall in this category.

Animal Studies: When pregnant rats, mice, and rabbits were treated with this drug, there was no evidence of fetal harm.

Human Studies: No controlled studies using this drug in pregnant women are available.

Remember: All pregnancies have a background risk of about 3% for a major birth defect, even when mom doesn't take a drug of any kind. If you are pregnant or planning a pregnancy, always let your doctor know before taking any drug, prescription or non-prescription, or herbal remedy.

. . . .

METOPROLOL

Brand Names: Lopressor, Toprol. This drug belongs to the beta-blocker family of drugs.

Drug Uses: This drug is approved by the FDA for the treatment of hypertension (high blood pressure), chest pain, and heart failure, alone or in combination with other drugs.

Pregnancy Risk Categories: This drug has been assigned two pregnancy risk categories: **C** when used in the first trimester, and **D** when used in the second and third trimesters. Approximately 12% of prescription drugs are assigned two pregnancy risk categories, depending on which trimester of pregnancy the drug is used.

> **Category C rating:** The FDA assigns a drug to Category **C** for one of two reasons: (1) Studies show evidence of fetal harm when using the drug in pregnant animals, but no controlled studies have been done using the drug in pregnant women, or (2) Studies using the drug in pregnant animals have not been done, and studies of pregnant women using the drug are insufficient to reach a conclusion. Thus, the drug should only be used if the potential benefit for mom is greater than the potential risk of fetal harm, which, in many cases, is unknown. Approximately 50% of prescription drugs fall in this category.

> **Category D rating:** The FDA assigns a drug to Category **D** when studies of pregnant women using the drug show evidence of fetal harm. Rarely, however, the potential benefit of using the drug in some life-threatening situations for mom may outweigh the potential risk of fetal harm. For example, when mom requires cancer treatment or when she has a serious disease for which safer drugs

cannot be used or are less effective. Approximately 11% of prescription drugs fall in this category.

Animal Studies: When pregnant rats and mice were treated with this drug, there was no evidence of fetal harm in the offspring.

Human Studies: There are no controlled studies in pregnant women taking this drug. However, since other members of the beta-blocker family of drugs have caused a decrease in fetal weight and placental weight when used in the second and third trimesters, this drug has been assigned a **D** rating for use during the second and third trimesters of pregnancy. All babies born to mothers taking this drug during the second and third trimesters should be closely observed for the first 24 to 48 hours after birth for signs of a low heart rate or other symptoms of withdrawal.

Remember: All pregnancies have a background risk of about 3% for a major birth defect, even when mom doesn't take a drug of any kind. If you are pregnant or planning a pregnancy, always let your doctor know before taking any drug, prescription or non-prescription, or herbal remedy.

METRONIDAZOLE

Brand Name: Flagyl

Drug Use: This drug is approved by the FDA for the treatment of trichomonis and a variety of bacterial infections during pregnancy.

Pregnancy Risk Category: B

Category B rating: The FDA assigns a drug to Category **B** for one of two reasons: (1) Studies show no evidence of fetal harm when using the drug in pregnant animals, but no controlled studies have been done using the drug in pregnant women, or

(2) Studies show evidence of fetal harm when using the drug in pregnant animals, but controlled studies using the drug in pregnant women do not show evidence of fetal harm. Approximately 21% of prescription drugs fall in this category.

Animal Studies: Pregnant mice and rats treated with this drug showed no evidence of fetal harm in the offspring.

Human Studies: There are no controlled studies using this drug in pregnant women.

Helpful Hints: Metronidazole gel is considerably less effective for the treatment of trichomoniasis (less than 50%) than oral preparations of metronidazole, according to the CDC. Thus, use of the gel is not recommended.

Remember: All pregnancies have a background risk of about 3% for a major birth defect, even when mom doesn't take a drug of any kind. If you are pregnant or planning a pregnancy, always let your doctor know before taking any drug, prescription or non-prescription, or herbal remedy.

MINOXIDIL

Brand Name: Loniten

Drug Use: This drug is approved by the FDA for the treatment of hypertension, which is high blood pressure.

Pregnancy Risk Category: C

Category C rating: The FDA assigns a drug to Category **C** for one of two reasons: (1) Studies show evidence of fetal harm when using the drug in pregnant animals, but no controlled studies have been done using the drug in pregnant women, or (2) Studies using the drug in pregnant animals have not been done, and studies of pregnant women using the drug are insufficient to reach a conclusion. Thus, the drug should only be used if the potential benefit for mom is greater than the potential risk of fetal harm, which, in many cases, is unknown. Approximately 50% of prescription drugs fall in this category.

Animal Studies: When pregnant rats and rabbits were treated with this drug, there was no evidence of birth defects in the offspring.

Human Studies: There are no controlled studies using this drug in pregnant women. In fact, this drug is rarely used in pregnancy.

Remember: All pregnancies have a background risk of about 3% for a major birth defect, even when mom doesn't take a drug of any kind. If you are pregnant or planning a pregnancy, always let your doctor know before taking any drug, prescription or non-prescription, or herbal remedy.

MISOPROSTOL

Brand Name: Cytotec

Drug Use: This drug is approved by the FDA to decrease the risk of non-steroidal anti-inflammatory drug-induced stomach ulcers.

Pregnancy Risk Category: X

> **Category X rating:** The FDA assigns a drug to Category **X** when studies have shown the risk of fetal harm clearly outweighs any potential maternal benefit from the drug. **Drugs in this category should not be used by pregnant women.** Approximately 5% of prescription drugs fall in this category.

Animal Studies: This drug does not cause birth defects in the offspring of pregnant rats and rabbits when they are treated at doses 625 and 63 times the human dose, respectively.

Human Studies: This drug has been shown to cause miscarriage when given to pregnant women. Thus, the medication labeling contains the following Black Box Warning:

"Misoprostol administration to women who are pregnant can cause abortion, premature birth, or birth defects.

It should not be taken by pregnant women to reduce the risk of ulcer induced by NSAIDs, which are the non-steroidal, anti-inflammatory drugs."

A Black Box Warning is the most serious prescription drug warning the FDA can require a drug company to issue.

Helpful Hints: When this drug is used later in pregnancy, especially during the third trimester, it has been shown effective for ripening the cervix in preparation for inducing labor.

Remember: All pregnancies have a background risk of about 3% for a major birth defect, even when mom doesn't take a drug of any kind. If you are pregnant or planning a pregnancy, always let your doctor know before taking any drug, prescription or non-prescription, or herbal remedy.

• •

MONTELUKAST

Brand Name: Singulair

Drug Use: This drug is approved by the FDA for the treatment of asthma, exercise-induced bronchoconstriction, and allergic rhinitis.

Pregnancy Risk Category: B

Category B rating: The FDA assigns a drug to Category **B** for one of two reasons: (1) Studies show no evidence of fetal harm when using the drug in pregnant animals, but no controlled studies have been done using the drug in pregnant women, or (2) Studies show evidence of fetal harm when using the drug in pregnant animals, but controlled studies using the drug in pregnant women do not show evidence of fetal harm. Approximately 21% of prescription drugs fall in this category.

Animal Studies: When pregnant rats and rabbits were treated with this drug, no birth defects were found in the offspring.

Human Studies: There are no controlled studies of pregnant women using this drug.

Helpful Hints: Merck & Company maintains a registry to monitor the pregnancy outcomes of women exposed to Singulair while pregnant. Healthcare providers are encouraged to report any prenatal exposure to Singulair by calling the pregnancy registry at 800-986-8999.

Remember: All pregnancies have a background risk of about 3% for a major birth defect, even when mom doesn't take a drug of any kind. If you are pregnant or planning a pregnancy, always let your doctor know before taking any drug, prescription or non-prescription, or herbal remedy.

· ·

MORPHINE

Brand Names: Astramorph, Avinza, Depodur, Kadian

Drug Use: This drug is approved by the FDA for the management of pain not responsive to non-narcotic drugs.

Pregnancy Risk Categories: This drug has been assigned two pregnancy risk categories: **C** if routinely used throughout pregnancy, but **D** if used for prolonged periods or near term. Approximately 12% of prescription drugs are assigned two pregnancy risk categories, depending on which trimester of pregnancy the drug is used.

> **Category C rating:** The FDA assigns a drug to Category **C** for one of two reasons: (1) Studies show evidence of fetal harm when

using the drug in pregnant animals, but no controlled studies have been done using the drug in pregnant women, or (2) Studies using the drug in pregnant animals have not been done, and studies of pregnant women using the drug are insufficient to reach a conclusion. Thus, the drug should only be used if the potential benefit for mom is greater than the potential risk of fetal harm, which, in many cases, is unknown. Approximately 50% of prescription drugs fall in this category.

Category D rating: The FDA assigns a drug to Category **D** when studies of pregnant women using the drug show evidence of fetal harm. Rarely, however, the potential benefit of using the drug in some life-threatening situations for mom may outweigh the potential risk of fetal harm. For example, when mom requires cancer treatment or when she has a serious disease for which safer drugs cannot be used or are less effective. Approximately 11% of prescription drugs fall in this category.

Animal Studies: When pregnant rats were treated with 35 times the usual human dose, morphine did not cause birth defects in the offspring.

Human Studies: There are no controlled studies of morphine use in pregnancy available. This drug should only be given to pregnant women when no other method for controlling pain is available and the means are at hand to manage the baby after birth. This means having the appropriate equipment and personnel available to intervene if the baby has significant respiratory depression in the delivery room.

Helpful Hints: This drug weakly interacts with grapefruit and grapefruit juice, which can cause harmful, and even life-threatening, side effects. Before taking this drug with grapefruit juice, or before consuming grapefruit or grapefruit juice during the day while taking this drug, first read the section "Grapefruit Juice–Drug Interactions Can Make You Sick" in the appendix of this book. Then discuss this with your pharmacist or the healthcare provider who prescribed this drug.

Remember: All pregnancies have a background risk of about 3% for a major birth defect, even when mom doesn't take a drug of any kind. If you are pregnant or planning a pregnancy, always let your doctor know before taking any drug, prescription or non-prescription, or herbal remedy.

. . . .

ADDITIONAL DRUGS AND THEIR FDA PREGNANCY RISK CATEGORIES

Since these additional drugs are uncommonly used in pregnancy, they are listed by generic name along with their FDA Pregnancy Risk Category without more detail:

Mannitol - C

Meclofenamate - B (D if used in third trimester or near delivery)

Mefloquine - C

Memantine - B

Meningococcal Vaccine - C

Meropenem - B

Mesna - B

Metaxalone - B

Methocarbamol - C

Methyltestosterone - X

Mexiletine - C

Micafungin - C

Miconazole - C

Midazolam - D

Midodrine - C

Mifepristone - X

Miglustat - X

Milrinone - C

Mineral Oil - C

Minocycline - D

Mirtazapine - C

Mitomycin - Not established

Mitotane - C

Mitoxantrone - D

Modafinil - C

Moexipril - C (D if used in second or third trimester)

Mometasone - C

Moxifloxacin - C

Mupirocin - B

Mycophenolate - D

N

NABUMETONE

Brand Name: Relafen

Drug Use: This drug is approved by the FDA for the treatment of osteoarthritis and rheumatoid arthritis. It belongs to the non-steroidal anti-inflammatory family of drugs (NSAIDs). (See Helpful Hints on next page.)

Pregnancy Risk Categories: This drug has been assigned two pregnancy risk categories: **C** when used in the first and second trimesters of pregnancy, and **D** when used in the third trimester or near the time of delivery. Approximately 12% of prescription drugs are assigned two pregnancy risk categories, depending on which trimester of pregnancy the drug is used.

Category C rating: The FDA assigns a drug to Category **C** for one of two reasons: (1) Studies show evidence of fetal harm when using the drug in pregnant animals, but no controlled studies have been done using the drug in pregnant women, or (2) Studies using the drug in pregnant animals have not been done, and studies of pregnant women using the drug are insufficient to reach a conclusion. Thus, the drug should only be used if the potential benefit for mom is greater than the potential risk of fetal harm, which, in many cases, is unknown. Approximately 50% of prescription drugs fall in this category.

Category D rating: The FDA assigns a drug to Category **D** when studies of pregnant women using the drug show evidence of fetal harm. Rarely, however, the potential benefit of using the drug in some life-threatening situations for mom may outweigh the potential risk of fetal harm. For example, when mom requires cancer treatment or when she has a serious disease for which safer drugs cannot be used or are less effective. Approximately 11% of prescription drugs fall in this category.

Animal Studies: When pregnant rats and rabbits were treated with this drug, there was no increased risk of birth defects in the offspring. However, delayed and prolonged labor was noted, as well as delayed fetal growth and decreased fetal survival. An increased risk of miscarriage was also seen in rats.

Human Studies: There are no controlled studies to date using this drug in pregnant women.

Helpful Hints: When taken in the third trimester of pregnancy, NSAIDs have seriously harmed the fetus, leading to life-threatening illness after birth and even death. These potential effects apply to all NSAIDs, whether purchased by prescription or over-the-counter without a prescription. They also explain why NSAIDs have been assigned a **D** pregnancy risk category. (See "Non-Steroidal, Anti-Inflammatory Drugs (NSAIDs) in Pregnancy" in the appendix for more details.)

Remember: All pregnancies have a background risk of about 3% for a major birth defect, even when mom doesn't take a drug of any kind. If you are pregnant or planning a pregnancy, always let your doctor know before taking any drug, prescription or non-prescription, or herbal remedy.

• •

NADOLOL

Brand Name: Corgard

Drug Uses: This drug is approved by the FDA for the treatment of high blood pressure, chest pain, heart irregularity, and for the prevention of certain types of headaches. Nadolol belongs to the beta-blocker family of drugs.

Pregnancy Risk Categories: This drug has been assigned two pregnancy risk categories: **C** when used in the first trimester, and **D** when used in the second or third trimesters. Approximately 12% of prescription drugs are assigned two pregnancy risk categories, depending on which trimester of pregnancy the drug is used.

Category C rating: The FDA assigns a drug to Category **C** for one of two reasons. (1) Studies show evidence of fetal harm when using the drug in pregnant animals, but no controlled studies have been done using the drug in pregnant women, or (2) Studies using the drug in pregnant animals have not been done, and studies of pregnant women using the drug are insufficient to reach a conclusion. Thus, the drug should only be used if the potential benefit for mom is greater than the potential risk of fetal harm, which, in many cases, is unknown. Approximately 50% of prescription drugs fall in this category.

Category D rating: The FDA assigns a drug to Category **D** when studies of pregnant women using the drug show evidence of fetal harm. Rarely, however, the potential benefit of using the drug in some life-threatening situations for mom may outweigh the potential risk of fetal harm. For example, when mom requires cancer treatment or when she has a serious disease for which safer drugs cannot be used or are less effective. Approximately 11% of prescription drugs fall in this category.

Animal Studies: No birth defects in the offspring were seen when this drug was given to pregnant rats or hamsters. In pregnant rabbits, however, there was an increased risk of fetal death.

Human Studies: There are no controlled studies in pregnant women using this drug. It is well known, however, that this family of drugs is associated with restricted growth of the fetus and reduced placental weight when taken during the second and third trimesters of pregnancy. This is why this drug has been assigned to a **D** category when used during this time.

Remember: All pregnancies have a background risk of about 3% for a major birth defect, even when mom

doesn't take a drug of any kind. If you are pregnant or planning a pregnancy, always let your doctor know before taking any drug, prescription or non-prescription, or herbal remedy.

NALIDIXIC ACID

Brand Name: Neggram

Drug Use: This drug is approved by the FDA for the treatment of urinary tract infections.

Pregnancy Risk Category: C

> **Category C rating:** The FDA assigns a drug to Category **C** for one of two reasons: (1) Studies show evidence of fetal harm when using the drug in pregnant animals, but no controlled studies have been done using the drug in pregnant women, or (2) Studies using the drug in pregnant animals have not been done, and studies of pregnant women using the drug are insufficient to reach a conclusion. Thus, the drug should only be used if the potential benefit for mom is greater than the potential risk of fetal harm, which, in many cases, is unknown. Approximately 50% of prescription drugs fall in this category.

Animal Studies: In pregnant animals treated with nalidixic acid, there was an increased risk of birth defects and early fetal death in the offspring.

Human Studies: This drug has seen limited use in pregnant women. Thus, it is difficult to draw any conclusions about its safety.

Remember: All pregnancies have a background risk of about 3% for a major birth defect, even when mom doesn't take a drug of any kind. If you are pregnant or planning a pregnancy, always let your doctor know before taking any drug, prescription or non-prescription, or herbal remedy.

. . . .

NALOXONE

Brand Name: Narcan

Drug Use: The FDA has approved naloxone for the treatment of narcotic overdose and to reverse the effects of narcotics given during labor or during surgery.

Pregnancy Risk Category: B

> **Category B rating:** The FDA assigns a drug to Category **B** for one of two reasons: (1) Studies show no evidence of fetal harm when using the drug in pregnant animals, but no controlled studies have been done using the drug in pregnant women, or (2) Studies show evidence of fetal harm when using the drug in pregnant animals, but controlled studies using the drug in pregnant women do not show evidence of fetal harm. Approximately 21% of prescription drugs fall in this category.

Animal Studies: Naloxone has not been associated with any fetal harm when given to pregnant rats and mice.

Human Studies: When used as indicated, there have been no documented adverse effects from using this drug in pregnancy.

Remember: All pregnancies have a background risk of about 3% for a major birth defect, even when mom doesn't take a drug of any kind. If you are pregnant or planning a pregnancy, always let your doctor know before taking any drug, prescription or non-prescription, or herbal remedy.

. . . .

NAPROXEN

Brand Names: Naproxen when given by prescription; Aleve when purchased over-the-counter

Drug Uses: This drug is approved by the FDA for the treatment of osteoarthritis, rheumatoid arthritis, ankylosing spondylitis, gout, cramps associated with menstrual periods, and generalized pain. Naproxen belongs to the nonsteroidal anti-inflammatory family of drugs (NSAIDs). (See Helpful Hint on next page.)

Pregnancy Risk Categories: This drug has been assigned two pregnancy risk categories: **C** when used in the first and second trimesters of pregnancy, and **D** when used in the third trimester or near the time of delivery. Approximately 12% of prescription drugs are assigned two pregnancy risk categories, depending on which trimester of pregnancy the drug is used.

> **Category C rating:** The FDA assigns a drug to Category **C** for one of two reasons: (1) Studies show evidence of fetal harm when using the drug in pregnant animals, but no controlled studies have been done using the drug in pregnant women, or (2) Studies using the drug in pregnant animals have not been done, and studies of pregnant women using the drug are insufficient to reach a conclusion. Thus, the drug should only be used if the potential benefit for mom is greater than the potential risk of fetal harm, which, in many cases, is unknown. Approximately 50% of prescription drugs fall in this category.

> **Category D rating:** The FDA assigns a drug to Category **D** when studies of pregnant women using the drug show evidence of fetal harm. Rarely, however, the potential benefit of using the drug in some life-threatening situations for mom may outweigh the potential risk of fetal harm. For example, when mom requires cancer treatment or when she has a serious disease for which safer drugs cannot be used or are less effective. Approximately 11% of prescription drugs fall in this category.

Animal Studies: When pregnant animals were treated with this drug, there was an increased risk of birth defects and miscarriage in the offspring. Also, this family of drugs has been associated with an increased risk of cleft palate (hole in the roof of the mouth) in pregnant mice.

Human Studies: There are no controlled studies of pregnant women using this drug.

Helpful Hints: When taken in the third trimester of pregnancy, NSAIDs have seriously harmed the fetus, leading to life-threatening illness after birth and even death. These potential effects apply to all NSAIDs, whether purchased by prescription or over-the-counter without a prescription. They also explain why NSAIDs have been assigned a D pregnancy risk category. (See "Non-Steroidal, Anti-Inflammatory Drugs (NSAIDs) in Pregnancy" in the appendix for more details.)

Remember: All pregnancies have a background risk of about 3% for a major birth defect, even when mom doesn't take a drug of any kind. If you are pregnant or planning a pregnancy, always let your doctor know before taking any drug, prescription or non-prescription, or herbal remedy.

. . . .

NEFADOZONE

Brand Name: Serzone

Drug Use: This drug is approved by the FDA for the treatment of depression.

Pregnancy Risk Category: C

> **Category C rating:** The FDA assigns a drug to Category C for one of two reasons: (1) Studies show evidence of fetal harm when using the drug in pregnant animals, but no controlled studies have been done using the drug in pregnant women, or (2) Studies using the drug in pregnant animals have not been done, and studies of pregnant women using the drug are insufficient to reach a conclusion. Thus, the drug should only be used if the potential benefit for mom is greater than the potential risk of fetal harm, which, in many cases, is unknown. Approximately 50% of prescription drugs fall in this category.

Animal Studies: When pregnant animals were treated with this drug, there was no increased risk of birth defects. At high doses, however, there was an increase in newborn deaths and lower birthweights.

Human Studies: There is limited information available about the use of this drug in pregnant women. This limited information suggests the drug is not associated with fetal harm.

Helpful Hints:

1. Studies show that antidepressants increase the risk of suicidal thinking and behavior in children, adolescents, and young adults. Anyone considering the use of this drug or any other antidepressant in these patients must balance that risk with the clinical need.

2. Almost all antidepressants carry some risk to the developing fetus. However, we also know depression in a pregnant woman carries potential risk for her health and for her unborn baby; for example, low birth weight and prematurity. The risks and benefits of medications and untreated depression must be weighed carefully. If you are pregnant and think you may have depression, or if you already know you do, talk with your doctor so the two of you can create the right plan for you and your unborn baby. (See "Antidepressants in Pregnancy" in the appendix for more details.)

Remember: All pregnancies have a background risk of about 3% for a major birth defect, even when mom doesn't take a drug of any kind. If you are pregnant or

planning a pregnancy, always let your doctor know before taking any drug, prescription or non-prescription, or herbal remedy.

. . . .

NICOTINE REPLACEMENT THERAPY

Brand Names: Nicotine replacement therapy has a number of brand names, including the following: Nicorette, which comes in the form of a gum; Nicoderm, which comes in the form of a skin patch, Nicotrol, which comes in the form of a skin patch and also in the form of a nasal spray; and Commit, which comes in the form of lozenges.

Drug Use: All of these drugs are designed and approved by the FDA to reduce withdrawal symptoms, including nicotine craving associated with quitting smoking.

Pregnancy Risk Category: D

> **Category D rating:** The FDA assigns a drug to Category **D** when studies of pregnant women using the drug show evidence of fetal harm. Rarely, however, the potential benefit of using the drug in some life-threatening situations for mom may outweigh the potential risk of fetal harm. For example, when mom requires cancer treatment or when she has a serious disease for which safer drugs cannot be used or are less effective. Approximately 11% of prescription drugs fall in this category.

Animal Studies: Studies in pregnant mice, rats, and rabbits showed widespread nicotine toxicity, including stillbirth, decreased body weight, birth defects, and decreased placental development. Overall, then, nicotine is toxic in experimental animals.

Human Studies: In one long retrospective study of pregnant women exposed to a variety of nicotine replacement therapies, the number of birth defects in women using these products during the first twelve weeks of pregnancy was greater than expected. Fetal risk for cigarette smoking is well known and includes an increased incidence of miscarriage, prematurity, stillbirth, and the possibility of sudden infant death syndrome (SIDS) later on.

Helpful Hints:

1. The American Heart Association makes the following statement: "While the use of replacement products during pregnancy is not risk-free, it is much less dangerous to you and your baby than smoking." Unfortunately, the reality of what often happens is that a pregnant woman finds that using the patches or some other method of nicotine replacement therapy does not completely stop her cravings and she winds up using the replacement therapy and smoking, also. Before a pregnant woman who smokes gets to this point, it is very helpful for her to have discussed the nicotine replacement therapy that appeals to her and developed a plan with her physician going forward.

   The American College of Obstetricians and Gynecologists (ACOG) has a very helpful smoking cessation program that many obstetricians use. Ideally, a woman who anticipates becoming pregnant and smokes should make a pre-pregnancy appointment with her doctor to discuss this or other programs that are available. Remember, if you decide to stop smoking, your future baby is not the only one who will benefit. You and your baby's father and all of your future children will benefit, also.

2. This drug weakly interacts with grapefruit and grapefruit juice, which can cause harmful, and even life-threatening, side effects. Before taking this drug with grapefruit juice, or before consuming grapefruit or grapefruit juice during the day while taking this drug, first read the section "Grapefruit Juice–Drug Interactions Can Make You Sick" in the appendix of this book. Then discuss this with your pharmacist or the healthcare provider who prescribed this drug.

Remember: All pregnancies have a background risk of about 3% for a major birth defect, even when mom doesn't take a drug of any kind. If you are pregnant or planning a pregnancy, always let your doctor know before taking any drug, prescription or non-prescription, or herbal remedy.

· ·

NIFEDIPINE

Brand Names: Adalat, Procardia

Drug Uses: This drug is approved by the FDA for the treatment of chest pain. It is also used to stop contractions in case of premature labor. However, this is an off-label, non-FDA approved, use.

Pregnancy Risk Category: C

Category C rating: The FDA assigns a drug to Category **C** for one of two reasons: (1) Studies show evidence of fetal harm when using the drug in pregnant animals, but no controlled studies have been done using the drug in pregnant women, or (2) Studies using the drug in pregnant animals have not been done, and studies of pregnant women using the drug are insufficient to reach a conclusion. Thus, the drug should only be used if the potential benefit for mom is greater than the potential risk of fetal harm, which, in many cases, is unknown. Approximately 50% of prescription drugs fall in this category.

Animal Studies: In pregnant rats and rabbits, the use of nifedipine has been associated with an increased risk of birth defects.

Human Studies: Limited studies in pregnant women show that the use of nifedipine has been associated with decreased infant birth weight. In addition, there are reports when nifedipine is taken with magnesium sulfate, another drug often used to treat premature labor, serious complications have occurred.

Helpful Hints: This drug weakly interacts with grapefruit and grapefruit juice, which can cause harmful, and even life-threatening, side effects. Before taking this drug with grapefruit juice, or before consuming grapefruit or grapefruit juice during the day while taking this drug, first read the section "Grapefruit Juice–Drug Interactions Can Make You Sick" in the appendix of this book. Then discuss this with your pharmacist or the healthcare provider who prescribed this drug.

Remember: All pregnancies have a background risk of about 3% for a major birth defect, even when mom doesn't take a drug of any kind. If you are pregnant or planning a pregnancy, always let your doctor know before taking any drug, prescription or non-prescription, or herbal remedy.

NITROFURANTOIN

Brand Name: Macrobid

Drug Use: This drug is approved by the FDA for the treatment of urinary tract infections.

Pregnancy Risk Category: B

> **Category B rating:** The FDA assigns a drug to Category **B** for one of two reasons: (1) Studies show no evidence of fetal harm

when using the drug in pregnant animals, but no controlled studies have been done using the drug in pregnant women, or (2) Studies show evidence of fetal harm when using the drug in pregnant animals, but controlled studies using the drug in pregnant women do not show evidence of fetal harm. Approximately 21% of prescription drugs fall in this category.

Animal Studies: Pregnant animals treated with this drug have not shown an increased risk of birth defects in their offspring.

Human Studies: When pregnant women have taken nitrofurantoin, there has been no increased risk of birth defects.

Remember: All pregnancies have a background risk of about 3% for a major birth defect, even when mom doesn't take a drug of any kind. If you are pregnant or planning a pregnancy, always let your doctor know before taking any drug, prescription or non-prescription, or herbal remedy.

. . . .

NITROGLYCERIN

Brand Names: Nitrobid, Nitrodur, Nitrostat, Nitroquick

Drug Uses: This drug is approved by the FDA for the treatment of chest pain, high blood pressure, and congestive heart failure.

Pregnancy Risk Category: **B**

Category B rating: The FDA assigns a drug to Category **B** for one of two reasons: (1) Studies show no evidence of fetal harm when using the drug in pregnant animals, but no controlled studies have been done using the drug in pregnant women, or (2) Studies show evidence of fetal harm when using the drug in pregnant animals, but controlled studies using the drug in pregnant women do not show evidence of fetal harm. Approximately 21% of prescription drugs fall in this category.

Animal Studies: When used in pregnant animals, this drug does not appear to be associated with fetal harm.

Human Studies: Information about the use of nitroglycerin in pregnant women is limited, especially for use during the first and second trimesters.

Remember: All pregnancies have a background risk of about 3% for a major birth defect, even when mom doesn't take a drug of any kind. If you are pregnant or planning a pregnancy, always let your doctor know before taking any drug, prescription or non-prescription, or herbal remedy.

· ·

NIZATIDINE

Brand Name: Axid

Drug Uses: This drug is approved by the FDA for the treatment of gastroesophageal reflux disease (GERD) and stomach ulcers.

Pregnancy Risk Category: B

> **Category B rating:** The FDA assigns a drug to Category **B** for one of two reasons: (1) Studies show no evidence of fetal harm when using the drug in pregnant animals, but no controlled studies have been done using the drug in pregnant women, or (2) Studies show evidence of fetal harm when using the drug in pregnant animals, but controlled studies using the drug in pregnant women do not show evidence of fetal harm. Approximately 21% of prescription drugs fall in this category.

Animal Studies: Pregnant animals treated with this drug have not shown a risk for fetal harm.

Human Studies: Controlled studies in pregnant women using this drug have not been done. However, no adverse fetal effects have been seen in uncontrolled studies.

Remember: All pregnancies have a background risk of about 3% for a major birth defect, even when mom doesn't take a drug of any kind. If you are pregnant or planning a pregnancy, always let your doctor know before taking any drug, prescription or non-prescription, or herbal remedy.

. . . .

NORTRIPTYLINE

Brand Name: Pamelor

Drug Use: This drug is approved by the FDA for the treatment of depression.

Pregnancy Risk Category: C

> **Category C rating:** The FDA assigns a drug to Category C for one of two reasons: (1) Studies show evidence of fetal harm when using the drug in pregnant animals, but no controlled studies have been done using the drug in pregnant women, or (2) Studies using the drug in pregnant animals have not been done, and studies of pregnant women using the drug are insufficient to reach a conclusion. Thus, the drug should only be used if the potential benefit for mom is greater than the potential risk of fetal harm, which, in many cases, is unknown. Approximately 50% of prescription drugs fall in this category.

Animal Studies: When pregnant animals have been treated with this drug, no adverse effects have been seen.

Human Studies: Controlled studies using this drug in pregnant women have not been done. However, in uncontrolled studies, there does not seem to be an increased risk of fetal harm.

Helpful Hints:

   1. Studies show that antidepressants increase the risk of suicidal thinking and behavior in children, adolescents, and young adults. Anyone considering

the use of this drug or any other antidepressant in these patients must balance that risk with the clinical need.

2. Almost all antidepressants carry some risk to the developing fetus. However, we also know depression in a pregnant woman carries potential risk for her health and for her unborn baby; for example, low birth weight and prematurity. The risks and benefits of medications and untreated depression must be weighed carefully. If you are pregnant and think you may have depression, or if you already know you do, talk with your doctor so the two of you can create the right plan for you and your unborn baby. (See "Antidepressants in Pregnancy" in the appendix for more details.)

Remember: All pregnancies have a background risk of about 3% for a major birth defect, even when mom doesn't take a drug of any kind. If you are pregnant or planning a pregnancy, always let your doctor know before taking any drug, prescription or non-prescription, or herbal remedy.

· ·

NYSTATIN

Brand Name: Mycostatin

Drug Use: This drug is approved by the FDA for the treatment of vaginal yeast infections.

Pregnancy Risk Category: C

> **Category C rating:** The FDA assigns a drug to Category C for one of two reasons: (1) Studies show evidence of fetal harm when using the drug in pregnant animals, but no controlled studies have been done using the drug in pregnant women, or (2) Studies using

the drug in pregnant animals have not been done, and studies of pregnant women using the drug are insufficient to reach a conclusion. Thus, the drug should only be used if the potential benefit for mom is greater than the potential risk of fetal harm, which, in many cases, is unknown. Approximately 50% of prescription drugs fall in this category.

Animal Studies: No adverse fetal effects have been seen in pregnant animals treated with this drug.

Human Studies: Similarly, no adverse fetal effects have been seen in pregnant women given this drug.

Remember: All pregnancies have a background risk of about 3% for a major birth defect, even when mom doesn't take a drug of any kind. If you are pregnant or planning a pregnancy, always let your doctor know before taking any drug, prescription or non-prescription, or herbal remedy.

ADDITIONAL DRUGS AND THEIR FDA PREGNANCY RISK CATEGORIES

Since these additional drugs are uncommonly used in pregnancy, they are listed by generic name along with their FDA Pregnancy Risk Category without more detail:

Nafcillin - B

Nalbuphine - B (D if used for long periods or in high doses before delivery)

Naltrexone - C

Naphazoline - C

Naratriptan - C

Natalizumab - C

Nateglinide - C

Nedocromil - B

Nelarabine - D

Nelfinavir - B

Neomycin - C

Nepafenac - C

Nesiritide - C

Nevirapine - C

Niacin - A (C if used in doses above the recommended daily allowance)

Nicardipine - C

Nilutamide - C

Nimodipine - C

Nisoldipine - C

Nitazoxanide - B

Nitric Oxide - C

Norepinephrine - C

Norfloxacin - C

O

OFLOXACIN

Brand Names: Approximately 70 different preparations containing this drug exist, including the brand names Cipro, Floxin, and Baytril.

Drug Use: This drug is approved by the FDA for the treatment of a variety of bacterial infections.

Pregnancy Risk Category: C

> **Category C rating:** The FDA assigns a drug to Category C for one of two reasons: (1) Studies show evidence of fetal harm when using the drug in pregnant animals, but no controlled studies have been done using the drug in pregnant women, or (2) Studies using the drug in pregnant animals have not been done, and studies of pregnant women using the drug are insufficient to reach a conclusion. Thus, the drug should only be used if the potential benefit for mom is greater than the potential risk of fetal harm, which, in many cases, is unknown. Approximately 50% of prescription drugs fall in this category.

Animal Studies: When pregnant rats and rabbits were treated with this drug, there was no increase in the number of birth defects in the offspring.

Human Studies: There are no controlled studies in pregnant women using this drug. Uncontrolled studies have revealed no increase in the incidence of birth defects.

Remember: All pregnancies have a background risk of about 3% for a major birth defect, even when mom doesn't take a drug of any kind. If you are pregnant or planning a pregnancy, always let your doctor know before taking any drug, prescription or non-prescription, or herbal remedy.

. . . .

OLANZAPINE

Brand Name: Zyprexa. This drug belongs to the "atypical antipsychotic" family of drugs.

Drug Uses: This drug is approved by the FDA for the treatment of schizophrenia and bipolar disorder.

Pregnancy Risk Category: C

> **Category C rating:** The FDA assigns a drug to Category C for one of two reasons: (1) Studies show evidence of fetal harm when using the drug in pregnant animals, but no controlled studies have been done using the drug in pregnant women, or (2) Studies using the drug in pregnant animals have not been done, and studies of pregnant women using the drug are insufficient to reach a conclusion. Thus, the drug should only be used if the potential benefit for mom is greater than the potential risk of fetal harm, which, in many cases, is unknown. Approximately 50% of prescription drugs fall in this category.

Animal Studies: When pregnant rats and rabbits were treated with this drug, the incidence of birth defects in their offspring was no greater than normally expected. However, there were toxic effects on their embryos.

Human Studies: There are no controlled studies using this drug in pregnant women.

Helpful Hints: Some experts recommend treating pregnant women taking a member of this drug family with ten times the normal daily intake of folic acid, which is normally .4 mg per day. This is done to reduce the risk of having a baby with a neural tube defect (open spine) due to an increased risk of folic acid deficiency. Thus, the new daily dose of folic acid would be 4 mg per day. This recommendation should be discussed with your doctor.

Remember: All pregnancies have a background risk of about 3% for a major birth defect, even when mom

doesn't take a drug of any kind. If you are pregnant or planning a pregnancy, always let your doctor know before taking any drug, prescription or non-prescription, or herbal remedy.

∙∙∙∙∙∙∙∙∙∙∙∙∙∙∙∙∙∙∙∙∙∙∙∙∙∙∙∙∙∙∙∙∙∙∙∙∙∙

OLSALAZINE

Brand Name: Dipentum

Drug Use: This drug is approved by the FDA for the maintenance of remission of ulcerative colitis in patients intolerant to sulfasalazine.

Pregnancy Risk Category: C

> **Category C rating:** The FDA assigns a drug to Category C for one of two reasons: (1) Studies show evidence of fetal harm when using the drug in pregnant animals, but no controlled studies have been done using the drug in pregnant women, or (2) Studies using the drug in pregnant animals have not been done, and studies of pregnant women using the drug are insufficient to reach a conclusion. Thus, the drug should only be used if the potential benefit for mom is greater than the potential risk of fetal harm, which, in many cases, is unknown. Approximately 50% of prescription drugs fall in this category.

Animal Studies: When this drug was given to pregnant rats in doses 5–20 times the human dose, it produced evidence of fetal toxicity consisting of decreased weight, delayed maturation of bones, and immaturity of organs.

Human Studies: There are no controlled studies using this drug in pregnant women.

Remember: All pregnancies have a background risk of about 3% for a major birth defect, even when mom doesn't take a drug of any kind. If you are pregnant or planning a pregnancy, always let your doctor know before taking any drug, prescription or non-prescription, or herbal remedy.

· ·

OMEPRAZOLE

Brand Names: Nexium, Prilosec

Drug Uses: This drug is approved by the FDA for the treatment of stomach and duodenal ulcers and other disorders associated with hypersecretion of gastric acid.

Pregnancy Risk Category: C

> **Category C rating:** The FDA assigns a drug to Category C for one of two reasons: (1) Studies show evidence of fetal harm when using the drug in pregnant animals, but no controlled studies have been done using the drug in pregnant women, or (2) Studies using the drug in pregnant animals have not been done, and studies of pregnant women using the drug are insufficient to reach a conclusion. Thus, the drug should only be used if the potential benefit for mom is greater than the potential risk of fetal harm, which, in many cases, is unknown. Approximately 50% of prescription drugs fall in this category.

Animal Studies: When pregnant rats and rabbits were treated with this drug, there was no evidence of an increase of birth defects.

Human Studies: Experts have concluded from analyzing a variety of uncontrolled human studies that therapeutic doses of this drug in human pregnancies are unlikely to cause birth defects. However, avoiding this drug during the first trimester of pregnancy is probably prudent.

Helpful Hints: This drug weakly interacts with grapefruit and grapefruit juice, which can cause harmful, and even life-threatening, side effects. Before taking this drug with grapefruit juice, or before consuming grapefruit or grapefruit juice during the day while taking this drug, first read the section "Grapefruit Juice–Drug Interactions Can Make You Sick" in the appendix of this book. Then discuss this with your pharmacist or the healthcare provider who prescribed this drug.

Remember: All pregnancies have a background risk of about 3% for a major birth defect, even when mom doesn't take a drug of any kind. If you are pregnant or planning a pregnancy, always let your doctor know before taking any drug, prescription or non-prescription, or herbal remedy.

• •

ONDANSETRON

Brand Names: Zofran, Zofran ODT (dissolves under the tongue)

Drug Use: This drug is used to prevent and treat nausea.

Pregnancy Risk Category: B

Category B rating: The FDA assigns a drug to Category **B** for one of two reasons: (1) Studies show no evidence of fetal harm when using the drug in pregnant animals, but no controlled studies have been done using the drug in pregnant women, or (2) Studies show evidence of fetal harm when using the drug in pregnant animals, but controlled studies using the drug in pregnant women do not show evidence of fetal harm. Approximately 21% of prescription drugs fall in this category.

Animal Studies: When pregnant rats and rabbits were treated with this drug, researchers found no evidence of fetal harm.

Human Studies: When this drug has been used by pregnant women, researchers have found no evidence of fetal harm.

Remember: All pregnancies have a background risk of about 3% for a major birth defect, even when mom doesn't take a drug of any kind. If you are pregnant or planning a pregnancy, always let your doctor know before taking any drug, prescription or non-prescription, or herbal remedy.

. . . .

OXACILLIN

Brand Name: Dicloxacillin

Drug Use: This antibiotic is approved by the FDA for the treatment of penicillin-resistant infections.

Pregnancy Risk Category: B

> **Category B rating:** The FDA assigns a drug to Category **B** for one of two reasons: (1) Studies show no evidence of fetal harm when using the drug in pregnant animals, but no controlled studies have been done using the drug in pregnant women, or (2) Studies show evidence of fetal harm when using the drug in pregnant animals, but controlled studies using the drug in pregnant women do not show evidence of fetal harm. Approximately 21% of prescription drugs fall in this category.

Animal Studies: When pregnant mice, rats, and rabbits were treated with this drug, there was no evidence of fetal harm.

Human Studies: There are no controlled studies in pregnant women.

Remember: All pregnancies have a background risk of about 3% for a major birth defect, even when mom doesn't take a drug of any kind. If you are pregnant or planning a pregnancy, always let your doctor know before taking any drug, prescription or non-prescription, or herbal remedy.

. . . .

OXAPROZIN

Brand Name: Daypro. This drug belongs to the non-steroidal anti-inflammatory family of drugs (NSAIDs). (See Helpful Hint on next page.)

Drug Use: This drug is approved by the FDA for the relief of pain in osteoarthritis and rheumatoid arthritis.

Pregnancy Risk Categories: This drug has been assigned two pregnancy risk categories: **C** when used in the first or second trimesters of pregnancy, and **D** when used in the third trimester or near term. Approximately 12% of prescription drugs are assigned two pregnancy risk categories, depending on which trimester of pregnancy the drug is used.

> **Category C rating:** The FDA assigns a drug to Category **C** for one of two reasons: (1) Studies show evidence of fetal harm when using the drug in pregnant animals, but no controlled studies have been done using the drug in pregnant women, or (2) Studies using the drug in pregnant animals have not been done, and studies of pregnant women using the drug are insufficient to reach a conclusion. Thus, the drug should only be used if the potential benefit for mom is greater than the potential risk of fetal harm, which, in many cases, is unknown. Approximately 50% of prescription drugs fall in this category.

> **Category D rating:** The FDA assigns a drug to Category **D** when studies of pregnant women using the drug show evidence of fetal harm. Rarely, however, the potential benefit of using the drug in some life-threatening situations for mom may outweigh the potential risk of fetal harm. For example, when mom requires cancer treatment or when she has a serious disease for which safer drugs cannot be used or are less effective. Approximately 11% of prescription drugs fall in this category.

Animal Studies: This drug produced infrequent birth defects when used in pregnant rabbits, but not in rats and mice.

Human Studies: There are no controlled studies using this drug in pregnant women.

Helpful Hints: When taken in the third trimester of pregnancy, NSAIDs have seriously harmed the fetus, leading to life-threatening illness after birth and even death. These potential effects apply to all NSAIDs, whether purchased by prescription or over-the-counter without a prescription. They also explain why NSAIDs have been assigned a **D** pregnancy risk category. (See "Non-Steroidal, Anti-Inflammatory Drugs (NSAIDs) in Pregnancy" in the appendix for more details.)

Remember: All pregnancies have a background risk of about 3% for a major birth defect, even when mom doesn't take a drug of any kind. If you are pregnant or planning a pregnancy, always let your doctor know before taking any drug, prescription or non-prescription, or herbal remedy.

· ·

OXAZEPAM

Brand Name: Oxazepam

Drug Use: This drug is approved by the FDA for the treatment of anxiety disorders. It is a member of the benzodiazepine family of drugs.

Pregnancy Risk Category: D

> **Category D rating:** The FDA assigns a drug to Category **D** when studies of pregnant women using the drug show evidence of fetal harm. Rarely, however, the potential benefit of using the drug in some life-threatening situations for mom may outweigh the potential risk of fetal harm. For example, when mom requires cancer treatment or when she has a serious disease for which safer drugs cannot be used or are less effective. Approximately 11% of prescription drugs fall in this category.

Animal Studies: No studies in pregnant animals could be located. However, other members of the benzodiazepine family of drugs are associated with an increased incidence of cleft palate in mice.

Human Studies: There are no controlled studies using this drug in pregnant women. The effects of this family of drugs on the human embryo and fetus are controversial. Some studies have concluded that members of this family of drugs are associated with birth defects, while other studies have not. For example, diazepam, a member of this family of drugs, has also been assigned a pregnancy risk category of **D**. Because the use of this drug is rarely a matter of urgency, its use during pregnancy should almost always be avoided, according to many experts.

Remember: All pregnancies have a background risk of about 3% for a major birth defect, even when mom doesn't take a drug of any kind. If you are pregnant or planning a pregnancy, always let your doctor know before taking any drug, prescription or non-prescription, or herbal remedy.

OXYCODONE

Brand Name: Oxycodone

Drug Use: This drug is approved by the FDA for the management of moderate to severe pain when a narcotic is appropriate. There are approximately 60 different preparations containing this drug in various combinations with other drugs, including acetaminophen.

Pregnancy Risk Categories: This drug has been assigned two pregnancy risk categories: **B** when used routinely throughout pregnancy. However, if it is used for prolonged periods or near term, its risk category is **D**. Approximately 12% of prescription drugs are assigned two pregnancy risk categories, depending on which trimester of pregnancy the drug is used.

Category B rating: The FDA assigns a drug to Category **B** for one of two reasons: (1) Studies show no evidence of fetal harm when using the drug in pregnant animals, but no controlled studies have been done using the drug in pregnant women, or (2) Studies show evidence of fetal harm when using the drug in pregnant animals, but controlled studies using the drug in pregnant women do not show evidence of fetal harm. Approximately 21% of prescription drugs fall in this category.

Category D rating: The FDA assigns a drug to Category **D** when studies of pregnant women using the drug show evidence of fetal harm. Rarely, however, the potential benefit of using the drug in some life-threatening situations for mom may outweigh the potential risk of fetal harm. For example, when mom requires cancer treatment or when she has a serious disease for which safer drugs cannot be used or are less effective. Approximately 11% of prescription drugs fall in this category.

Animal Studies: When pregnant rats and rabbits were treated with this drug, there was no evidence of fetal harm in the offspring.

Human Studies: There are no controlled studies in pregnant women. However, newborns whose mothers have taken oxycodone chronically may suffer respiratory depression and/or withdrawal symptoms either at birth or in the nursery.

Helpful Hints: Oxycodone is not recommended for use in pregnant women during or immediately prior to labor. Newborns whose mothers have received the drug during labor should be observed closely for signs of respiratory depression. A specific narcotic antagonist, naloxone, should be readily available in the delivery room and in the nursery in case it is needed to reverse the respiratory depressive effects of this drug.

Remember: All pregnancies have a background risk of about 3% for a major birth defect, even when mom doesn't take a drug of any kind. If you are pregnant or planning a pregnancy, always let your doctor know before taking any drug, prescription or non-prescription, or herbal remedy.

. . . .

ADDITIONAL DRUGS AND THEIR FDA PREGNANCY RISK CATEGORIES

Since these additional drugs are uncommonly used in pregnancy, they are listed by generic name along with their FDA Pregnancy Risk Category without more detail:

Octreotide - B

Olmesartan - C (D if used in the second or third trimester)

Olopatadine - C

Omalizumab - B

Orlistat - B

Oseltamivir - C

Oxaliplatin - D

Oxcarbazepine - C

Oxiconazole - B

Oxybutynin - B

Oxymetazoline - C

P

PAROXETINE

Brand Name: Paxil

Drug Uses: This drug is approved by the FDA for the treatment of depression, obsessive compulsive disorder, panic disorder, and social anxiety disorder. This drug is a member of the selective serotonin reuptake inhibitor (SSRI) family of drugs.

Pregnancy Risk Category: D

> **Category D rating:** The FDA assigns a drug to Category **D** when studies of pregnant women using the drug show evidence of fetal harm. Rarely, however, the potential benefit of using the drug in some life-threatening situations for mom may outweigh the potential risk of fetal harm. For example, when mom requires cancer treatment or when she has a serious disease for which safer drugs cannot be used or are less effective. Approximately 11% of prescription drugs fall in this category.

Animal Studies: When pregnant rats and rabbits were given paroxetine, there was no evidence of fetal birth defects. However, one study did show an increase in newborn deaths when the drug was given in the third trimester and continued throughout lactation. When pregnant mice were treated with paroxetine, the only ill effect was lower birth weights.

Human Studies: There are no controlled studies of pregnant women taking paroxetine. However, uncontrolled studies and case reports involving paroxetine and other members of the SSRI family of drugs have found the following:

1. Women who stop taking their antidepressants (mainly SSRIs) during pregnancy were roughly

five times more likely to relapse during their pregnancy than women who continued taking their antidepressant medicine while pregnant.

2. In another study, pregnant women who took an SSRI antidepressant after the 20th week of pregnancy (second half) were six times more likely to have a baby with persistent pulmonary hypertension—a serious and sometimes life-threatening disorder in which a baby has high pressure in their lung blood vessels, resulting in breathing problems and the need for respirator support—than babies of mothers who did not take an antidepressant.

3. More directly related to paroxetine, the pregnancy risk category for paroxetine was recently changed by the FDA to **D** throughout pregnancy from **C** during the first half and **D** for the second half because yet another study suggested that taking the drug in the first trimester of pregnancy may be associated with an increased risk of fetal heart defects.

Helpful Hints:

1. Studies show that antidepressants increase the risk of suicidal thinking and behavior in children, adolescents, and young adults. Anyone considering the use of this drug or any other antidepressant in these patients must balance that risk with the clinical need.

2. Almost all antidepressants carry some risk to the developing fetus. However, we also know depression in a pregnant woman carries potential risk for her health and for her unborn baby; for

example, low birth weight and prematurity. The risks and benefits of medications and untreated depression must be weighed carefully. If you are pregnant and think you may have depression, or if you already know you do, talk with your doctor so the two of you can create the right plan for you and your unborn baby. (See "Antidepressants in Pregnancy" in the appendix for more details.)

Remember: All pregnancies have a background risk of about 3% for a major birth defect, even when mom doesn't take a drug of any kind. If you are pregnant or planning a pregnancy, always let your doctor know before taking any drug, prescription or non-prescription, or herbal remedy.

. . . .

PENICILLIN

Brand Name: Penicillin

Drug Use: The FDA has approved penicillin to treat various bacterial infections.

Pregnancy Risk Category: B

> **Category B rating:** The FDA assigns a drug to Category **B** for one of two reasons: (1) Studies show no evidence of fetal harm when using the drug in pregnant animals, but no controlled studies have been done using the drug in pregnant women, or (2) Studies show evidence of fetal harm when using the drug in pregnant animals, but controlled studies using the drug in pregnant women do not show evidence of fetal harm. Approximately 21% of prescription drugs fall in this category.

Animal Studies: Pregnant animals treated with penicillin have shown no evidence of fetal harm.

Human Studies: Extensive use of this drug in pregnant women has shown no evidence of fetal harm.

Remember: All pregnancies have a background risk of about 3% for a major birth defect, even when mom doesn't take a drug of any kind. If you are pregnant or planning a pregnancy, always let your doctor know before taking any drug, prescription or non-prescription, or herbal remedy.

. . . .

PENTAZOCINE

Brand Name: Talwin

Drug Use: This drug is approved by the FDA for the treatment of moderate to severe pain. It belongs to the narcotic family of pain relievers.

Pregnancy Risk Categories: This drug has been assigned two risk categories: **C** and then **D** if used for prolonged periods or in high doses near the time of delivery. Approximately 12% of prescription drugs are assigned two pregnancy risk categories, depending on which trimester of pregnancy the drug is used.

Category C rating: The FDA assigns a drug to Category **C** for one of two reasons: (1) Studies show evidence of fetal harm when using the drug in pregnant animals, but no controlled studies have been done using the drug in pregnant women, or (2) Studies using the drug in pregnant animals have not been done, and studies of pregnant women using the drug are insufficient to reach a conclusion. Thus, the drug should only be used if the potential benefit for mom is greater than the potential risk of fetal harm, which, in many cases, is unknown. Approximately 50% of prescription drugs fall in this category.

Category D rating: The FDA assigns a drug to Category **D** when studies of pregnant women using the drug show evidence of fetal harm. Rarely, however, the potential benefit of using the drug in some life-threatening situations for mom may outweigh the potential risk of fetal harm. For example, when mom requires cancer treatment or when she has a serious disease for which safer drugs cannot be used or are less effective. Approximately 11% of prescription drugs fall in this category.

Animal Studies: When pregnant animals have been treated with this drug, there has been no evidence of fetal harm.

Human Studies: When taken by pregnant women in the third trimester of pregnancy and close to the time of delivery, withdrawal symptoms have been seen in some of these babies. These symptoms include trembling, jitteriness, increased irritability, hyperactivity, sweating, diarrhea, and vomiting. Also, behavioral changes, such as decreased interaction, have been described.

Remember: All pregnancies have a background risk of about 3% for a major birth defect, even when mom doesn't take a drug of any kind. If you are pregnant or planning a pregnancy, always let your doctor know before taking any drug, prescription or non-prescription, or herbal remedy.

PERMETHRIN

Brand Names: Nix, Elimite

Drug Use: This drug is approved by the FDA for the treatment of scabies and lice.

Pregnancy Risk Category: B

> **Category B rating:** The FDA assigns a drug to Category **B** for one of two reasons: (1) Studies show no evidence of fetal harm when using the drug in pregnant animals, but no controlled studies have been done using the drug in pregnant women, or (2) Studies show evidence of fetal harm when using the drug in pregnant animals, but controlled studies using the drug in pregnant women do not show evidence of fetal harm. Approximately 21% of prescription drugs fall in this category.

Animal Studies: When given by mouth to pregnant animals, no evidence of fetal harm was seen.

Human Studies: When used by pregnant women, there has also been no evidence of fetal harm seen.

Helpful Hints: This drug is used topically to treat scabies and lice. Since it is only applied to the skin or the scalp, there is very little exposure, if any, of this drug to the fetus.

Remember: All pregnancies have a background risk of about 3% for a major birth defect, even when mom doesn't take a drug of any kind. If you are pregnant or planning a pregnancy, always let your doctor know before taking any drug, prescription or non-prescription, or herbal remedy.

. . . .

PHENOBARBITAL

Brand Name: Phenobarbital

Drug Uses: This drug is approved by the FDA for the treatment of seizures and for sedation.

Pregnancy Risk Category: D

> **Category D rating:** The FDA assigns a drug to Category **D** when studies of pregnant women using the drug show evidence of fetal harm. Rarely, however, the potential benefit of using the drug in some life-threatening situations for mom may outweigh the potential risk of fetal harm. For example, when mom requires cancer treatment or when she has a serious disease for which safer drugs cannot be used or are less effective. Approximately 11% of prescription drugs fall in this category.

Animal Studies: No relevant animal studies are available.

Human Studies: In pregnant women, phenobarbital is associated with an increased risk of birth defects, as well as an increased risk of bleeding in the newborn at birth. Several studies have also shown development delays in babies exposed to phenobarbital during pregnancy.

Helpful Hints: Phenobarbital therapy in the pregnant woman suffering from epilepsy presents a risk to the fetus for major and minor birth defects, hemorrhage at birth, and addiction. On the other hand, the risk to the mother may be greater if the drug is withheld and seizure control is not maintained. The risk-to-benefit ratio, in this case, may favor continued use of the drug during pregnancy at the lowest possible dose to control seizures. This decision requires consultation with your doctor.

Remember: All pregnancies have a background risk of about 3% for a major birth defect, even when mom doesn't take a drug of any kind. If you are pregnant or planning a pregnancy, always let your doctor know before taking any drug, prescription or non-prescription, or herbal remedy.

PHENYTOIN

Brand Name: Dilantin

Drug Use: This drug is approved by the FDA for the treatment of seizure disorders. This drug is a member of the folic acid antagonist family of drugs.

Pregnancy Risk Category: D

> **Category D rating:** The FDA assigns a drug to Category **D** when studies of pregnant women using the drug show evidence of fetal harm. Rarely, however, the potential benefit of using the drug in some life-threatening situations for mom may outweigh the potential risk of fetal harm. For example, when mom requires cancer treatment or when she has a serious disease for which safer drugs cannot be used or are less effective. Approximately 11% of prescription drugs fall in this category.

Animal Studies: There are no relevant study results from pregnant animals treated with this drug.

Human Studies: The use of phenytoin during pregnancy involves significant risk to the fetus for major and minor birth defects and hemorrhage.

Helpful Hints:

1. Folic acid antagonists are drugs that limit the effectiveness of folic acid, making it more likely that a baby born to a mom taking one of these drugs might have a serious birth defect, such as an open spine. If you are taking a folic acid antagonist and trying to become pregnant, discuss the possibility of increasing your folic acid intake with your clinician before becoming pregnant. (See "Folic Acid Antagonist Drugs in Pregnancy" in the Appendix for more details.)

2. In pregnant women with epilepsy, the first priority is to prevent seizures. This can be difficult because many seizure medications do not work quite as well during pregnancy. Sometimes the dose has to be increased or other medications added just to prevent seizures. Regardless, the healthiest situation for both mom and unborn baby is to have the fewest seizures possible.

Remember: All pregnancies have a background risk of about 3% for a major birth defect, even when mom doesn't take a drug of any kind. If you are pregnant or planning a pregnancy, always let your doctor know before taking any drug, prescription or non-prescription, or herbal remedy.

PINDOLOL

Brand Name: Visken

Drug Use: This drug is approved by the FDA for the treatment of hypertension (high blood pressure), alone or in combination with other anti-hypertension drugs. This drug belongs to the beta-blocker family of drugs.

Pregnancy Risk Categories: This drug has been assigned two pregnancy risk categories: a **B** rating when used in the first trimester (first 12 weeks of pregnancy), and a **D** rating when used in the second or third trimesters. Approximately 12% of prescription drugs are assigned two pregnancy risk categories, depending on which trimester of pregnancy the drug is used.

> **Category B rating:** The FDA assigns a drug to Category **B** for one of two reasons: (1) Studies show no evidence of fetal harm when using the drug in pregnant animals, but no controlled studies have been done using the drug in pregnant women, or (2) Studies show evidence of fetal harm when using the drug in pregnant animals, but controlled studies using the drug in pregnant women do not show evidence of fetal harm. Approximately 21% of prescription drugs fall in this category.

> **Category D rating:** The FDA assigns a drug to Category **D** when studies of pregnant women using the drug show evidence of fetal harm. Rarely, however, the potential benefit of using the drug in some life-threatening situations for mom may outweigh the potential risk of fetal harm. For example, when mom requires cancer treatment or when she has a serious disease for which safer drugs cannot be used or are less effective. Approximately 11% of prescription drugs fall in this category.

Animal Studies: When pregnant rats and rabbits were treated with this drug, there was no evidence of fetal harm.

Human Studies: There are no controlled studies in pregnant women taking this drug. However, some drugs in this beta-blocker family of drugs are associated with decreased fetal and placental weight when taken during the second and third trimesters. That is mainly why this drug has been assigned a Category **D** rating if used in the second or third trimesters.

Helpful Hints: This drug should only be taken during the second and third trimesters after consulting with your doctor to see if the benefits of using the drug may out-weigh the potential risk of fetal harm.

Remember: All pregnancies have a background risk of about 3% for a major birth defect, even when mom doesn't take a drug of any kind. If you are pregnant or planning a pregnancy, always let your doctor know before taking any drug, prescription or non-prescription, or herbal remedy.

PIROXICAM

Brand Name: Feldane. This drug is a member of the non-steroidal anti-inflammatory family of drugs (NSAIDs). (See Helpful Hint on next page.)

Drug Use: This drug is approved by the FDA for the re-lief of pain from osteoarthritis and rheumatoid arthritis.

Pregnancy Risk Categories: This drug has been as-signed two pregnancy risk categories: **C** when used in the first and second trimesters of pregnancy, and **D** when used during the third trimester or at term. Approximately 12% of prescription drugs are assigned two pregnancy risk cat-egories, depending on which trimester of pregnancy the drug is used.

Category C rating: The FDA assigns a drug to Category **C** for one of two reasons: (1) Studies show evidence of fetal harm when using the drug in pregnant animals, but no controlled studies have been done using the drug in pregnant women, or (2) Studies using the drug in pregnant animals have not been done, and studies of pregnant women using the drug are insufficient to reach a conclu-sion. Thus, the drug should only be used if the potential benefit for mom is greater than the potential risk of fetal harm, which, in many cases, is unknown. Approximately 50% of prescription drugs fall in this category.

Category D rating: The FDA assigns a drug to Category **D** when studies of pregnant women using the drug show evidence of fetal harm. Rarely, however, the potential benefit of using the drug in some life-threatening situations for mom may outweigh the potential risk of fetal harm. For example, when mom requires cancer treatment or when she has a serious disease for which safer drugs cannot be used or are less effective. Approximately 11% of prescription drugs fall in this category.

Animal Studies: When pregnant rats and rabbits were treated with this drug, there was no evidence of fetal birth defects.

Human Studies: There are no controlled studies of using this drug in pregnant women.

Helpful Hints: When taken in the third trimester of pregnancy, NSAIDs have seriously harmed the fetus, leading to life-threatening illness after birth and even death. These potential effects apply to all NSAIDs, whether purchased by prescription or over-the-counter without a prescription. They also explain why NSAIDs have been assigned a **D** pregnancy risk category. (See "Non-Steroidal, Anti-Inflammatory Drugs (NSAIDs) in Pregnancy" in the appendix for more details.)

Remember: All pregnancies have a background risk of about 3% for a major birth defect, even when mom doesn't take a drug of any kind. If you are pregnant or planning a pregnancy, always let your doctor know before taking any drug, prescription or non-prescription, or herbal remedy.

POTASSIUM CHLORIDE

Brand Name: Potassium Chloride

Drug Use: This drug is approved by the FDA as a replacement therapy for patients with low serum potassium levels.

Pregnancy Risk Category: **A**

> **Category A rating:** The FDA assigns a drug to Category **A** when controlled studies using the drug in pregnant women do not show harmful fetal effects throughout pregnancy. Approximately 1% of prescription drugs fall in this category.

Animal Studies: Studies using this medication in pregnant animals have not been done.

Human Studies: There are no controlled studies available.

Remember: All pregnancies have a background risk of about 3% for a major birth defect, even when mom doesn't take a drug of any kind. If you are pregnant or planning a pregnancy, always let your doctor know before taking any drug, prescription or non-prescription, or herbal remedy.

POTASSIUM IODIDE

Brand Names: Pima, SSKI

Drug Uses: This drug is approved by the FDA for several purposes: preparation for thyroid surgery, to protect the thyroid in a radiation emergency, and as an active ingredient in an expectorant to loosen mucus.

Pregnancy Risk Category: **D**

> **Category D rating:** The FDA assigns a drug to Category **D** when studies of pregnant women using the drug show evidence of fetal harm. Rarely, however, the potential benefit of using the drug in some life-threatening situations for mom may outweigh the potential risk of fetal harm. For example, when mom requires cancer treatment or when she has a serious disease for which safer drugs cannot be used or are less effective. Approximately 11% of prescription drugs fall in this category.

Animal Studies: Studies using this drug in pregnant animals could not be located.

Human Studies: There are no controlled studies using this drug in pregnant women. However, case reports indicate that this drug has produced goiter (an enlarged thyroid) in the fetus and hypothyroidism, which is decreased thyroid function. These findings account for potassium iodide being assigned to a pregnancy risk category of **D**.

Remember: All pregnancies have a background risk of about 3% for a major birth defect, even when mom doesn't take a drug of any kind. If you are pregnant or planning a pregnancy, always let your doctor know before taking any drug, prescription or non-prescription, or herbal remedy.

PRAVASTATIN

Brand Name: Pravachol

Drug Use: This drug is approved by the FDA to lower elevated serum cholesterol and to reduce the risk of a heart attack. It is a member of the "statin" family of drugs.

Pregnancy Risk Category: X

> **Category X rating:** The FDA assigns a drug to Category **X** when studies have shown the risk of fetal harm clearly outweighs any potential maternal benefit from the drug. **Drugs in this category should not be used by pregnant women.** Approximately 5% of prescription drugs fall in this category.

Animal Studies: Studies using this drug in pregnant animals could not be located.

Human Studies: There are no controlled studies using this drug in pregnant women.

Helpful Hints:

1. Drugs that belong to the statin family of drugs, such as this one, should only be prescribed for women of childbearing age when they are highly

unlikely to conceive and have been informed of the potential hazards, according to the FDA. Why? Because cholesterol is essential for normal fetal development, and anything that lowers the serum level of cholesterol—which is what statins do—might adversely affect fetal development. If a woman becomes pregnant while taking this drug, or any member of the statin family of drugs, it should be discontinued immediately and she should be told of the potential hazard to her unborn baby.

2. This drug weakly interacts with grapefruit and grapefruit juice, which can cause harmful, and even life-threatening, side effects. Before taking this drug with grapefruit juice, or before consuming grapefruit or grapefruit juice during the day while taking this drug, first read the section "Grapefruit Juice–Drug Interactions Can Make You Sick" in the appendix of this book. Then discuss this with your pharmacist or the health-care provider who prescribed this drug.

Remember: All pregnancies have a background risk of about 3% for a major birth defect, even when mom doesn't take a drug of any kind. If you are pregnant or planning a pregnancy, always let your doctor know before taking any drug, prescription or non-prescription, or herbal remedy.

PREDNISONE

Brand Name: Deltasone

Drug Uses: Prednisone is approved by the FDA for use to treat dozens of disorders, including rheumatoid arthritis, lupus, psoriasis, asthma, sarcoidosis, leukemia, and multiple sclerosis.

Pregnancy Risk Categories: This drug has been assigned two pregnancy risk categories: **D** when used in the first trimester, and **C** when used in the second and third trimesters. Approximately 12% of prescription drugs are assigned two pregnancy risk categories, depending on which trimester of pregnancy the drug is used.

> **Category D rating:** The FDA assigns a drug to Category **D** when studies of pregnant women using the drug show evidence of fetal harm. Rarely, however, the potential benefit of using the drug in some life-threatening situations for mom may outweigh the potential risk of fetal harm. For example, when mom requires cancer treatment or when she has a serious disease for which safer drugs cannot be used or are less effective. Approximately 11% of prescription drugs fall in this category.

> **Category C rating:** The FDA assigns a drug to Category C for one of two reasons: (1) Studies show evidence of fetal harm when using the drug in pregnant animals, but no controlled studies have been done using the drug in pregnant women, or (2) Studies using the drug in pregnant animals have not been done, and studies of pregnant women using the drug are insufficient to reach a conclusion. Thus, the drug should only be used if the potential benefit for mom is greater than the potential risk of fetal harm, which, in many cases, is unknown. Approximately 50% of prescription drugs fall in this category.

Animal Studies: Birth defects have been reported in the offspring of pregnant mice, rabbits, and rats treated with prednisone.

Human Studies: Controlled studies using this drug in pregnant women have not been done. Most experts recommend avoiding this drug during the first trimester of pregnancy, and limiting its use to the second and third trimesters. This explains why the drug has been assigned to the **D** pregnancy risk category when used in the first trimester.

Helpful Hints: This drug weakly interacts with grape-fruit and grapefruit juice, which can cause harmful, and even life-threatening, side effects. Before taking this drug with grapefruit juice, or before consuming grapefruit or grapefruit juice during the day while taking this drug, first read the section "Grapefruit Juice–Drug Interactions Can Make You Sick" in the appendix of this book. Then discuss this with your pharmacist or the healthcare provider who prescribed this drug.

Remember: All pregnancies have a background risk of about 3% for a major birth defect, even when mom doesn't take a drug of any kind. If you are pregnant or planning a pregnancy, always let your doctor know before taking any drug, prescription or non-prescription, or herbal remedy.

PRIMIDONE

Brand Name: Mysoline

Drug Use: This drug is approved by the FDA for the treatment of seizures, when used alone or in combination with other anticonvulsants.This drug is a member of the folic acid antagonist family of drugs. (See Helpful Hint on next page.)

Pregnancy Risk Category: D

Category D rating: The FDA assigns a drug to Category **D** when studies of pregnant women using the drug show evidence of fetal harm. Rarely, however, the potential benefit of using the drug in some life-threatening situations for mom may outweigh the potential risk of fetal harm. For example, when mom requires cancer treatment or when she has a serious disease for which safer drugs cannot be used or are less effective. Approximately 11% of prescription drugs fall in this category.

Animal Studies: No studies using this drug in pregnant animals were located.

Human Studies: There are no controlled studies using this drug in pregnant women. However, uncontrolled studies in pregnant women suggest an increased risk of fetal birth defects. The great majority of pregnant women taking this anticonvulsant medication deliver normal infants.

Helpful Hints:

1. Folic acid antagonists are drugs that limit the effectiveness of folic acid, making it more likely that a baby born to a mom taking one of these drugs might have a serious birth defect, such as an open spine. If you are taking a folic acid antagonist and trying to become pregnant, discuss the possibility of increasing your folic acid intake with your clinician before becoming pregnant. (See "Folic Acid Antagonist Drugs in Pregnancy" in the appendix for more details.)

2. There are other potential complications associated with using primidone during pregnancy. Neonatal hemorrhage with primidone alone or in combination with other anticonvulsants has been reported. This may be due to suppression of clotting factors which depend on vitamin K. Thus, when mom is receiving this drug, taking vitamin K preventatively immediately after birth is recommended by some experts.

3. In pregnant women with epilepsy, the first priority is to prevent seizures. This can be difficult because many seizure medications do not work quite as well during pregnancy. Sometimes the dose has to be increased or other medications added just to prevent seizures. Regardless, the

healthiest situation for both mom and unborn baby is to have the fewest seizures possible.

Remember: All pregnancies have a background risk of about 3% for a major birth defect, even when mom doesn't take a drug of any kind. If you are pregnant or planning a pregnancy, always let your doctor know before taking any drug, prescription or non-prescription, or herbal remedy.

. . . .

PROCAINAMIDE

Brand Name: Pronestyl

Drug Use: This drug is approved by the FDA for the treatment of heart arrhythmias.

Pregnancy Risk Category: C

Category C rating: The FDA assigns a drug to Category C for one of two reasons: (1) Studies show evidence of fetal harm when using the drug in pregnant animals, but no controlled studies have been done using the drug in pregnant women, or (2) Studies using the drug in pregnant animals have not been done, and studies of pregnant women using the drug are insufficient to reach a conclusion. Thus, the drug should only be used if the potential benefit for mom is greater than the potential risk of fetal harm, which, in many cases, is unknown. Approximately 50% of prescription drugs fall in this category.

Animal Studies: Studies using this drug in pregnant animals are not available.

Human Studies: Although controlled studies in pregnant women using this drug have not been done, this drug's limited use in pregnant women has not been associated with birth defects or other evidence of fetal harm.

Remember: All pregnancies have a background risk of about 3% for a major birth defect, even when mom doesn't

take a drug of any kind. If you are pregnant or planning a pregnancy, always let your doctor know before taking any drug, prescription or non-prescription, or herbal remedy.
. . . .

PROCHLORPERAZINE

Brand Name: Compazine. This drug is a member of the piperazine phenothiazine family of drugs.

Drug Uses: This drug is approved by the FDA for the control of nausea and vomiting, and the treatment of schizophrenia.

Pregnancy Risk Category: C

> **Category C rating:** The FDA assigns a drug to Category C for one of two reasons: (1) Studies show evidence of fetal harm when using the drug in pregnant animals, but no controlled studies have been done using the drug in pregnant women, or (2) Studies using the drug in pregnant animals have not been done, and studies of pregnant women using the drug are insufficient to reach a conclusion. Thus, the drug should only be used if the potential benefit for mom is greater than the potential risk of fetal harm, which, in many cases, is unknown. Approximately 50% of prescription drugs fall in this category.

Animal Studies: When pregnant rats were treated with this drug, an increase in birth defects was noted.

Human Studies: There are no controlled studies in pregnant women receiving this drug. However, there are isolated case reports of birth defects in children exposed to this drug in utero. Taken all together, most of the evidence suggests this drug is safe for mom and baby, according to experts.

Remember: All pregnancies have a background risk of about 3% for a major birth defect, even when mom doesn't take a drug of any kind. If you are pregnant or planning a pregnancy, always let your doctor know

before taking any drug, prescription or non-prescription, or herbal remedy.

. . . .

PROMETHAZINE

Brand Name: Phenergan

Drug Uses: This drug is approved by the FDA for the treatment of allergic rhinitis, conjunctivitis, the prevention of nausea and vomiting associated with surgery, the treatment of motion sickness, and nausea and vomiting in pregnancy.

Pregnancy Risk Category: C

> **Category C rating:** The FDA assigns a drug to Category C for one of two reasons: (1) Studies show evidence of fetal harm when using the drug in pregnant animals, but no controlled studies have been done using the drug in pregnant women, or (2) Studies using the drug in pregnant animals have not been done, and studies of pregnant women using the drug are insufficient to reach a conclusion. Thus, the drug should only be used if the potential benefit for mom is greater than the potential risk of fetal harm, which, in many cases, is unknown. Approximately 50% of prescription drugs fall in this category.

Animal Studies: When pregnant rats were treated with this drug, there was no increase in birth defects in the offspring.

Human Studies: There are no controlled studies in pregnant women. However, when phenergan tablets and suppositories are administered to pregnant women within two weeks of delivery, they may inhibit platelet aggregation, meaning the ability to aid in clotting, in the newborn. Limited data suggests that the use of phenergan during labor and delivery does not appreciably affect the duration of labor or delivery, and does not increase the risk for intervention in the newborn.

Remember: All pregnancies have a background risk of about 3% for a major birth defect, even when mom doesn't take a drug of any kind. If you are pregnant or planning a pregnancy, always let your doctor know before taking any drug, prescription or non-prescription, or herbal remedy.

· ·

PROPOXYPHENE

Brand Names: Darvon, Darvocet contains propoxyphene and acetaminophen

Drug Use: This drug is approved by the FDA for the relief of mild to moderate pain.

Pregnancy Risk Categories: This drug has been assigned two pregnancy risk categories: **C** when used for short periods during pregnancy and **D** if used for prolonged periods or in high doses near term. Approximately 12% of prescription drugs are assigned two pregnancy risk categories, depending on which trimester of pregnancy the drug is used.

Category C rating: The FDA assigns a drug to Category **C** for one of two reasons: (1) Studies show evidence of fetal harm when using the drug in pregnant animals, but no controlled studies have been done using the drug in pregnant women, or (2) Studies using the drug in pregnant animals have not been done, and studies of pregnant women using the drug are insufficient to reach a conclusion. Thus, the drug should only be used if the potential benefit for mom is greater than the potential risk of fetal harm, which, in many cases, is unknown. Approximately 50% of prescription drugs fall in this category.

Category D rating: The FDA assigns a drug to Category **D** when studies of pregnant women using the drug show evidence of fetal harm. Rarely, however, the potential benefit of using the drug in some life-threatening situations for mom may outweigh the potential risk of fetal harm. For example, when mom requires cancer treatment or when she has a serious disease for which safer drugs cannot be used or are less effective. Approximately 11% of prescription drugs fall in this category.

Animal Studies: Adequate studies of pregnant animals using this drug have not been done. However, pregnant rats and rabbits treated with this drug showed no evidence of an increased risk of birth defects.

Human Studies: There are no controlled studies in pregnant women. Neonates whose mothers have received this drug chronically in pregnancy may have respiratory depression or withdrawal symptoms at birth. Delivery room personnel should anticipate this possibility and be prepared to respond accordingly.

Remember: All pregnancies have a background risk of about 3% for a major birth defect, even when mom doesn't take a drug of any kind. If you are pregnant or planning a pregnancy, always let your doctor know before taking any drug, prescription or non-prescription, or herbal remedy.

PROPRANOLOL

Brand Name: Inderal

Drug Use: This drug has been used for a variety of purposes including the treatment of maternal hypertension (high blood pressure).

Pregnancy Risk Category: C

Category C rating: The FDA assigns a drug to Category C for one of two reasons: (1) Studies show evidence of fetal harm when using the drug in pregnant animals, but no controlled studies have been done using the drug in pregnant women, or (2) Studies using the drug in pregnant animals have not been done, and studies of pregnant women using the drug are insufficient to reach a conclusion. Thus, the drug should only be used if the potential benefit for mom is greater than the potential risk of fetal harm, which, in many cases, is unknown. Approximately 50% of prescription drugs fall in this category.

Animal Studies: When pregnant rats and rabbits were treated with this drug, they showed no evidence of an increase in birth defects in the offspring.

Human Studies: There are no controlled studies of this drug in pregnant women. There are, however, reports of growth restriction, small placentas, and birth defects when women received propranolol in pregnancy. Neonates whose mothers have received this drug before birth have shown low heart rates, low blood sugar, and respiratory depression after birth.

Remember: All pregnancies have a background risk of about 3% for a major birth defect, even when mom doesn't take a drug of any kind. If you are pregnant or planning a pregnancy, always let your doctor know before taking any drug, prescription or non-prescription, or herbal remedy.

PROPYLTHIOURACIL

Brand Name: Propylthiouracil

Drug Use: This drug is approved by the FDA for the treatment of hyperthyroidism. Some experts consider this drug the drug of choice for this condition.

Pregnancy Risk Category: D

> **Category D rating:** The FDA assigns a drug to Category **D** when studies of pregnant women using the drug show evidence of fetal harm. Rarely, however, the potential benefit of using the drug in some life-threatening situations for mom may outweigh the potential risk of fetal harm. For example, when mom requires cancer treatment or when she has a serious disease for which safer drugs cannot be used or are less effective. Approximately 11% of prescription drugs fall in this category.

Animal Studies: Relevant studies in pregnant animals are not available.

Human Studies: This drug crosses the placenta and may cause fetal harm in pregnant women by inducing a goiter and hypothyroidism in the developing fetus. This is why the drug has been assigned to pregnancy risk category **D**.

Remember: All pregnancies have a background risk of about 3% for a major birth defect, even when mom doesn't take a drug of any kind. If you are pregnant or planning a pregnancy, always let your doctor know before taking any drug, prescription or non-prescription, or herbal remedy.

PSEUDOEPHEDRINE

Brand Name: Advil Cold & Sinus, as well as 30 other preparations which contain this drug as an active ingredient.

Drug Use: This drug is approved by the FDA for the treatment of nasal congestion due to the common cold and hay fever.

Pregnancy Risk Category: C

> **Category C rating:** The FDA assigns a drug to Category **C** for one of two reasons: (1) Studies show evidence of fetal harm when using the drug in pregnant animals, but no controlled studies have been done using the drug in pregnant women, or (2) Studies using the drug in pregnant animals have not been done, and studies of pregnant women using the drug are insufficient to reach a conclusion. Thus, the drug should only be used if the potential benefit for mom is greater than the potential risk of fetal harm, which, in many cases, is unknown. Approximately 50% of prescription drugs fall in this category.

Animal Studies: This drug may cause birth defects in the offspring of some pregnant animals, but so far, not in humans.

Human Studies: No controlled studies have been done in pregnant women. Since the drug is often used in combination with other ingredients, it is often difficult to identify which ingredient is responsible for a certain defect, if at all. Studies have suggested that this drug may be linked to several intestinal birth defects, including gastroschisis, which is a condition characterized by part of the intestine developing outside the abdomen, and small bowel atresia, which is a congenital block of the small bowel. These findings, however, remain to be confirmed. Until this is done, it may be best to avoid this drug during the first trimester of pregnancy.

Remember: All pregnancies have a background risk of about 3% for a major birth defect, even when mom doesn't take a drug of any kind. If you are pregnant or planning a pregnancy, always let your doctor know before taking any drug, prescription or non-prescription, or herbal remedy.

PYRIDOSTIGMINE

Brand Names: Mestinon, Regonol

Drug Use: This drug is approved by the FDA for the treatment of myasthenia gravis.

Pregnancy Risk Category: C

> **Category C rating:** The FDA assigns a drug to Category **C** for one of two reasons: (1) Studies show evidence of fetal harm when using the drug in pregnant animals, but no controlled studies have been done using the drug in pregnant women, or (2) Studies using the drug in pregnant animals have not been done, and studies of pregnant women using the drug are insufficient to reach a conclusion. Thus, the drug should only be used if the potential benefit for mom is greater than the potential risk of fetal harm, which, in many cases, is unknown. Approximately 50% of prescription drugs fall in this category.

Animal Studies: When pregnant rats were treated with this drug, there was no increase in the incidence of birth defects.

Human Studies: No controlled studies of this drug in pregnant women have been done. Numerous reports, however, have described the safe use of this drug when taken by pregnant women. There was one case of microcephaly and other defects published in 2000 in which the authors attributed the defects to this drug.

Remember: All pregnancies have a background risk of about 3% for a major birth defect, even when mom doesn't take a drug of any kind. If you are pregnant or planning a pregnancy, always let your doctor know before taking any drug, prescription or non-prescription, or herbal remedy.

PYRIDOXINE

Brand Name: Pyridoxine

Drug Uses: This drug is vitamin B6 and is approved by the FDA to prevent and treat pyridoxine deficiency and to treat nausea and vomiting in pregnancy.

Pregnancy Risk Category: A

> **Category A rating:** The FDA assigns a drug to Category **A** when controlled studies using the drug in pregnant women do not show harmful fetal effects throughout pregnancy. Approximately 1% of prescription drugs fall in this category.

Animal Studies: Pyridoxine deficiency in pregnant animals is associated with cleft palate. When taken within reasonable doses, pyridoxine itself is not associated with birth defects in animals or humans.

Human Studies: Pyridoxine deficiency is a common problem in unsupplemented pregnant women. Pyridoxine supplementation with the recommended daily allowance is, in itself, not a cause of birth defects or toxicity in pregnant females or their newborns.

Remember: All pregnancies have a background risk of about 3% for a major birth defect, even when mom doesn't take a drug of any kind. If you are pregnant or planning a pregnancy, always let your doctor know before taking any drug, prescription or non-prescription, or herbal remedy.

∙ ∙

PYRIMETHAMINE

Brand Name: Daraprim

Drug Use: This drug is approved by the FDA for the treatment of toxoplasmosis and malaria in combination with other drugs. This drug is a member of the folic acid antagonist family of drugs. (See Helpful Hint on next page.)

Pregnancy Risk Category: C

> **Category C rating:** The FDA assigns a drug to Category C for one of two reasons: (1) Studies show evidence of fetal harm when using the drug in pregnant animals, but no controlled studies have been done using the drug in pregnant women, or (2) Studies using the drug in pregnant animals have not been done, and studies of pregnant women using the drug are insufficient to reach a conclusion. Thus, the drug should only be used if the potential benefit for mom is greater than the potential risk of fetal harm, which, in many cases, is unknown. Approximately 50% of prescription drugs fall in this category.

Animal Studies: In pregnant rats the drug was associated with a variety of birth defects when doses two to seven times that used in humans were used. The drug also causes birth defects in pregnant hamsters and small pigs.

Human Studies: No controlled studies have been done in pregnant women.

Helpful Hints: Folic acid antagonists are drugs that limit the effectiveness of folic acid, making it more likely that a baby born to a mom taking one of these drugs might have a serious birth defect, such as an open spine. If you are taking a folic acid antagonist and trying to become pregnant, discuss the possibility of increasing your folic acid intake with your clinician before becoming pregnant. (See "Folic Acid Antagonist Drugs in Pregnancy" in the appendix for more details.)

Remember: All pregnancies have a background risk of about 3% for a major birth defect, even when mom doesn't take a drug of any kind. If you are pregnant or planning a pregnancy, always let your doctor know before taking any drug, prescription or non-prescription, or herbal remedy.

. . . .

ADDITIONAL DRUGS AND THEIR FDA PREGNANCY RISK CATEGORIES

Since these additional drugs are uncommonly used in pregnancy, they are listed by generic name along with their FDA Pregnancy Risk Category without more detail:

Paliperidone - C	**Pegaptanib** - B
Palonosetron - B	**Pegaspargase** - C
Pamidronate - D	**Pegfilgrastim** - C
Pancuronium - C	**Pegvisomant** - B
Pantoprazole - B	**Pentamidine** - C

Pentoxifylline - C

Pergolide - B

Perindopril - C (D if used in the second or third trimester)

Phenazopyridine-B

Phentermine-C

Phentolamine - C

Phenylephrine - C

Physostigmine - C

Phytonadione - C

Pilocarpine - C

Pimecrolimus - C

Pimozide - C

Pioglitazone - C

Piperacillin - B

Podofilox - C

Polymyxin B - B

Posaconazole - C

Pramipexole - C

Pramlintide - C

Prazosin - C

Prednisolone - C (D if used in the first trimester)

Pregabalin - C

Primaquine - C

Procarbazine - D

Procyclidine - C

Propafenone - C

Propofol - B

Prussian Blue - C

Q

QUINAPRIL

Brand Name: Accupril. This drug belongs to the ACE inhibitor family of drugs. (See Helpful Hint on next page.)

Drug Use: This drug is approved by the FDA for the treatment of hypertension, which is high blood pressure.

Pregnancy Risk Categories: This drug has been assigned two pregnancy risk categories: **C** when used in the first trimester, and **D** when used in the second and third trimesters. Approximately 12% of prescription drugs are assigned two pregnancy risk categories, depending on which trimester of pregnancy the drug is used.

Category C rating: The FDA assigns a drug to Category **C** for one of two reasons: (1) Studies show evidence of fetal harm when using the drug in pregnant animals, but no controlled studies have been done using the drug in pregnant women, or (2) Studies using the drug in pregnant animals have not been done, and studies of pregnant women using the drug are insufficient to reach a conclusion. Thus, the drug should only be used if the potential benefit for mom is greater than the potential risk of fetal harm, which, in many cases, is unknown. Approximately 50% of prescription drugs fall in this category.

Category D rating: The FDA assigns a drug to Category **D** when studies of pregnant women using the drug show evidence of fetal harm. Rarely, however, the potential benefit of using the drug in some life-threatening situations for mom may outweigh the potential risk of fetal harm. For example, when mom requires cancer treatment or when she has a serious disease for which safer drugs cannot be used or are less effective. Approximately 11% of prescription drugs fall in this category.

Animal Studies: When pregnant rats and rabbits were treated with this drug, there was no increase in birth defects found.

Human Studies: No controlled studies in pregnant women have been done. However, the FDA has issued the following Black Box Warning:

"When used in pregnancy during the second and third trimesters, ACE inhibitors can cause injury and even death in the developing fetus. When pregnancy is detected, Accupril should be discontinued as soon as possible."

A Black Box Warning is the most serious prescription drug warning the FDA can require a drug company to issue.

Helpful Hints: The ACE inhibitor family of drugs are commonly used to treat hypertension, which is high blood pressure. The labels for these drugs have long included a Black Box Warning that women who become pregnant should be taken off ACE inhibitor drugs as soon as possible to avoid exposing the fetus in the second and third trimesters, when they are known to cause fetal birth defects, especially related to the kidneys. In addition, these drugs have been assigned a pregnancy risk category of **D** for the last six months, and **C** for the first three months of pregnancy.

Now, a more recent study has raised doubt about the safety of these drugs when taken during the first trimester of pregnancy. The uncontrolled study, published in 2006, showed that babies whose mothers had taken an ACE inhibitor during the first three months of pregnancy had an increased risk of birth defects when compared with babies whose mothers did not take any drugs for high blood pressure.

The FDA has not changed the first trimester of pregnancy risk category of C for these drugs. However, it has urged providers to take this information into account when prescribing one of these drugs for women of childbearing age. The FDA has also reiterated the need for providers to discontinue an ACE inhibitor as soon as possible if a patient taking one of these drugs becomes pregnant, (See "ACE Inhibitor Drugs in Pregnancy" in the appendix for more details.)

Remember: All pregnancies have a background risk of about 3% for a major birth defect, even when mom doesn't take a drug of any kind. If you are pregnant or planning a pregnancy, always let your doctor know before taking any drug, prescription or non-prescription, or herbal remedy.

QUINIDINE

Brand Name: Quinidine

Drug Use: This drug is approved by the FDA to restore a normal heart rhythm in patients with atrial fibrillation or flutter, and in patients with other ventricular arrhythmias.

Pregnancy Risk Category: C

Category C rating: The FDA assigns a drug to Category C for one of two reasons: (1) Studies show evidence of fetal harm when using the drug in pregnant animals, but no controlled studies have been done using the drug in pregnant women, or (2) Studies using the drug in pregnant animals have not been done, and studies of pregnant women using the drug are insufficient to reach a conclusion. Thus, the drug should only be used if the potential benefit for mom is greater than the potential risk of fetal harm, which, in many cases, is unknown. Approximately 50% of prescription drugs fall in this category.

Animal Studies: No studies using this drug in pregnant animals were found.

Human Studies: No controlled studies using this drug in pregnant women have been done. This drug has been used in pregnancy for some 90 years. In therapeutic doses, it is considered relatively safe for the fetus by most experts.

Helpful Hints: This drug weakly interacts with grapefruit and grapefruit juice, which can cause harmful, and even life-threatening, side effects. Before taking this drug with grapefruit juice, or before consuming grapefruit or grapefruit juice during the day while taking this drug, first read the section "Grapefruit Juice–Drug Interactions Can Make You Sick" in the appendix of this book. Then discuss this with your pharmacist or the healthcare provider who prescribed this drug.

Remember: All pregnancies have a background risk of about 3% for a major birth defect, even when mom doesn't take a drug of any kind. If you are pregnant or planning a pregnancy, always let your doctor know before taking any drug, prescription or non-prescription, or herbal remedy.

ADDITIONAL DRUGS AND THEIR FDA PREGNANCY RISK CATEGORIES

Since these additional drugs are uncommonly used in pregnancy, they are listed by generic name along with their FDA Pregnancy Risk Category without more detail:

Quetiapine - C
Quinine - D (X according to manufacturer, Merrell Dow)
Quinupristin - B

R

RALOXIFENE

Brand Name: Evista

Drug Uses: This drug is approved by the FDA for the prevention of osteoporosis in post-menopausal women, as well as to prevent breast cancer.

Pregnancy Risk Category: X

> **Category X rating:** The FDA assigns a drug to Category **X** when studies have shown the risk of fetal harm clearly outweighs any potential maternal benefit from the drug. **Drugs in this category should not be used by pregnant women.** Approximately 5% of prescription drugs fall in this category.

Animal Studies: When pregnant animals were treated with this drug, significant fetal birth defects were found in the offspring as well as miscarriages in the pregnancies. As a result, the drug was assigned to pregnancy risk category **X**.

Human Studies: No studies have been done in pregnant women treated with this medication and compared to untreated pregnant women.

Helpful Hints: In pregnant animal studies using raloxifene, the drug caused a range of problems, from miscarriages and birth defects to delayed labor and delivery. As a result, the FDA assigned the drug to pregnancy risk category **X**, meaning it should never be taken by a pregnant woman. If you are taking raloxifene and pregnancy occurs, it is important that you notify your healthcare provider right away.

Remember: All pregnancies have a background risk of about 3% for a major birth defect, even when mom doesn't take a drug of any kind. If you are pregnant or planning a pregnancy, always let your doctor know before taking any drug, prescription or non-prescription, or herbal remedy.

• •

RAMIPRIL

Brand Name: Altace

Drug Use: This drug is approved by the FDA for the treatment of hypertension. It is a member of the ACE inhibitor family of drugs. (See Helpful Hint on next page.)

Pregnancy Risk Categories: This drug has been assigned two pregnancy risk categories: **C** when used in the first trimester, and **D** when used in the second and third trimesters. Approximately 12% of prescription drugs are assigned two pregnancy risk categories, depending on which trimester of pregnancy the drug is used.

Category C rating: The FDA assigns a drug to Category **C** for one of two reasons: (1) Studies show evidence of fetal harm when using the drug in pregnant animals, but no controlled studies have been done using the drug in pregnant women, or (2) Studies using the drug in pregnant animals have not been done, and studies of pregnant women using the drug are insufficient to reach a conclusion. Thus, the drug should only be used if the potential benefit for mom is greater than the potential risk of fetal harm, which, in many cases, is unknown. Approximately 50% of prescription drugs fall in this category.

Category D rating: The FDA assigns a drug to Category **D** when studies of pregnant women using the drug show evidence of fetal harm. Rarely, however, the potential benefit of using the drug in some life-threatening situations for mom may outweigh the potential risk of fetal harm. For example, when mom requires cancer treatment or when she has a serious disease for which safer drugs cannot be used or are less effective. Approximately 11% of prescription drugs fall in this category.

Animal Studies: When pregnant rats, rabbits, and monkeys were treated with this drug, there was no increase in the incidence of birth defects.

Human Studies: There have been no studies in which pregnant women were treated with this drug and compared to untreated pregnant women. There is, however, the following Black Box Warning:

"When used in pregnancy during the second and third trimesters, ACE inhibitors can cause injury and even death to the developing fetus. When pregnancy is detected, Altace should be discontinued as soon as possible."

A Black Box Warning is the most serious prescription drug warning the FDA can require a drug company to issue.

Helpful Hints: The ACE inhibitor family of drugs is commonly used to treat hypertension, which is high blood pressure. The labels for these drugs have long included a Black Box Warning mentioned above. In addition, these drugs are assigned a pregnancy risk category of **D** for the last six months of pregnancy, and **C** for the first three months of pregnancy.

Now, a more recent study has raised doubt about the safety of these drugs when taken during the first trimester of pregnancy. The uncontrolled study, published in 2006, showed that babies whose mothers had taken an ACE inhibitor during the first three months of pregnancy had an increased risk of birth defects when compared with babies whose mothers did not take any drugs for high blood pressure.

The FDA has not changed the first trimester pregnancy risk category of **C** for these drugs. However, it has urged providers to take this information into account when prescribing one of these drugs for women of childbearing age. The FDA has also reiterated the need for providers to discontinue an ACE inhibitor as soon as possible if a patient taking one of these drugs becomes pregnant. (See "ACE Inhibitor Drugs in Pregnancy" in the appendix for more details.)

Remember: All pregnancies have a background risk of about 3% for a major birth defect, even when mom doesn't take a drug of any kind. If you are pregnant or planning a pregnancy, always let your doctor know before taking any drug, prescription or non-prescription, or herbal remedy.

• •

RANITIDINE

Brand Name: Zantac

Drug Use: This drug is approved by the FDA for maintenance therapy and active treatment of duodenal ulcers, stomach ulcers, and erosive esophagitis.

Pregnancy Risk Category: B

> **Category B rating:** The FDA assigns a drug to Category **B** for one of two reasons: (1) Studies show no evidence of fetal harm when using the drug in pregnant animals, but no controlled studies have been done using the drug in pregnant women, or (2) Studies show evidence of fetal harm when using the drug in pregnant animals, but controlled studies using the drug in pregnant women do not show evidence of fetal harm. Approximately 21% of prescription drugs fall in this category.

Animal Studies: When pregnant rats and rabbits were treated with this drug, there was no evidence of impaired fertility or an increase in birth defects in the offspring.

Human Studies: No studies have been done in which pregnant women were treated with this drug and compared to pregnant women not treated with this drug.

Remember: All pregnancies have a background risk of about 3% for a major birth defect, even when mom doesn't take a drug of any kind. If you are pregnant or planning a pregnancy, always let your doctor know before taking any drug, prescription or non-prescription, or herbal remedy.

. . . .

RIBAVIRIN

Brand Names: Virazole, Copegus, Rebetol

Drug Use: In combination with the drug Pegasys, this drug is used to treat adults with chronic hepatitis C.

Pregnancy Risk Category: X

> **Category X rating:** The FDA assigns a drug to Category **X** when studies have shown the risk of fetal harm clearly outweighs any potential maternal benefit from the drug. **Drugs in this category should not be used by pregnant women.** Approximately 5% of prescription drugs fall in this category.

Animal Studies: When various pregnant animal species were treated with this drug, it caused birth defects in the offspring. This also occurred even when doses as low as 120th the human dose of ribarvirin was used.

Human Studies: There have been no studies of pregnant women treated with this drug and compared to pregnant women not treated with this drug.

Helpful Hints: The FDA has issued the following Black Box Warning:

"Ribavirin may cause birth defects and/or death of the exposed fetus. Extreme care must be taken to avoid pregnancy in female patients and in female partners of male patients. Ribavirin has demonstrated significant teratogenic effects, meaning it causes birth defects and/or embryocidal effects, meaning it destroys the embryo in all animal studies that have been conducted. These effects occurred at doses as low as 120th of the recommended human dose of Ribavirin. Copegus therapy should not be started unless a report of a negative pregnancy test has been obtained immediately prior to planned initiation of therapy. Patients should be instructed to use at least two forms of effective contraception during treatment and for six months after treatment has been stopped. Pregnancy testing should occur monthly during Copegus therapy and for six months after therapy has stopped."

A Black Box Warning is the most serious warning the FDA can issue, short of withdrawing a drug from the market.

Remember: All pregnancies have a background risk of about 3% for a major birth defect, even when mom doesn't take a drug of any kind. If you are pregnant or planning a pregnancy, always let your doctor know before taking any drug, prescription or non-prescription, or herbal remedy.

• •

RIFAMPIN

Brand Name: Rifadin

Drug Uses: This drug is approved by the FDA for use in treating all forms of tuberculosis and for the treatment of carriers of meningococcus to eliminate the bacteria from the throat.

Pregnancy Risk Category: C

> **Category C rating:** The FDA assigns a drug to Category C for one of two reasons: (1) Studies show evidence of fetal harm when using the drug in pregnant animals, but no controlled studies have been done using the drug in pregnant women, or (2) Studies using the drug in pregnant animals have not been done, and studies of pregnant women using the drug are insufficient to reach a conclusion. Thus, the drug should only be used if the potential benefit for

mom is greater than the potential risk of fetal harm, which, in many cases, is unknown. Approximately 50% of prescription drugs fall in this category.

Animal Studies: When pregnant mice and rats were treated with this drug, an increased number of cleft palates were noted in the mice offspring and spina bifida (open spine) in rat offspring. Toxic effects were also reported in pregnant rabbits treated with this drug.

Human Studies: There have been no studies of pregnant women treated with this drug and compared to pregnant women not treated with this drug. However, isolated cases of fetal malformations have been reported.

When administered during the last few weeks of pregnancy, rifampin can cause post-natal hemorrhages in the mother and infant for which treatment with vitamin K may be indicated.

Remember: All pregnancies have a background risk of about 3% for a major birth defect, even when mom doesn't take a drug of any kind. If you are pregnant or planning a pregnancy, always let your doctor know before taking any drug, prescription or non-prescription, or herbal remedy.

RIFAXIMIN

Brand Name: Xifaxan

Drug Use: This antibiotic is approved by the FDA for the treatment of patients with travelers' diarrhea.

Pregnancy Risk Category: C

Category C rating: The FDA assigns a drug to Category **C** for one of two reasons: (1) Studies show evidence of fetal harm when using the drug in pregnant animals, but no controlled studies have been done using the drug in pregnant women, or (2) Studies using the drug in pregnant animals have not been done, and studies of pregnant women using the drug are insufficient to reach a conclusion. Thus, the drug should only be used if the potential benefit for mom is greater than the potential risk of fetal harm, which, in many cases, is unknown. Approximately 50% of prescription drugs fall in this category.

Animal Studies: When pregnant rats and rabbits were treated with this drug, a variety of birth defects were noted in some of the offspring.

Human Studies: There are no studies in which pregnant women have been treated with this drug and compared to pregnant women not treated with this drug.

Remember: All pregnancies have a background risk of about 3% for a major birth defect, even when mom doesn't take a drug of any kind. If you are pregnant or planning a pregnancy, always let your doctor know before taking any drug, prescription or non-prescription, or herbal remedy.

∙ ∙

RISPERIDONE

Brand Name: Risperdal

Drug Use: This antipsychotic drug is approved by the FDA for the treatment of schizophrenia. This drug is a member of the folic acid antagonist family of drugs. (See Helpful Hint on next page.)

Pregnancy Risk Category: C

Category C rating: The FDA assigns a drug to Category **C** for one of two reasons: (1) Studies show evidence of fetal harm when using the drug in pregnant animals, but no controlled studies have been done using the drug in pregnant women, or (2) Studies using the drug in pregnant animals have not been done, and studies of pregnant women using the drug are insufficient to reach a conclusion. Thus, the drug should only be used if the potential benefit for mom is greater than the potential risk of fetal harm, which, in many cases, is unknown. Approximately 50% of prescription drugs fall in this category.

Animal Studies: When pregnant animals were treated with this drug there was no increased incidence of birth defects in the offspring. However, stillbirths and pup toxicity have occurred.

Human Studies: There have been no studies of pregnant women treated with this drug and compared to pregnant women not treated with this drug.

Helpful Hints: Folic acid antagonists like risperidone are drugs that limit the effectiveness of folic acid, making it more likely that a baby born to a mom taking one of these drugs might have a serious birth defect, such as an open spine. If you are taking a folic acid antagonist and trying to become pregnant, discuss the possibility of increasing your folic acid intake with your clinician before becoming pregnant. (See "Folic Acid Antagonist Drugs in Pregnancy" in the appendix for more details.)

Remember: All pregnancies have a background risk of about 3% for a major birth defect, even when mom doesn't take a drug of any kind. If you are pregnant or planning a pregnancy, always let your doctor know before taking any drug, prescription or non-prescription, or herbal remedy.

ROFECOXIB

Brand Name: Vioxx

Drug Use: This drug is approved by the FDA for the treatment of pain from osteoarthritis and rheumatoid arthritis. It is a member of the non-steroidal anti-inflammatory family of drugs (NSAIDs). (See Helpful Hint on next page.)

Pregnancy Risk Categories: This drug has been assigned two pregnancy risk categories: **C** when used in the first and second trimesters, and **D** when used in the third trimester or near delivery. Approximately 12% of prescription drugs are assigned two pregnancy risk categories, depending on which trimester of pregnancy the drug is used.

Category C rating: The FDA assigns a drug to Category **C** for one of two reasons: (1) Studies show evidence of fetal harm when using the drug in pregnant animals, but no controlled studies have been done using the drug in pregnant women, or (2) Studies using the drug in pregnant animals have not been done, and studies of pregnant women using the drug are insufficient to reach a conclusion. Thus, the drug should only be used if the potential benefit for mom is greater than the potential risk of fetal harm, which, in many cases, is unknown. Approximately 50% of prescription drugs fall in this category.

Category D rating: The FDA assigns a drug to Category **D** when studies of pregnant women using the drug show evidence of fetal harm. Rarely, however, the potential benefit of using the drug in some life-threatening situations for mom may outweigh the potential risk of fetal harm. For example, when mom requires cancer treatment or when she has a serious disease for which safer drugs cannot be used or are less effective. Approximately 11% of prescription drugs fall in this category.

Animal Studies: When pregnant rats and rabbits were treated with this drug, no increase in the incidence of birth defects in the offspring was noted.

Human Studies: There have been no studies in pregnant women taking this drug and compared to pregnant women not taking this drug.

Helpful Hints:

1. This drug was voluntarily withdrawn from the market on September 30, 2004. However, it may still be available for special use through the manufacturer.

2. When taken in the third trimester of pregnancy, NSAIDs have seriously harmed the fetus, leading to life-threatening illness after birth and

even death. These potential effects apply to all NSAIDs, whether purchased by prescription or over-the-counter without a prescription. They also explain why NSAIDs have been assigned a **D** pregnancy risk category. (See "Non-Steroidal, Anti-Inflammatory Drugs (NSAIDs) in Pregnancy" in the appendix for more details.)

Remember: All pregnancies have a background risk of about 3% for a major birth defect, even when mom doesn't take a drug of any kind. If you are pregnant or planning a pregnancy, always let your doctor know before taking any drug, prescription or non-prescription, or herbal remedy.

ADDITIONAL DRUGS AND THEIR FDA PREGNANCY RISK CATEGORIES

Since these additional drugs are uncommonly used in pregnancy, they are listed by generic name along with their FDA Pregnancy Risk Category without more detail:

Rabeprazole - B	**Risedronate** - C
Rabies Vaccine - C	**Ritonavir** - B
Ramelteon - C	**Rituximab** - C
Ranolazine - C	**Rivastigmine** - B
Rasagiline - C	**Rizatriptan** - C
Rasburicase - C	**Rocuronium** - C
Repaglinide - C	**Ropinirole** - C
Reteplase - C	**Rosiglitazone** - C
Riluzole - C	**Rosuvastatin** - X
Rimantadine - C	

S

SALMETEROL

Brand Names: Serevent, Advair (when used in combination with fluticasone)

Drug Uses: This drug is approved by the FDA for the treatment of asthma and chronic obstructive pulmonary disease.

Pregnancy Risk Category: C

Category C rating: The FDA assigns a drug to Category **C** for one of two reasons: (1) Studies show evidence of fetal harm when using the drug in pregnant animals, but no controlled studies have been done using the drug in pregnant women, or (2) Studies using the drug in pregnant animals have not been done, and studies of pregnant women using the drug are insufficient to reach a conclusion. Thus, the drug should only be used if the potential benefit for mom is greater than the potential risk of fetal harm, which, in many cases, is unknown. Approximately 50% of prescription drugs fall in this category.

Animal Studies: When pregnant rats were treated with this drug, no fetal harm was found in the offspring. However, when pregnant rabbits were treated, toxic effects were found when 50 times the maximum human dose was used.

Human Studies: There have been no studies in pregnant women in which they were treated with this drug and compared to pregnant women not treated with this drug. Because of the potential for interference with the ability of the uterus to contract in labor, use of this drug during labor should be restricted to those patients in whom the benefit clearly is greater than the risk.

Remember: All pregnancies have a background risk of about 3% for a major birth defect, even when mom doesn't take a drug of any kind. If you are pregnant or planning a pregnancy, always let your doctor know before taking any drug, prescription or non-prescription, or herbal remedy.

· ·

SCOPOLAMINE

Brand Name: Transderm Scop

Drug Use: This drug is approved by the FDA for the prevention and treatment of nausea and vomiting associated with motion sickness and recovery from surgery and anesthesia.

Pregnancy Risk Category: C

> **Category C rating:** The FDA assigns a drug to Category C for one of two reasons: (1) Studies show evidence of fetal harm when using the drug in pregnant animals, but no controlled studies have been done using the drug in pregnant women, or (2) Studies using the drug in pregnant animals have not been done, and studies of pregnant women using the drug are insufficient to reach a conclusion. Thus, the drug should only be used if the potential benefit for mom is greater than the potential risk of fetal harm, which, in many cases, is unknown. Approximately 50% of prescription drugs fall in this category.

Animal Studies: When pregnant rats were treated with this drug, no evidence of fetal harm was found in the offspring. In addition, when pregnant rabbits were treated with this drug, there was marginal harm to the embryo when the dose reached 100 times the maximum human dose.

Human Studies: During a clinical study among women undergoing cesarean section treated with scopolamine in conjunction with epidural anesthesia and opiate analgesia, no evidence of central nervous system depression

358 *Secobarbital*

was found in the newborns. There are no other controlled studies using this drug in pregnant women.

Helpful Hints: This drug weakly interacts with grapefruit and grapefruit juice, which can cause harmful, and even life-threatening, side effects. Before taking this drug with grapefruit juice, or before consuming grapefruit or grapefruit juice during the day while taking this drug, first read the section "Grapefruit Juice–Drug Interactions Can Make You Sick" in the appendix of this book. Then discuss this with your pharmacist or the healthcare provider who prescribed this drug.

Remember: All pregnancies have a background risk of about 3% for a major birth defect, even when mom doesn't take a drug of any kind. If you are pregnant or planning a pregnancy, always let your doctor know before taking any drug, prescription or non-prescription, or herbal remedy.

SECOBARBITAL

Brand Name: Seconal

Drug Uses: This drug is approved by the FDA as a sedative for short-term treatment for insomnia and as a pre-anesthestic. This drug is a member of the barbiturate family of drugs.

Pregnancy Risk Category: D

> **Category D rating:** The FDA assigns a drug to Category **D** when studies of pregnant women using the drug show evidence of fetal harm. Rarely, however, the potential benefit of using the drug in some life-threatening situations for mom may outweigh the potential risk of fetal harm. For example, when mom requires cancer treatment or when she has a serious disease for which safer drugs cannot be used or are less effective. Approximately 11% of prescription drugs fall in this category.

Animal Studies: There have been no reports linking secobarbital with birth defects in animals.

Human Studies: There have been no studies in pregnant women in which a group of pregnant women were treated with this drug and compared to a group of pregnant women not treated with this drug.

Helpful Hints: The main reason this drug has been assigned to pregnancy risk category **D** is because administration of drugs in the barbiturate family of drugs to the mother during labor has resulted in respiratory depression in the newborn. Premature infants are particularly susceptible to these depressant effects. If a barbiturate such as Seconal is used during labor and delivery, resuscitation equipment and trained personnel should be available to deal with any problems. Moreover, there are reports of infants suffering from long-term barbiturate exposure in utero which have resulted in acute withdrawal featuring seizures and increased irritability from birth or with a delayed onset for up to 14 days after birth.

Remember: All pregnancies have a background risk of about 3% for a major birth defect, even when mom doesn't take a drug of any kind. If you are pregnant or planning a pregnancy, always let your doctor know before taking any drug, prescription or non-prescription, or herbal remedy.

SERTRALINE

Brand Name: Zoloft. This drug belongs to the selective serotonin reuptake inhibitor (SSRI) family of drugs.

Drug Uses: This drug is approved by the FDA for the treatment of major depressive disorder in adults, obsessive-compulsive disorder, panic disorder, post traumatic stress disorder, premenstrual problems, and social anxiety disorder.

Pregnancy Risk Categories: This drug has been assigned two pregnancy risk categories: **C** when used in the first half of pregnancy, and **D** when used in the second half of pregnancy. Approximately 12% of prescription drugs are assigned two pregnancy risk categories, depending on which trimester of pregnancy the drug is used.

> **Category C rating:** The FDA assigns a drug to Category **C** for one of two reasons: (1) Studies show evidence of fetal harm when using the drug in pregnant animals, but no controlled studies have been done using the drug in pregnant women, or (2) Studies using the drug in pregnant animals have not been done, and studies of pregnant women using the drug are insufficient to reach a conclusion. Thus, the drug should only be used if the potential benefit for mom is greater than the potential risk of fetal harm, which, in many cases, is unknown. Approximately 50% of prescription drugs fall in this category.

> **Category D rating:** The FDA assigns a drug to Category **D** when studies of pregnant women using the drug show evidence of fetal harm. Rarely, however, the potential benefit of using the drug in some life-threatening situations for mom may outweigh the potential risk of fetal harm. For example, when mom requires cancer treatment or when she has a serious disease for which safer drugs cannot be used or are less effective. Approximately 11% of prescription drugs fall in this category.

Animal Studies: Studies using this drug in pregnant animals suggest the drug is not a significant cause of birth defects in animals.

Human Studies: There are no controlled studies using this drug in pregnant women. However, there are numerous case reports involving SSRIs which have led to the **D** pregnancy risk category for this family of drugs when used in second half of pregnancy.

Newborns exposed to members of the SSRI family of drugs in the second half of pregnancy have developed complications immediately after birth. These complications have required hospitalization, respiratory support, and tube feeding. These features are consistent with either a direct toxic effect of the drug or, possibly, abrupt withdrawal from the drug which occurs at birth, once the umbilical cord is cut. When treating a woman with a SSRI during the second half of pregnancy, the physician should carefully weigh these potential risks to the baby and the benefits of treatment to the mother.

Helpful Hints:

1. Studies show that antidepressants increase the risk of suicidal thinking and behavior in children, adolescents, and young adults. Anyone considering the use of this drug or any other antidepressant in these patients must balance that risk with the clinical need.

2. Almost all antidepressants carry some risk to the developing fetus. However, we also know depression in a pregnant woman carries potential risk for her health and for her unborn baby; for example, low birth weight and prematurity. The risks and benefits of medications and untreated depression must be weighed carefully. If you are pregnant and think you may have depression, or if you already know you do, talk with your doctor so the two of you can create the right plan for you and your unborn baby. (See "Antidepressants in Pregnancy" in the appendix for more details.)

3. This drug weakly interacts with grapefruit and grapefruit juice, which can cause harmful, and even

life-threatening, side effects. Before taking this drug with grapefruit juice, or before consuming grapefruit or grapefruit juice during the day while taking this drug, first read the section "Grapefruit Juice–Drug Interactions Can Make You Sick" in the appendix of this book. Then discuss this with your pharmacist or the healthcare provider who prescribed this drug.

Remember: All pregnancies have a background risk of about 3% for a major birth defect, even when mom doesn't take a drug of any kind. If you are pregnant or planning a pregnancy, always let your doctor know before taking any drug, prescription or non-prescription, or herbal remedy.

SIMVASTATIN

Brand Name: Zocor. This drug is a member of the statin family of drugs.

Drug Uses: This drug is approved by the FDA for lowering serum cholesterol and lowering the risk of coronary heart disease.

Pregnancy Risk Category: X

> **Category X rating:** The FDA assigns a drug to Category **X** when studies have shown the risk of fetal harm clearly outweighs any potential maternal benefit from the drug. **Drugs in this category should not be used by pregnant women.** Approximately 5% of prescription drugs fall in this category.

Animal Studies: Pregnant rats and rabbits treated with simvastatin showed no evidence of fetal harm. However, skeletal malformations have been identified in the offspring of pregnant rats and mice treated with other members of the statin family of drugs.

Human Studies: There are no studies in which pregnant women were treated with this drug and compared to pregnant women not treated with this drug.

Helpful Hints:

1. Drugs that belong to the statin family of drugs, such as this one, should only be prescribed for women of childbearing age when they are highly unlikely to conceive and have been informed of the potential hazards, according to the FDA. Why? Because cholesterol is essential for normal fetal development, and anything that lowers the serum level of cholesterol—which is what statins do—might adversely affect fetal development. If a woman becomes pregnant while taking this drug, or any member of the statin family of drugs, it should be discontinued immediately and she should be told of the potential hazard to her unborn baby.

2. This drug strongly interacts with grapefruit and grapefruit juice, which can cause harmful, and even life-threatening, side effects. Before taking this drug with grapefruit juice, or before consuming grapefruit or grapefruit juice during the day while taking this drug, first read the section "Grapefruit Juice–Drug Interactions Can Make You Sick" in the appendix of this book. Then discuss this with your pharmacist or the healthcare provider who prescribed this drug.

Remember: All pregnancies have a background risk of about 3% for a major birth defect, even when mom doesn't take a drug of any kind. If you are pregnant or planning a pregnancy, always let your doctor know

before taking any drug, prescription or non-prescription, or herbal remedy.

. . . .

SPIRONOLACTONE

Brand Name: Aldactone

Drug Use: This drug is approved by the FDA for use as a diuretic to treat hypertension, or high blood pressure.

Pregnancy Risk Categories: This drug has been assigned two pregnancy risk categories: **C** if not used for the treatment of gestational hypertension, and **D** if used for the treatment of gestational hypertension. Why? Because diuretics are not recommended for treating gestational hypertension since these women have a low blood volume already and the use of a diuretic will only deplete their blood volume further. Approximately 12% of prescription drugs are assigned two pregnancy risk categories, depending on which trimester of pregnancy the drug is used.

Category C rating: The FDA assigns a drug to Category **C** for one of two reasons: (1) Studies show evidence of fetal harm when using the drug in pregnant animals, but no controlled studies have been done using the drug in pregnant women, or (2) Studies using the drug in pregnant animals have not been done, and studies of pregnant women using the drug are insufficient to reach a conclusion. Thus, the drug should only be used if the potential benefit for mom is greater than the potential risk of fetal harm, which, in many cases, is unknown. Approximately 50% of prescription drugs fall in this category.

Category D rating: The FDA assigns a drug to Category **D** when studies of pregnant women using the drug show evidence of fetal harm. Rarely, however, the potential benefit of using the drug in some life-threatening situations for mom may outweigh the potential risk of fetal harm. For example, when mom requires cancer treatment or when she has a serious disease for which safer drugs cannot be used or are less effective. Approximately 11% of prescription drugs fall in this category.

Animal Studies: When pregnant mice were treated with this drug, the findings revealed no adverse effects in the offspring. However, when pregnant rabbits were treated with this drug, a lower number of live fetuses were observed. In addition, the drug caused feminization of male rat fetuses.

Human Studies: There are no studies in which pregnant women were treated with this drug and compared to pregnant women not treated with this drug. However, because of the findings in pregnant animals, the use of spironolactone in pregnant women requires that the anticipated benefit be weighed against the possible hazards to the fetus. Otherwise, there are no reports linking the drug with human birth defects.

Remember: All pregnancies have a background risk of about 3% for a major birth defect, even when mom doesn't take a drug of any kind. If you are pregnant or planning a pregnancy, always let your doctor know before taking any drug, prescription or non-prescription, or herbal remedy.

. . . .

STREPTOMYCIN

Brand Name: Streptomycin. This drug belongs to the aminoglycoside family of antibiotics.

Drug Use: This drug is approved by the FDA for use in treating a variety of bacterial infections.

Pregnancy Risk Category: **D**

Category D rating: The FDA assigns a drug to Category **D** when studies of pregnant women using the drug show evidence of fetal harm. Rarely, however, the potential benefit of using the drug in some life-threatening situations for mom may outweigh the potential risk of fetal harm. For example, when mom requires cancer treatment or when she has a serious disease for which safer drugs cannot be used or are less effective. Approximately 11% of prescription drugs fall in this category.

Animal Studies: No reports of pregnant animals treated with this drug could be located.

Human Studies: Although members of the aminoglycoside family of drugs have caused hearing impairment in the fetus when used during pregnancy, based on uncontrolled studies in pregnant women, the risk of hearing impairment happening with this drug appears to be lower than that of other members of the aminoglycoside family of drugs.

Remember: All pregnancies have a background risk of about 3% for a major birth defect, even when mom doesn't take a drug of any kind. If you are pregnant or planning a pregnancy, always let your doctor know before taking any drug, prescription or non-prescription, or herbal remedy.

· ·

SULBACTAM

Brand Name: Unasyn, which is the combination of ampicillin and sulbactam

Drug Use: When used alone, this drug lacks effective anti-bacterial activity. However, when combined with ampicillin, its activity is significantly extended.

Pregnancy Risk Category: B

Category B rating: The FDA assigns a drug to Category **B** for one of two reasons: (1) Studies show no evidence of fetal harm when using the drug in pregnant animals, but no controlled studies have been done using the drug in pregnant women, or (2) Studies show evidence of fetal harm when using the drug in pregnant animals, but controlled studies using the drug in pregnant women do not show evidence of fetal harm. Approximately 21% of prescription drugs fall in this category.

Animal Studies: When pregnant rats, mice, and rabbits were treated with approximately ten times the human dose of this drug, there was no evidence of fetal harm in the offspring.

Human Studies: There have been no studies in which pregnant women were treated with this drug and compared to pregnant women not treated with this drug.

Remember: All pregnancies have a background risk of about 3% for a major birth defect, even when mom doesn't take a drug of any kind. If you are pregnant or planning a pregnancy, always let your doctor know before taking any drug, prescription or non-prescription, or herbal remedy.

SULFASALAZINE

Brand Name: Azulfidine

Drug Use: This drug is approved by the FDA for the treatment of ulcerative colitis. This drug is a member of the folic acid antagonist family of drugs. (See Helpful Hint on next page.)

Pregnancy Risk Categories: This drug has been assigned two pregnancy risk categories: **B** when used throughout most of pregnancy, and **D** if given near term. Approximately 12% of prescription drugs are assigned two pregnancy risk categories, depending on which trimester of pregnancy the drug is used.

> **Category B rating:** The FDA assigns a drug to Category **B** for one of two reasons: (1) Studies show no evidence of fetal harm when using the drug in pregnant animals, but no controlled studies have been done using the drug in pregnant women, or (2) Studies show evidence of fetal harm when using the drug in pregnant animals, but controlled studies using the drug in pregnant women do not show evidence of fetal harm. Approximately 21% of prescription drugs fall in this category.

Category D rating: The FDA assigns a drug to Category **D** when studies of pregnant women using the drug show evidence of fetal harm. Rarely, however, the potential benefit of using the drug in some life-threatening situations for mom may outweigh the potential risk of fetal harm. For example, when mom requires cancer treatment or when she has a serious disease for which safer drugs cannot be used or are less effective. Approximately 11% of prescription drugs fall in this category.

Animal Studies: Pregnant rats and rabbits treated with this drug at 6 times the human dose showed no evidence of fetal harm in the offspring.

Human Studies: There have been no controlled studies in pregnant women in which one group was treated with this drug and compared to another group not treated with this drug. Since sulfasalazine is a member of the sulfonamide family of drugs, and other members of the family have caused jaundice in the newborn when the drug has been given near term, and this level of jaundice in the newborn can reach high levels, this mainly accounts for the assignment of this drug to category **D** if taken near term.

Helpful Hints: Folic acid antagonists like sulfasalazine are drugs that limit the effectiveness of folic acid, making it more likely that a baby born to a mom taking one of these drugs might have a serious birth defect, such as an open spine. If you are taking a folic acid antagonist and trying to become pregnant, discuss the possibility of increasing your folic acid intake with your clinician before becoming pregnant. (See "Folic Acid Antagonist Drugs in Pregnancy" in the appendix for more details.)

Remember: All pregnancies have a background risk of about 3% for a major birth defect, even when mom

doesn't take a drug of any kind. If you are pregnant or planning a pregnancy, always let your doctor know before taking any drug, prescription or non-prescription, or herbal remedy.

. . . .

SULFISOXAZOLE

Brand Name: Gantrisin

Drug Use: This antibiotic is approved by the FDA for the treatment of middle ear infections. This drug is a member of the folic acid antagonist family of drugs. (See Helpful Hint on next page.)

Pregnancy Risk Categories: This drug has been assigned two pregnancy risk categories: **C** when used throughout pregnancy, and **D** when used near term, as are all members of the sulfonamide family of drugs. Approximately 12% of prescription drugs are assigned two pregnancy risk categories, depending on which trimester of pregnancy the drug is used.

> **Category C rating:** The FDA assigns a drug to Category **C** for one of two reasons: (1) Studies show evidence of fetal harm when using the drug in pregnant animals, but no controlled studies have been done using the drug in pregnant women, or (2) Studies using the drug in pregnant animals have not been done, and studies of pregnant women using the drug are insufficient to reach a conclusion. Thus, the drug should only be used if the potential benefit for mom is greater than the potential risk of fetal harm, which, in many cases, is unknown. Approximately 50% of prescription drugs fall in this category.
>
> **Category D rating:** The FDA assigns a drug to Category **D** when studies of pregnant women using the drug show evidence of fetal harm. Rarely, however, the potential benefit of using the drug in some life-threatening situations for mom may outweigh the potential risk of fetal harm. For example, when mom requires cancer treatment or when she has a serious disease for which safer drugs cannot be used or are less effective. Approximately 11% of prescription drugs fall in this category.

Animal Studies: No studies in pregnant animals treated with this drug could be located.

Human Studies: This drug is a member of the sulfonamide family of drugs. Since other family members have caused an increased level of jaundice in the newborn when used near term, this drug has been assigned to pregnancy risk category **D** when used near term.

Helpful Hints: Folic acid antagonists are drugs that limit the effectiveness of folic acid, making it more likely that a baby born to a mom taking one of these drugs might have a serious birth defect, such as an open spine. If you are taking a folic acid antagonist like this one and trying to become pregnant, discuss the possibility of increasing your folic acid intake with your clinician before becoming pregnant. (See "Folic Acid Antagonist Drugs in Pregnancy" in the appendix for more details.)

Remember: All pregnancies have a background risk of about 3% for a major birth defect, even when mom doesn't take a drug of any kind. If you are pregnant or planning a pregnancy, always let your doctor know before taking any drug, prescription or non-prescription, or herbal remedy.

SULINDAC

Brand Name: Clinoril

Drug Use: This drug is approved by the FDA for the treatment of pain. It is a member of the non-steroidal anti-inflammatory (NSAID) family of drugs. (See Helpful Hint on next page.)

Pregnancy Risk Categories: This drug has been assigned two pregnancy risk categories: **B** when used in the first and second trimesters, and **D** when used in the third trimester or near term. Approximately 12% of prescription drugs are assigned two pregnancy risk categories, depending on which trimester of pregnancy the drug is used.

Category B rating: The FDA assigns a drug to Category **B** for one of two reasons: (1) Studies show no evidence of fetal harm when using the drug in pregnant animals, but no controlled studies have been done using the drug in pregnant women, or (2) Studies show evidence of fetal harm when using the drug in pregnant animals, but controlled studies using the drug in pregnant women do not show evidence of fetal harm. Approximately 21% of prescription drugs fall in this category.

Category D rating: The FDA assigns a drug to Category **D** when studies of pregnant women using the drug show evidence of fetal harm. Rarely, however, the potential benefit of using the drug in some life-threatening situations for mom may outweigh the potential risk of fetal harm. For example, when mom requires cancer treatment or when she has a serious disease for which safer drugs cannot be used or are less effective. Approximately 11% of prescription drugs fall in this category.

Animal Studies: Studies in pregnant rats and rabbits treated with this drug showed no evidence of fetal harm in the offspring.

Human Studies: There have been no studies in which pregnant women were treated with this drug and compared to pregnant women not treated with this drug.

Helpful Hints: When taken in the third trimester of pregnancy, NSAIDs have seriously harmed the fetus, leading to life-threatening illness after birth and even death. These potential effects apply to all NSAIDs, whether purchased by prescription or over-the-counter without a prescription. They also explain why NSAIDs have been assigned a **D** pregnancy risk category. (See "Non-Steroidal, Anti-Inflammatory Drugs (NSAIDs) in Pregnancy" in the appendix for more details.)

Remember: All pregnancies have a background risk of about 3% for a major birth defect, even when mom doesn't take a drug of any kind. If you are pregnant or planning a pregnancy, always let your doctor know before taking any drug, prescription or non-prescription, or herbal remedy.

• •

SUMATRIPTAN

Brand Name: Imitrex

Drug Uses: This drug is approved by the FDA for the treatment of migraine headaches and is also used to treat cluster headaches.

Pregnancy Risk Category: C

> **Category C rating:** The FDA assigns a drug to Category C for one of two reasons: (1) Studies show evidence of fetal harm when using the drug in pregnant animals, but no controlled studies have been done using the drug in pregnant women, or (2) Studies using the drug in pregnant animals have not been done, and studies of pregnant women using the drug are insufficient to reach a conclusion. Thus, the drug should only be used if the potential benefit for mom is greater than the potential risk of fetal harm, which, in many cases, is unknown. Approximately 50% of prescription drugs fall in this category.

Animal Studies: Pregnant rabbits treated intravenously during the early stages of pregnancy with this drug showed no evidence of harm to their embryos. Pregnant rats treated continuously with this drug throughout pregnancy also showed no evidence of fetal harm.

Human Studies: There have been no studies in which pregnant women were treated with this drug and compared to pregnant women not treated with this drug. However, there has been no evidence linking this drug to birth defects in babies of women taking the drug.

Remember: All pregnancies have a background risk of about 3% for a major birth defect, even when mom doesn't take a drug of any kind. If you are pregnant or planning a pregnancy, always let your doctor know before taking any drug, prescription or non-prescription, or herbal remedy.

- -

ADDITIONAL DRUGS AND THEIR FDA PREGNANCY RISK CATEGORIES

Since these additional drugs are uncommonly used in pregnancy, they are listed by generic name along with their FDA Pregnancy Risk Category without more detail:

Salsalate - C (D if used in third trimester or near delivery)

Saquinavir - B

Sargramostim - C

Selegiline - C

Sertaconazole - C

Sevelamer - C

Shingles (Zoster) Vaccine - C

Sibutramine - C

Sildenafil - B

Simethicone - C

Sirolimus - C

Sitagliptin - B

Sodium Bicarbonate - C

Sodium Ferric Gluconate - B

Sodium Nitroprusside - C

Sodium Oxybate - B

Sodium Polystyrene

Solifenacin - C

Sotalol - B (D if used in second or third trimester)

Spectinomycin - C

Stavudine - C

Succinylcholine - C

Sufentanil - C (D if used for prolonged periods or in high doses near delivery)

Sulconazole - C

Sulfacetamide - C

Sulfonate - C

Sunitinib - D

T

TAMOXIFEN

Brand Name: Nolvadex

Drug Use: This drug is approved by the FDA for the treatment of breast cancer in women and men.

Pregnancy Risk Category: D

> **Category D rating:** The FDA assigns a drug to Category **D** when studies of pregnant women using the drug show evidence of fetal harm. Rarely, however, the potential benefit of using the drug in some life-threatening situations for mom may outweigh the potential risk of fetal harm. For example, when mom requires cancer treatment or when she has a serious disease for which safer drugs cannot be used or are less effective. Approximately 11% of prescription drugs fall in this category.

Animal Studies: When pregnant rats were treated with this drug, reversible skeletal changes occurred in some of their offspring. In addition, in fertility studies in pregnant rats and rabbits, when they were treated with this drug there was a lower incidence of embryo implantation and a higher incidence of fetal death or retarded growth in utero. When several pregnant marmosets were treated with this drug, no birth defects were seen.

In rodent models of fetal reproductive tract development, this drug caused changes in both sexes that are similar to those cause by diethylstilbestrol (DES). The clinical relevance of these changes in humans is unknown.

Human Studies: There have been no studies in pregnant women who were treated with this drug and compared to pregnant women not treated with this drug. However, there have been a small number of reports of vaginal bleeding, spontaneous abortions, birth defects, and fetal deaths in pregnant women treated with this drug. If this drug is used during pregnancy, or the patient becomes pregnant while taking this drug, or becomes pregnant within two months after discontinuing therapy, the patient should be warned of the potential risk to the fetus, including the potential long-term risk of a DES-like syndrome.

Helpful Hints: Tamoxifen may cause fetal harm when administered to a pregnant woman. Women should be advised not to become pregnant while taking tamoxifen or within two months of discontinuing tamoxifen and should use barrier or non-hormonal contraceptive measures if sexually active.

Remember: All pregnancies have a background risk of about 3% for a major birth defect, even when mom doesn't take a drug of any kind. If you are pregnant or planning a pregnancy, always let your doctor know before taking any drug, prescription or non-prescription, or herbal remedy.

TEGASEROD

Brand Name: Zelnorm

Drug Use: This drug is approved by the FDA as a laxative to treat women with irritable bowel syndrome whose primary symptom is constipation.

Pregnancy Risk Category: B

> **Category B rating:** The FDA assigns a drug to Category **B** for one of two reasons: (1) Studies show no evidence of fetal harm when using the drug in pregnant animals, but no controlled studies have been done using the drug in pregnant women, or (2) Studies show evidence of fetal harm when using the drug in pregnant animals,

but controlled studies using the drug in pregnant women do not show evidence of fetal harm. Approximately 21% of prescription drugs fall in this category.

Animal Studies: When pregnant rats and rabbits were treated with doses of this drug equivalent to 51 times the maximum human dose (in rats) and 15 times the maximum human dose (in rabbits), they showed no evidence of fetal harm.

Human Studies: There are no studies in which pregnant women were treated with this drug and compared to pregnant women not treated with this drug.

Remember: All pregnancies have a background risk of about 3% for a major birth defect, even when mom doesn't take a drug of any kind. If you are pregnant or planning a pregnancy, always let your doctor know before taking any drug, prescription or non-prescription, or herbal remedy.

TEMAZEPAM

Brand Name: Restoril. This drug is a member of the benzodiazepine family of drugs.

Drug Use: This drug is approved by the FDA for the treatment of insomnia.

Pregnancy Risk Category: X

Category X rating: The FDA assigns a drug to Category **X** when studies have shown the risk of fetal harm clearly outweighs any potential maternal benefit from the drug. **Drugs in this category should not be used by pregnant women.** Approximately 5% of prescription drugs fall in this category.

Animal Studies: When pregnant rats and rabbits were treated with this drug, there was an increase in fetal deaths in one study and variation in rib formation in a second study. In rabbits, a variety of malformations were noted.

Human Studies: The benzodiazepine family of drugs may cause fetal harm when administered to a pregnant woman. For example, an increased risk of congenital malformations has been associated with the use of diazepam and chlordiazepoxide during the first trimester of pregnancy in several studies. Also, depression of breathing in the newborn has followed with women taking a benzodiazepine drug during the last weeks of pregnancy. For all these reasons, as well as the results of animal studies on using temazepam, this drug should not be taken during pregnancy.

Helpful Hints: The primary reason this drug was assigned a pregnancy risk category of **X** is because it belongs to the benzodiazepine family of drugs, and several members of that family have been found to cause major birth defects and be associated with depressed respiration in the newborn when the drug was taken during the last week or so of pregnancy. These findings have not been found specifically for temazepam. Nevertheless, the FDA has assigned the drug to category **X** because it belongs to this family of drugs.

Remember: All pregnancies have a background risk of about 3% for a major birth defect, even when mom doesn't take a drug of any kind. If you are pregnant or planning a pregnancy, always let your doctor know before taking any drug, prescription or non-prescription, or herbal remedy.

TERBINAFINE

Brand Name: Lamasil AT

Drug Use: This drug is approved by the FDA for use in treating fungal infections involving the toenail and fingernail.

Pregnancy Risk Category: **B**

Category B rating: The FDA assigns a drug to Category **B** for one of two reasons: (1) Studies show no evidence of fetal harm when using the drug in pregnant animals, but no controlled studies have been done using the drug in pregnant women, or (2) Studies show evidence of fetal harm when using the drug in pregnant animals, but controlled studies using the drug in pregnant women do not show evidence of fetal harm. Approximately 21% of prescription drugs fall in this category.

Animal Studies: When pregnant rats and rabbits were treated with this drug, no fetal harm was noted in the offspring.

Human Studies: There are no studies in which pregnant women were treated with this drug and compared to pregnant women not treated with this drug.

Remember: All pregnancies have a background risk of about 3% for a major birth defect, even when mom doesn't take a drug of any kind. If you are pregnant or planning a pregnancy, always let your doctor know before taking any drug, prescription or non-prescription, or herbal remedy.

TERBUTALINE

Brand Name: Terbutaline

Drug Uses: This drug is approved by the FDA for the prevention and treatment of bronchospasm in patients 12 years of age and older with asthma. It is also used as a tocolytic agent to stop premature labor.

Pregnancy Risk Category: **B**

Category B rating: The FDA assigns a drug to Category **B** for one of two reasons: (1) Studies show no evidence of fetal harm when using the drug in pregnant animals, but no controlled studies have been done using the drug in pregnant women, or (2) Studies show evidence of fetal harm when using the drug in pregnant animals, but controlled studies using the drug in pregnant women do not show evidence of fetal harm. Approximately 21% of prescription drugs fall in this category.

Animal Studies: When pregnant rats and rabbits were treated with this drug, there was no evidence of fetal harm in the offspring.

Human Studies: There are no studies in which pregnant women were treated with this drug and compared to pregnant women not treated with this drug.

Remember: All pregnancies have a background risk of about 3% for a major birth defect, even when mom doesn't take a drug of any kind. If you are pregnant or planning a pregnancy, always let your doctor know before taking any drug, prescription or non-prescription, or herbal remedy.

· ·

TETRACYCLINE

Brand Name: Sumycin

Drug Use: This antibiotic is approved by the FDA for the treatment of a variety of infections. This drug is a member of the tetracycline family of antibiotics.

Pregnancy Risk Category: D

Category D rating: The FDA assigns a drug to Category **D** when studies of pregnant women using the drug show evidence of fetal harm. Rarely, however, the potential benefit of using the drug in some life-threatening situations for mom may outweigh the potential risk of fetal harm. For example, when mom requires cancer treatment or when she has a serious disease for which safer drugs cannot be used or are less effective. Approximately 11% of prescription drugs fall in this category.

Animal Studies: Animal studies have shown this drug crosses the placenta and can have harmful effects on the developing fetus, often related to slowing development of the skeleton. Also, when animals have been treated early in pregnancy, this drug has had toxic effects on the developing embryo.

Human Studies: When pregnant women have been treated with members of this family of drugs during the last half of pregnancy, the drug has caused permanent discoloration of fetal teeth as well as underdevelopment of tooth enamel. For these reasons and the results of animal studies, this family of drugs has been assigned to pregnancy risk category **D**. Thus, its use is contraindicated in pregnancy.

Remember: All pregnancies have a background risk of about 3% for a major birth defect, even when mom doesn't take a drug of any kind. If you are pregnant or planning a pregnancy, always let your doctor know before taking any drug, prescription or non-prescription, or herbal remedy.

. . . .

THALIDOMIDE

Brand Name: Thalomid

Drug Uses: This drug is used as an immunologic agent in the treatment of leprosy and multiple myeloma.

Pregnancy Risk Category: X

> **Category X rating:** The FDA assigns a drug to Category **X** when studies have shown the risk of fetal harm clearly outweighs any potential maternal benefit from the drug. **Drugs in this category should not be used by pregnant women.** Approximately 5% of prescription drugs fall in this category.

Animal Studies: When used in pregnant animals such as mice, rats, rabbits and monkeys, this drug has produced a variety of birth defects, including major abnormalities of the limbs.

Human Studies: This drug has probably caused more severe defects in humans than any other drug. Its use is contraindicated in pregnant women or in women of childbearing age capable of becoming pregnant since it is known to cause major birth defects even following a single dose.

Women of childbearing age who are taking this drug are advised to abstain continuously from sexual contact or to use two methods of reliable birth control, including at least one highly effective method and one additional effective method, beginning four weeks prior to starting treatment with thalidomide, during treatment with thalidomide, and continuing for four weeks following stopping the drug.

Because thalidomide is present in the semen of patients receiving the drug, males receiving thalidomide must always use a latex condom during any sexual contact with women of childbearing potential. The risk to the fetus from the semen of male patients taking thalidomide is unknown.

Remember: All pregnancies have a background risk of about 3% for a major birth defect, even when mom doesn't take a drug of any kind. If you are pregnant or planning a pregnancy, always let your doctor know before taking any drug, prescription or non-prescription, or herbal remedy.

THEOPHYLLINE

Brand Name: Theolair

Drug Use: This drug is approved by the FDA for the treatment of asthma and chronic obstructive pulmonary disease (COPD).

Pregnancy Risk Category: C

> **Category C rating:** The FDA assigns a drug to Category C for one of two reasons: (1) Studies show evidence of fetal harm when using the drug in pregnant animals, but no controlled studies have been done using the drug in pregnant women, or (2) Studies using the drug in pregnant animals have not been done, and studies of pregnant women using the drug are insufficient to reach a conclusion. Thus, the drug should only be used if the potential benefit for mom is greater than the potential risk of fetal harm, which, in many cases, is unknown. Approximately 50% of prescription drugs fall in this category.

Animal Studies: When pregnant mice and rats were treated with theophylline, no fetal harm was noted in the offspring.

Human Studies: There have been no published reports of birth defects linked to pregnant women taking this drug during pregnancy. However, there was one case report of theophylline withdrawal in a newborn that had been exposed throughout pregnancy to this drug. Apneic spells (short delays in breathing) developed in the baby at 28 hours after delivery and became progressively worse over the next four days. Treatment with theophylline resolved the spells.

Helpful Hints: This drug weakly interacts with grapefruit and grapefruit juice, which can cause harmful, and even life-threatening, side effects. Before taking this drug with grapefruit juice, or before consuming grapefruit or grapefruit juice during the day while taking this drug, first read the section "Grapefruit Juice–Drug Interactions Can Make You Sick" in the appendix of this book. Then discuss this with your pharmacist or the healthcare provider who prescribed this drug.

Remember: All pregnancies have a background risk of about 3% for a major birth defect, even when mom

doesn't take a drug of any kind. If you are pregnant or planning a pregnancy, always let your doctor know before taking any drug, prescription or non-prescription, or herbal remedy.

. . . .

THIORIDAZINE

Brand Name: Thioridazine

Drug Use: This drug is approved by the FDA for the treatment of schizophrenia after trials of treatment with other antipsychotic drugs have failed.

Pregnancy Risk Category: C

> **Category C rating:** The FDA assigns a drug to Category C for one of two reasons: (1) Studies show evidence of fetal harm when using the drug in pregnant animals, but no controlled studies have been done using the drug in pregnant women, or (2) Studies using the drug in pregnant animals have not been done, and studies of pregnant women using the drug are insufficient to reach a conclusion. Thus, the drug should only be used if the potential benefit for mom is greater than the potential risk of fetal harm, which, in many cases, is unknown. Approximately 50% of prescription drugs fall in this category.

Animal Studies: The drug apparently does not cause birth defects in animals. However, this statement by one expert did not specify which species was tested.

Human Studies: There is minimal human data concerning pregnant women taking this drug. In a Michigan Medicaid population, there was no increased risk of birth defects associated with pregnant women taking this drug.

Remember: All pregnancies have a background risk of about 3% for a major birth defect, even when mom doesn't take a drug of any kind. If you are pregnant or planning a pregnancy, always let your doctor know

before taking any drug, prescription or non-prescription, or herbal remedy.

. . . .

TICARCILLIN

Brand Name: Timentin, which is a combination of ticarcillin and clavulanate

Drug Use: This antibiotic is approved by the FDA for the treatment of a variety of bacterial infections.

Pregnancy Risk Category: B

> **Category B rating:** The FDA assigns a drug to Category **B** for one of two reasons: (1) Studies show no evidence of fetal harm when using the drug in pregnant animals, but no controlled studies have been done using the drug in pregnant women, or (2) Studies show evidence of fetal harm when using the drug in pregnant animals, but controlled studies using the drug in pregnant women do not show evidence of fetal harm. Approximately 21% of prescription drugs fall in this category.

Animal Studies: When pregnant rats were treated with this drug, no fetal harm was noted in the offspring.

Human Studies: There are no studies in which pregnant women were treated with this drug and the results compared to pregnant women not treated with this drug.

Remember: All pregnancies have a background risk of about 3% for a major birth defect, even when mom doesn't take a drug of any kind. If you are pregnant or planning a pregnancy, always let your doctor know before taking any drug, prescription or non-prescription, or herbal remedy.

. . . .

TIMOLOL

Brand Names: Timoptic, Betimol, Blocadren. These drugs belong to the beta blocker family of drugs.

Drug Uses: This drug is approved by the FDA for the treatment of hypertension, migraine headaches, and myocardial infarction.

Pregnancy Risk Categories: This drug has been assigned two pregnancy risk categories: **C** when used in the first trimester, and **D** when used in the second and third trimesters. Approximately 12% of prescription drugs are assigned two pregnancy risk categories, depending on which trimester of pregnancy the drug is used.

> **Category C rating:** The FDA assigns a drug to Category **C** for one of two reasons: (1) Studies show evidence of fetal harm when using the drug in pregnant animals, but no controlled studies have been done using the drug in pregnant women, or (2) Studies using the drug in pregnant animals have not been done, and studies of pregnant women using the drug are insufficient to reach a conclusion. Thus, the drug should only be used if the potential benefit for mom is greater than the potential risk of fetal harm, which, in many cases, is unknown. Approximately 50% of prescription drugs fall in this category.

> **Category D rating:** The FDA assigns a drug to Category **D** when studies of pregnant women using the drug show evidence of fetal harm. Rarely, however, the potential benefit of using the drug in some life-threatening situations for mom may outweigh the potential risk of fetal harm. For example, when mom requires cancer treatment or when she has a serious disease for which safer drugs cannot be used or are less effective. Approximately 11% of prescription drugs fall in this category.

Animal Studies: When pregnant mice, rats, and rabbits were treated with this drug at doses up to 40 times the maximum recommended human dose, there was no evidence of an increase in birth defects in their offspring.

Human Studies: There are no studies in which pregnant women were treated with this drug and compared to pregnant women not treated with this drug. This drug was assigned two risk categories because timolol is a member of the beta blocker family of drugs.

Helpful Hints: Use of drugs in the beta blocker family during pregnancy may cause delayed growth in the fetus and reduced placental weight. The use of some drugs in this family has resulted in symptoms consisting primarily of a slow heart rate, which is known as bradycardia, usually within the first 48 hours after birth. For all these reasons, slow growth in utero, reduced placental weight, and bradycardia after birth, the drug has been assigned to a pregnancy risk category of **D** if used in the second and third trimesters.

Remember: All pregnancies have a background risk of about 3% for a major birth defect, even when mom doesn't take a drug of any kind. If you are pregnant or planning a pregnancy, always let your doctor know before taking any drug, prescription or non-prescription, or herbal remedy.

- -

TOBRAMYCIN

Brand Name: Tobrex

Drug Use: This antibiotic is approved by the FDA for the treatment of serious bacterial infections. The drug is a member of the aminoglycoside family of antibiotics.

Pregnancy Risk Categories: **C** according to the FDA (**D** according to Eli Lilly, the manufacturer)

> **Category C rating:** The FDA assigns a drug to Category C for one of two reasons: (1) Studies show evidence of fetal harm when using the drug in pregnant animals, but no controlled studies have been done using the drug in pregnant women, or (2) Studies using the drug in pregnant animals have not been done, and studies of pregnant women using the drug are insufficient to reach a conclusion. Thus, the drug should only be used if the potential benefit for mom is greater than the potential risk of fetal harm, which, in many cases, is unknown. Approximately 50% of prescription drugs fall in this category.

Category D rating: The FDA assigns a drug to Category **D** when studies of pregnant women using the drug show evidence of fetal harm. Rarely, however, the potential benefit of using the drug in some life-threatening situations for mom may outweigh the potential risk of fetal harm. For example, when mom requires cancer treatment or when she has a serious disease for which safer drugs cannot be used or are less effective. Approximately 11% of prescription drugs fall in this category.

Animal Studies: Studies in pregnant rats and rabbits treated with this drug showed no increase in birth defects in the offspring.

Human Studies: There are no studies in which pregnant women were treated with this drug and the results compared to pregnant women not treated with this drug. There have also been no reports linking this drug to birth defects. However, there have been several reports of total, bilateral congenital deafness in children whose mothers received streptomycin, another aminoglycoside family member, during pregnancy. However, there have been no similar reports in pregnant women treated with tobramycin.

Remember: All pregnancies have a background risk of about 3% for a major birth defect, even when mom doesn't take a drug of any kind. If you are pregnant or planning a pregnancy, always let your doctor know before taking any drug, prescription or non-prescription, or herbal remedy.

· ·

TOLBUTAMIDE

Brand Name: Tolbutamide

Drug Use: This drug is approved by the FDA for the oral treatment of Type 2 diabetes.

Pregnancy Risk Category: **C**

Category C rating: The FDA assigns a drug to Category **C** for one of two reasons: (1) Studies show evidence of fetal harm when using the drug in pregnant animals, but no controlled studies have been done using the drug in pregnant women, or (2) Studies using the drug in pregnant animals have not been done, and studies of pregnant women using the drug are insufficient to reach a conclusion. Thus, the drug should only be used if the potential benefit for mom is greater than the potential risk of fetal harm, which, in many cases, is unknown. Approximately 50% of prescription drugs fall in this category.

Animal Studies: When pregnant rats were treated with this drug using doses 25 to 100 times the human dose, an increased incidence of birth defects was found. Similar studies in pregnant rabbits, however, have not shown these effects.

Human Studies: There are no studies in which pregnant women were treated with this drug and compared to pregnant women not treated with this drug. According to the The American College of Obstetricians and Gynecologists (ACOG), this drug is not indicated in pregnancy. Insulin is preferred for the treatment of diabetes in pregnancy instead.

Remember: All pregnancies have a background risk of about 3% for a major birth defect, even when mom doesn't take a drug of any kind. If you are pregnant or planning a pregnancy, always let your doctor know before taking any drug, prescription or non-prescription, or herbal remedy.

TOPIRAMATE

Brand Name: Topamax

Drug Uses: This drug is approved by the FDA for the treatment of seizures and migraine headaches. This drug is a member of the folic acid antagonist family of drugs. (See Helpful Hint below.)

Pregnancy Risk Category: C

Category C rating: The FDA assigns a drug to Category C for one of two reasons: (1) Studies show evidence of fetal harm when using the drug in pregnant animals, but no controlled studies have been done using the drug in pregnant women, or (2) Studies using the drug in pregnant animals have not been done, and studies of pregnant women using the drug are insufficient to reach a conclusion. Thus, the drug should only be used if the potential benefit for mom is greater than the potential risk of fetal harm, which, in many cases, is unknown. Approximately 50% of prescription drugs fall in this category.

Animal Studies: Studies in pregnant mice, rats, and rabbits treated with this drug have shown toxic effects in the mother and birth defects in their offspring. However, experience in human pregnancy is too limited to determine if similar effects also occur in human pregnancies.

Human Studies: There is limited data in pregnant women treated with this drug. There are no studies in which pregnant women were treated with this drug and compared to pregnant women not treated with this drug.

Helpful Hints:

1. Folic acid antagonists like topiramate are drugs that limit the effectiveness of folic acid, making it more likely that a baby born to a mom taking one of these drugs might have a serious birth defect, such as an open spine. If you are taking a folic acid antagonist and trying to become pregnant, discuss the possibility of increasing your folic acid intake with your clinician before becoming pregnant. (See "Folic Acid Antagonist Drugs in Pregnancy" in the appendix for more details.)

2. In pregnant women with epilepsy, the first priority is to prevent seizures. This can be difficult because many seizure medications do not work quite as well during pregnancy. Sometimes the dose has to be increased or other medications added just to prevent seizures. Regardless, the healthiest situation for both mom and unborn baby is to have the fewest seizures possible.

Remember: All pregnancies have a background risk of about 3% for a major birth defect, even when mom doesn't take a drug of any kind. If you are pregnant or planning a pregnancy, always let your doctor know before taking any drug, prescription or non-prescription, or herbal remedy.

· ·

TRAMADOL

Brand Name: Ryzolt and Ultram. Ultracet when acetaminophen is added.

Drug Use: This drug is approved by the FDA for the relief of pain.

Pregnancy Risk Category: C

Category C rating: The FDA assigns a drug to Category C for one of two reasons: (1) Studies show evidence of fetal harm when using the drug in pregnant animals, but no controlled studies have been done using the drug in pregnant women, or (2) Studies using the drug in pregnant animals have not been done, and studies of pregnant women using the drug are insufficient to reach a conclusion. Thus, the drug should only be used if the potential benefit for mom is greater than the potential risk of fetal harm, which, in many cases, is unknown. Approximately 50% of prescription drugs fall in this category.

Animal Studies: Studies in pregnant mice, rats, and rabbits treated with this drug have shown toxic effects on the embryo and fetal offspring.

Human Studies: There are no studies in which pregnant women were treated with this drug and the results compared to pregnant women not treated with this drug. There have been reports of neonatal withdrawal symptoms in babies of mothers who have been treated with this drug.

Remember: All pregnancies have a background risk of about 3% for a major birth defect, even when mom doesn't take a drug of any kind. If you are pregnant or planning a pregnancy, always let your doctor know before taking any drug, prescription or non-prescription, or herbal remedy.

TRIAMCINOLONE

Brand Names: Aristopan, Aristocort. This drug is a member of the corticosteroid family of drugs.

Drug Uses: This drug is approved by the FDA for the treatment of a variety of disorders, including asthma.

Pregnancy Risk Categories: This drug has been assigned two pregnancy risk categories: **C** when used in the second and third trimester, and **D** when used in the first trimester. Approximately 12% of prescription drugs are assigned two pregnancy risk categories, depending on which trimester of pregnancy the drug is used.

> **Category C rating:** The FDA assigns a drug to Category **C** for one of two reasons: (1) Studies show evidence of fetal harm when using the drug in pregnant animals, but no controlled studies have been done using the drug in pregnant women, or (2) Studies using the drug in pregnant animals have not been done, and studies of pregnant women using the drug are insufficient to reach a conclusion. Thus, the drug should only be used if the potential benefit for mom is greater than the potential risk of fetal harm, which, in many cases, is unknown. Approximately 50% of prescription drugs fall in this category.

Category D rating: The FDA assigns a drug to Category **D** when studies of pregnant women using the drug show evidence of fetal harm. Rarely, however, the potential benefit of using the drug in some life-threatening situations for mom may outweigh the potential risk of fetal harm. For example, when mom requires cancer treatment or when she has a serious disease for which safer drugs cannot be used or are less effective. Approximately 11% of prescription drugs fall in this category.

Animal Studies: Animal studies in which this family of drugs has been given to pregnant mice, rats, and rabbits have produced an increased incidence of cleft palate (hole in the roof of the mouth) of the offspring. For these reasons, the drug has been assigned to category **D** when used in the first trimester.

Human Studies: There are no studies in which pregnant women were treated with this drug and the results compared to pregnant women not treated with this drug.

Remember: All pregnancies have a background risk of about 3% for a major birth defect, even when mom doesn't take a drug of any kind. If you are pregnant or planning a pregnancy, always let your doctor know before taking any drug, prescription or non-prescription, or herbal remedy.

· ·

TRIAMTERENE

Brand Name: Dyrenium

Drug Use: This drug is approved by the FDA for use as a diuretic (water pill) for treating edema. This drug is a member of the folic acid antagonist family of drugs.

Pregnancy Risk Categories: This drug has been assigned two pregnancy risk categories: **C** for all of pregnancy, and **D** if the drug is used for the treatment of gestational hypertension. Approximately 12% of prescription drugs are assigned two pregnancy risk categories, depending on which trimester of pregnancy the drug is used.

> **Category C rating:** The FDA assigns a drug to Category **C** for one of two reasons: (1) Studies show evidence of fetal harm when using the drug in pregnant animals, but no controlled studies have been done using the drug in pregnant women, or (2) Studies using the drug in pregnant animals have not been done, and studies of pregnant women using the drug are insufficient to reach a conclusion. Thus, the drug should only be used if the potential benefit for mom is greater than the potential risk of fetal harm, which, in many cases, is unknown. Approximately 50% of prescription drugs fall in this category.

> **Category D rating:** The FDA assigns a drug to Category **D** when studies of pregnant women using the drug show evidence of fetal harm. Rarely, however, the potential benefit of using the drug in some life-threatening situations for mom may outweigh the potential risk of fetal harm. For example, when mom requires cancer treatment or when she has a serious disease for which safer drugs cannot be used or are less effective. Approximately 11% of prescription drugs fall in this category.

Animal Studies: Pregnant rats treated with 20 times the maximum human dose have produced no evidence of increased risk of birth defects in the offspring.

Human Studies: There are no studies in which pregnant women were treated with this drug and compared to pregnant women not treated with this drug. The drug is not recommended for the treatment of gestational hypertension associated with toxemia since those patients already have a low blood volume, a contraindication for diuretic treatment. If the drug is used to treat gestational hypertension, it is assigned a pregnancy risk rating of **D**.

Helpful Hints: Folic acid antagonists are drugs that limit the effectiveness of folic acid, making it more likely that a baby born to a mom taking one of these drugs might have a serious birth defect, such as an open spine. If you are taking a folic acid antagonist and trying to become pregnant, discuss the possibility of increasing your folic acid intake with your clinician before becoming pregnant. (See "Folic Acid Antagonist Drugs in Pregnancy" in the Appendix for more details.)

Remember: All pregnancies have a background risk of about 3% for a major birth defect, even when mom doesn't take a drug of any kind. If you are pregnant or planning a pregnancy, always let your doctor know before taking any drug, prescription or non-prescription, or herbal remedy.

TRICHLORMETHIAZIDE

Brand Name: Triflumen

Drug Use: This drug is approved by the FDA for the treatment of edema associated with heart failure and high blood pressure. It is a member of the thiazide family of diuretics.

Pregnancy Risk Categories: This drug has been assigned two pregnancy risk categories: **C** when used throughout pregnancy, and **D** if used during pregnancy for the treatment of gestational hypertension. Approximately 12% of prescription drugs are assigned two pregnancy risk categories, depending on which trimester of pregnancy the drug is used.

> **Category C rating:** The FDA assigns a drug to Category **C** for one of two reasons: (1) Studies show evidence of fetal harm when using the drug in pregnant animals, but no controlled studies have been done using the drug in pregnant women, or (2) Studies using the drug in pregnant animals have not been done, and studies of pregnant women using the drug are insufficient to reach a conclusion. Thus, the drug should only be used if the potential benefit for mom is greater than the potential risk of fetal harm, which, in many cases, is unknown. Approximately 50% of prescription drugs fall in this category.

Category D rating: The FDA assigns a drug to Category **D** when studies of pregnant women using the drug show evidence of fetal harm. Rarely, however, the potential benefit of using the drug in some life-threatening situations for mom may outweigh the potential risk of fetal harm. For example, when mom requires cancer treatment or when she has a serious disease for which safer drugs cannot be used or are less effective. Approximately 11% of prescription drugs fall in this category.

Animal Studies: When pregnant mice, rats, and rabbits were treated using members of this family of drugs, there was no evidence of fetal harm.

Human Studies: There are no studies in which pregnant women were treated with this drug and the results compared to pregnant women not treated with this drug. Low platelet counts in newborns have been reported following the near term use of some thiazide diuretics. Other studies have not confirmed this finding.

Remember: All pregnancies have a background risk of about 3% for a major birth defect, even when mom doesn't take a drug of any kind. If you are pregnant or planning a pregnancy, always let your doctor know before taking any drug, prescription or non-prescription, or herbal remedy.

TRIFLUOPERAZINE

Brand Name: Trifluoperazine

Drug Uses: This drug is approved by the FDA for the treatment of nausea and vomiting in pregnancy and for the treatment of schizophrenia. It is a member of the phenothiazine family of drugs.

Pregnancy Risk Category: C

Category C rating: The FDA assigns a drug to Category **C** for one of two reasons: (1) Studies show evidence of fetal harm when using the drug in pregnant animals, but no controlled studies have been done using the drug in pregnant women, or (2) Studies using the drug in pregnant animals have not been done, and studies of pregnant women using the drug are insufficient to reach a conclusion. Thus, the drug should only be used if the potential benefit for mom is greater than the potential risk of fetal harm, which, in many cases, is unknown. Approximately 50% of prescription drugs fall in this category.

Animal Studies: When pregnant rats, rabbits, and monkeys were treated with a dose of this drug that was greater than 600 times the maximum human dose, an increased risk of birth defects in the offspring was noted. But when the dose was reduced in half, those effects vanished.

Human Studies: Although some reports have tried to link this drug with birth defects, the bulk of the evidence suggests the drug is safe for mom and low-risk for the fetus, according to experts. However, there are reports of this family of drugs causing prolonged jaundice in the newborn when a member of this family of drugs has been used near the time of delivery. In some instances, the level of jaundice has gotten high enough to cause neurologic symptoms.

Remember: All pregnancies have a background risk of about 3% for a major birth defect, even when mom doesn't take a drug of any kind. If you are pregnant or planning a pregnancy, always let your doctor know before taking any drug, prescription or non-prescription, or herbal remedy.

. . . .

TRIMETHOBENZAMIDE

Brand Name: Tigan

Drug Uses: This drug is approved by the FDA for the prevention of post-operative nausea and vomiting and nausea associated with gastroenteritis.

Pregnancy Risk Category: C

Category C rating: The FDA assigns a drug to Category C for one of two reasons: (1) Studies show evidence of fetal harm when using the drug in pregnant animals, but no controlled studies have been done using the drug in pregnant women, or (2) Studies using the drug in pregnant animals have not been done, and studies of pregnant women using the drug are insufficient to reach a conclusion. Thus, the drug should only be used if the potential benefit for mom is greater than the potential risk of fetal harm, which, in many cases, is unknown. Approximately 50% of prescription drugs fall in this category.

Animal Studies: When pregnant rats and rabbits were treated with this drug, there was no increase in the incidence of birth defects in the offspring.

Human Studies: There are no studies in which pregnant women were treated with this drug and the results compared to pregnant women not treated with this drug. However, the drug has been used in pregnancy to treat nausea and vomiting. No adverse effects on the fetus were observed.

Remember: All pregnancies have a background risk of about 3% for a major birth defect, even when mom doesn't take a drug of any kind. If you are pregnant or planning a pregnancy, always let your doctor know before taking any drug, prescription or non-prescription, or herbal remedy.

∙ ∙

TRIMETHOPRIM

Brand Names: Proloprin when used singularly. Bactrim when used in combination with sulfamethoxazole.

Drug Use: This antibiotic is approved by the FDA to treat urinary tract infections caused by susceptible bacteria. This drug is a member of the folic acid antagonist family of drugs. (See Helpful Hint on next page.)

Pregnancy Risk Category: **C**

Category C rating: The FDA assigns a drug to Category **C** for one of two reasons: (1) Studies show evidence of fetal harm when using the drug in pregnant animals, but no controlled studies have been done using the drug in pregnant women, or (2) Studies using the drug in pregnant animals have not been done, and studies of pregnant women using the drug are insufficient to reach a conclusion. Thus, the drug should only be used if the potential benefit for mom is greater than the potential risk of fetal harm, which, in many cases, is unknown. Approximately 50% of prescription drugs fall in this category.

Animal Studies: When pregnant rats were treated with 40 times the maximum human dose of this drug, the results did show an increased risk of birth defects in the offspring.

Human Studies: There are no studies in which pregnant women were treated with this drug and the results compared to pregnant women not treated with this drug. However, in a retrospective study of pregnant women receiving a placebo or trimethoprim plus sulfamethoxazole, there was no increased incidence of birth defects in the treated group.

Helpful Hints: Folic acid antagonists like trimethoprim are drugs that limit the effectiveness of folic acid, making it more likely that a baby born to a mom taking one of these drugs might have a serious birth defect, such as an open spine. If you are taking a folic acid antagonist and trying to become pregnant, discuss the possibility of increasing your folic acid intake with your clinician before becoming pregnant. (See "Folic Acid Antagonist Drugs in Pregnancy" in the appendix for more details.)

Remember: All pregnancies have a background risk of about 3% for a major birth defect, even when mom doesn't take a drug of any kind. If you are pregnant or

planning a pregnancy, always let your doctor know before taking any drug, prescription or non-prescription, or herbal remedy.

• •

TRIPROLIDINE

Brand Name: Pseudodine C (a combination of triprolidine, pseudoephedrine, and codeine)

Drug Use: This drug is approved by the FDA for the relief of coughs and upper respiratory symptoms, including nasal congestion associated with allergies or the common cold.

Pregnancy Risk Category: C

> **Category C rating:** The FDA assigns a drug to Category C for one of two reasons: (1) Studies show evidence of fetal harm when using the drug in pregnant animals, but no controlled studies have been done using the drug in pregnant women, or (2) Studies using the drug in pregnant animals have not been done, and studies of pregnant women using the drug are insufficient to reach a conclusion. Thus, the drug should only be used if the potential benefit for mom is greater than the potential risk of fetal harm, which, in many cases, is unknown. Approximately 50% of prescription drugs fall in this category.

Animal Studies: No animal studies of triprolidine have been published using all three ingredients together. However, animal studies of the three ingredients individually showed no fetal harm in any of those studies.

Human Studies: There are no studies in which pregnant women were treated with this drug and the results compared to pregnant women not treated with this drug.

Helpful Hints: Some cough syrups contain ethanol (alcohol). Be sure to check the label on the bottle to see if ethanol is listed as an ingredient. Alcohol is known to cause birth defects in developing fetuses.

Remember: All pregnancies have a background risk of about 3% for a major birth defect, even when mom doesn't take a drug of any kind. If you are pregnant or planning a pregnancy, always let your doctor know before taking any drug, prescription or non-prescription, or herbal remedy.

. . . .

ADDITIONAL DRUGS AND THEIR FDA PREGNANCY RISK CATEGORIES

Since these additional drugs are uncommonly used in pregnancy, they are listed by generic name along with their FDA Pregnancy Risk Category without more detail:

Tacrine - C

Tacrolimus - C

Tadalafil - B

Talc - B

Tamsulosin - B

Tazarotene - X

Telithromycin - C

Telmisartan - C (D if used in the second or third trimesters)

Temozolomide - D

Tenecteplase - C

Teniposide - D

Tenofovir - B

Terazosin - C

Terconazole - C

Teriparatide - C

Testosterone - X

Tetnus and Diphtheria Vaccine - C

Tetnus, Diphtheria, and Pertussis Vaccine - C

Thioguanine - D

Thiopental - C

Thrombin - C

Tiagabine - C

Ticlopidine - B

Tigecycline - D

Tinidazole - C

Tinzaparin - B

Tioconazole - C

Tiotropium - C

Tipranavir - C

Tirofiban - B

Tizanidine - C

Tolcapone - C

Tolmetin - C (D if used in third trimester or near delivery)

Tolnaftate - C

Tolterodine - C

Topotecan - D

Toremifene - D

Torsemide - B

Tositumomab - X

Trandolapril - C (D if used in the second or third trimester)

Trastuzumab - B

Travoprost - C

Trazodone - C

Treprostinil - B

Tretinoin - C (Topical use); D (Systemic use)

Triazolam - X

Trifluridine - C

Trihexyphenidyl - C

Triptorelin - X

Tromethamine - C

Trospium - C

Typhoid Vaccine - C

U

UROKINASE

Brand Name: Kinlytic

Drug Use: This drug is approved by the FDA for the treatment of pulmonary embolism, which means it helps break up massive clots in the lung which are obstructing blood flow to a portion of the lung.

Pregnancy Risk Category: B

Category B rating: The FDA assigns a drug to Category **B** for one of two reasons: (1) Studies show no evidence of fetal harm when using the drug in pregnant animals, but no controlled studies have been done using the drug in pregnant women, or (2) Studies show evidence of fetal harm when using the drug in pregnant animals, but controlled studies using the drug in pregnant women do not show evidence of fetal harm. Approximately 21% of prescription drugs fall in this category.

Animal Studies: When pregnant mice and rats were treated with this drug using up to 1,000 times the maximum human dose, there was no evidence of fetal harm in the offspring.

Human Studies: There have been no studies in pregnant women using this drug and comparing the results to pregnant women not using the drug.

Remember: All pregnancies have a background risk of about 3% for a major birth defect, even when mom doesn't take a drug of any kind. If you are pregnant or planning a pregnancy, always let your doctor know before taking any drug, prescription or non-prescription, or herbal remedy.

V

VALACYCLOVIR

Brand Name: Valtrex

Drug Uses: This antiviral medication is used to treat herpes zoster (shingles), herpes labialis (cold sores), and genital herpes.

Pregnancy Risk Category: B

> **Category B rating:** The FDA assigns a drug to Category **B** for one of two reasons: (1) Studies show no evidence of fetal harm when using the drug in pregnant animals, but no controlled studies have been done using the drug in pregnant women, or (2) Studies show evidence of fetal harm when using the drug in pregnant animals, but controlled studies using the drug in pregnant women do not show evidence of fetal harm. Approximately 21% of prescription drugs fall in this category.

Animal Studies: When pregnant rats and rabbits were treated with this drug, researchers found no evidence of harm in their offspring.

Human Studies: When this drug has been used by pregnant women, researchers have found no harm to the fetus.

Helpful Hints:

1. Valacyclovir is actually a cousin of acyclovir. It is broken down by the body into acyclovir, the active form of the drug.

2. For the management of herpes in pregnancy, either valacyclovir or acyclovir is recommended, but only acyclovir is recommended for severe or wide-spread infection with the herpes virus.

3. It is very important for a pregnant woman to tell her doctor if she has had herpes infections in the past or if she thinks she might have a herpes infection during her current pregnancy. If the baby passes through the birth canal and is exposed to an active herpes lesion, there is a risk the baby might develop a herpes infection. Herpes infection in the newborn can be very serious, even fatal.

Remember: All pregnancies have a background risk of about 3% for a major birth defect, even when mom doesn't take a drug of any kind. If you are pregnant or planning a pregnancy, always let your doctor know before taking any drug, prescription or non-prescription, or herbal remedy.

VALPROIC ACID

Brand Names: Depakene, Valproic

Drug Use: This drug is approved by the FDA as an anti-convulsant for the treatment of seizures. This drug belongs to the folic acid antagonist family of drugs.

Pregnancy Risk Category: D

Category D rating: The FDA assigns a drug to Category **D** when studies of pregnant women using the drug show evidence of fetal harm. Rarely, however, the potential benefit of using the drug in some life-threatening situations for mom may outweigh the potential risk of fetal harm. For example, when mom requires cancer treatment or when she has a serious disease for which safer drugs cannot be used or are less effective. Approximately 11% of prescription drugs fall in this category.

Animal Studies: When pregnant mice, rats, rabbits, and monkeys were treated with valproic acid, an increased incidence of birth defects were produced in all of the animals.

Human Studies: The FDA has issued a Black Box Warning for valproic acid as follows:

"Valproic acid can produce teratogenic effects (birth defects). Data suggests that there is an increased incidence of congenital malformations associated with the use of this drug by women with seizure disorders during pregnancy when compared to the incidence of women with seizure disorders who do not use anti-epileptic drugs during pregnancy. Therefore, valproic acid should be considered for women of childbearing potential only after the risks have been thoroughly discussed with the patient and weighed against the potential benefits of treatment."

"There are multiple reports in the clinical literature that indicate the use of anti-epileptic drugs during pregnancy results in an increased incidence of congenital malformations in offspring. Anti-epileptic drugs, including valproic acid, should be administered to women of childbearing potential only if they are clearly shown to be essential in the management of their medical condition."

"The strongest association of maternal valproic acid with congenital malformations is with neural tube defects, or open spine. However, other congenital anomalies such as cranio facial defects, cardiovascular malformations, and anomalies involving various body systems compatible and incompatible with life have been reported."

"The incidence of neural tube defects is increased in mothers receiving valproic acid during the first trimester of pregnancy. The CDC has estimated the risk of valproic acid exposed women having children with spina bifida (open spine) to be approximately one to two percent. In comparison, the American College of Obstetricians and Gynecologists estimate the general population risk for congenital neural tube defects as .14 percent to .2 percent."

"Patients taking valproic acid may develop clotting abnormalities. Patients taking valproic acid may also develop liver failure. Fatal liver failures, in a newborn and in an infant, have been reported following the maternal use of valproic acid during pregnancy."

A Black Box Warning is the most serious prescription drug warning the FDA can require a drug company to issue.

Helpful Hints:

1. In pregnant women with epilepsy, the first priority is to prevent seizures. This can be difficult because many seizure medications do not work quite as well during pregnancy. Sometimes the dose has to be increased or other medications added just to prevent seizures. Regardless, the healthiest situation for both mom and unborn baby is to have the fewest seizures possible.

2. Do not discontinue this drug or any other anticonvulsant drug abruptly. This may precipitate a seizure crisis which may be life-threatening to mom and her unborn baby.

3. Folic acid antagonists like valproic acid are drugs that limit the effectiveness of folic acid, making it more likely that a baby born to a mom taking one of these drugs might have a serious birth defect, such as an open spine. If you are taking a folic acid antagonist and trying to become pregnant, discuss the possibility of increasing your folic acid intake with your clinician before becoming pregnant. (See "Folic Acid Antagonist

Drugs in Pregnancy" in the Appendix for more details.)

Remember: All pregnancies have a background risk of about 3% for a major birth defect, even when mom doesn't take a drug of any kind. If you are pregnant or planning a pregnancy, always let your doctor know before taking any drug, prescription or non-prescription, or herbal remedy.

• •

VANCOMYCIN

Brand Name: Vancocin

Drug Use: This antibiotic is approved by the FDA to treat bacterial infections.

Pregnancy Risk Category: B

> **Category B rating:** The FDA assigns a drug to Category **B** for one of two reasons: (1) Studies show no evidence of fetal harm when using the drug in pregnant animals, but no controlled studies have been done using the drug in pregnant women, or (2) Studies show evidence of fetal harm when using the drug in pregnant animals, but controlled studies using the drug in pregnant women do not show evidence of fetal harm. Approximately 21% of prescription drugs fall in this category.

Animal Studies: When pregnant rats and rabbits were treated with this drug, there was no evidence of fetal harm in the offspring.

Human Studies: No fetal kidney damage or hearing loss was found in a controlled clinical study of vancomycin given intravenously to pregnant women for serious staphylococcal infections complicating intravenous drug abuse.

Remember: All pregnancies have a background risk of about 3% for a major birth defect, even when mom

doesn't take a drug of any kind. If you are pregnant or planning a pregnancy, always let your doctor know before taking any drug, prescription or non-prescription, or herbal remedy.

· ·

VARICELLA VACCINE

Brand Name: Varivax

Drug Use: Varicella vaccine is used to prevent varicella (chicken pox) infection.

Pregnancy Category: C

> **Category C rating:** The FDA assigns a drug to Category **C** for one of two reasons: (1) Studies show evidence of fetal harm when using the drug in pregnant animals, but no controlled studies have been done using the drug in pregnant women, or (2) Studies using the drug in pregnant animals have not been done, and studies of pregnant women using the drug are insufficient to reach a conclusion. Thus, the drug should only be used if the potential benefit for mom is greater than the potential risk of fetal harm, which, in many cases, is unknown. Approximately 50% of prescription drugs fall in this category.

Animal Studies: No studies of pregnant animals using this vaccine have been done.

Human Studies: There have been no studies of pregnant women using this vaccine, so the effects of the vaccine on pregnant women remain unknown.

Helpful Hints:

1. The manufacturer states that women should not be vaccinated with this vaccine within three months before conception or during pregnancy. In comparison, the Advisory Committee on Immunization Practices and the American Academy of Pediatrics recommends that women should not be vaccinated with this vaccine within one

month before conception or during pregnancy. The American College of Obstetricians and Gynecologists advises not to vaccinate women with this vaccine during pregnancy.

2. It is permissible to vaccinate a child with varicella vaccine when the child's mother, or any household member, is pregnant.

3. If you are pregnant and think you may be developing chicken pox, contact your healthcare provider right away. Chicken pox infection can be especially serious in pregnancy (not just for the fetus but for you, too).

Remember: All pregnancies have a background risk of about 3% for a major birth defect, even when mom doesn't take a drug of any kind. If you are pregnant or planning a pregnancy, always let your doctor know before taking any drug, prescription or non-prescription, or herbal remedy.

VENLAFAXINE

Brand Name: Effexor XR

Drug Uses: This drug is approved by the FDA for multiple purposes, including the treatment of depression, generalized and social anxiety, and panic disorder. Although this drug is not a member of the SSRI family of anti-depressants, its mode of action is quite similar.

Pregnancy Risk Categories: This drug has been assigned two pregnancy risk categories: **C** when used in the first half of pregnancy, and **D** if taken in the second half of pregnancy. Approximately 12% of prescription drugs are assigned two pregnancy risk categories, depending on which trimester of pregnancy the drug is used.

Category C rating: The FDA assigns a drug to Category **C** for one of two reasons: (1) Studies show evidence of fetal harm when using the drug in pregnant animals, but no controlled studies have been done using the drug in pregnant women, or (2) Studies using the drug in pregnant animals have not been done, and studies of pregnant women using the drug are insufficient to reach a conclusion. Thus, the drug should only be used if the potential benefit for mom is greater than the potential risk of fetal harm, which, in many cases, is unknown. Approximately 50% of prescription drugs fall in this category.

Category D rating: The FDA assigns a drug to Category **D** when studies of pregnant women using the drug show evidence of fetal harm. Rarely, however, the potential benefit of using the drug in some life-threatening situations for mom may outweigh the potential risk of fetal harm. For example, when mom requires cancer treatment or when she has a serious disease for which safer drugs cannot be used or are less effective. Approximately 11% of prescription drugs fall in this category.

Animal Studies: This drug did not cause an increased incidence of birth defects in the offspring of pregnant rats or rabbits treated with two and a half times the maximum human dose in rats, and four times the maximum human dose in rabbits.

Human Studies: There are no well-controlled studies of pregnant women using this drug. However, uncontrolled studies have shown that some newborns exposed to venlafaxine late in the third trimester have developed complications requiring prolonged hospitalization, respirator support, and tube feeding. However, these studies have not shown an increased risk of birth defects.

Helpful Hints:

1. Studies show that antidepressants increase the risk of suicidal thinking and behavior in children, adolescents, and young adults. Anyone considering the use of this drug or any other antidepressant in these patients must balance that risk with the clinical need.

2. Almost all antidepressants carry some risk to the developing fetus. However, we also know depression in a pregnant woman carries potential risk for her health and for her unborn baby; for example, low birth weight and prematurity. The risks and benefits of medications and untreated depression must be weighed carefully. If you are pregnant and think you may have depression, or if you already know you do, talk with your doctor so the two of you can create the right plan for you and your unborn baby.

(See "Antidepressants in Pregnancy" in the appendix for more information.)

Remember: All pregnancies have a background risk of about 3% for a major birth defect, even when mom doesn't take a drug of any kind. If you are pregnant or planning a pregnancy, always let your doctor know before taking any drug, prescription or non-prescription, or herbal remedy.

· ·

VERAPAMIL

Brand Name: Calan

Drug Uses: This drug is approved by the FDA for the treatment of heart rhythm disturbances, angina (chest pain), and hypertension.

Pregnancy Risk Category: C

Category C rating: The FDA assigns a drug to Category C for one of two reasons: (1) Studies show evidence of fetal harm when using the drug in pregnant animals, but no controlled studies have been done using the drug in pregnant women, or (2) Studies using the drug in pregnant animals have not been done, and studies of pregnant women using the drug are insufficient to reach a conclusion. Thus, the drug should only be used if the potential benefit for

mom is greater than the potential risk of fetal harm, which, in many cases, is unknown. Approximately 50% of prescription drugs fall in this category.

Animal Studies: When pregnant rats and rabbits were treated with this drug, there was no evidence of an increased risk of birth defects found in the offspring.

Human Studies: There have been no studies in pregnant women using this drug and comparing the results to pregnant women not using the drug.

Helpful Hints: This drug weakly interacts with grapefruit and grapefruit juice, which can cause harmful, and even life-threatening, side effects. Before taking this drug with grapefruit juice, or before consuming grapefruit or grapefruit juice during the day while taking this drug, first read the section "Grapefruit Juice–Drug Interactions Can Make You Sick" in the appendix of this book. Then discuss this with your pharmacist or the healthcare provider who prescribed this drug.

Remember: All pregnancies have a background risk of about 3% for a major birth defect, even when mom doesn't take a drug of any kind. If you are pregnant or planning a pregnancy, always let your doctor know before taking any drug, prescription or non-prescription, or herbal remedy.

VINCRISTINE

Brand Name: Vincristine

Drug Uses: This drug is approved by the FDA for the treatment of acute leukemia and in combination with other drugs to treat Hodgkins disease, non-Hodgkins malignant lymphoma, and Wilm's tumor.

Pregnancy Risk Category: **D**

> **Category D rating:** The FDA assigns a drug to Category **D** when studies of pregnant women using the drug show evidence of fetal harm. Rarely, however, the potential benefit of using the drug in some life-threatening situations for mom may outweigh the potential risk of fetal harm. For example, when mom requires cancer treatment or when she has a serious disease for which safer drugs cannot be used or are less effective. Approximately 11% of prescription drugs fall in this category.

Animal Studies: When pregnant mice, hamsters, and monkeys were treated with this drug, their offspring showed an increased risk of fetal malformations.

Human Studies: There have been no studies in pregnant women using this drug and comparing the results to pregnant women not using the drug.

Helpful Hints: This drug moderately interacts with grapefruit and grapefruit juice, which can cause harmful, and even life-threatening, side effects. Before taking this drug with grapefruit juice, or before consuming grapefruit or grapefruit juice during the day while taking this drug, first read the section "Grapefruit Juice–Drug Interactions Can Make You Sick" in the appendix of this book. Then discuss this with your pharmacist or the healthcare provider who prescribed this drug.

Remember: All pregnancies have a background risk of about 3% for a major birth defect, even when mom doesn't take a drug of any kind. If you are pregnant or planning a pregnancy, always let your doctor know before taking any drug, prescription or non-prescription, or herbal remedy.

. . . .

ADDITIONAL DRUGS AND THEIR FDA PREGNANCY RISK CATEGORIES

Since these additional drugs are uncommonly used in pregnancy, they are listed by generic name along with their FDA Pregnancy Risk Category without more detail:

Valganciclovir - C

Valproate - D

Valsartan - C (D if used in the second or third trimesters)

Vardenafil - B

Varenicline - C

Vasopressin - B

Vecuronium - C

Verteporfin - C

Vinblastine - D

Voriconazole - D

W

WARFARIN

Brand Name: Coumadin

Drug Use: This drug is approved by the FDA as an anti-coagulant (blood thinner) for the prevention and treatment of venous thrombosis and pulmonary embolism; to prevent and treat thromboembolic complications associated with heart rhythm abnormalities; and to reduce the risk of death, recurrent myocardial infarction, and events such as stroke or embolization after a heart attack. This drug is a member of the coumarin family of anticoagulants.

Pregnancy Risk Categories: The FDA assigned this drug to Category **D** however, the manufacturer assigned the drug to Category **X**.

> **Category D rating:** The FDA assigns a drug to Category **D** when studies of pregnant women using the drug show evidence of fetal harm. Rarely, however, the potential benefit of using the drug in some life-threatening situations for mom may outweigh the potential risk of fetal harm. For example, when mom requires cancer treatment or when she has a serious disease for which safer drugs cannot be used or are less effective. Approximately 11% of prescription drugs fall in this category.
>
> **Category X rating:** The FDA assigns a drug to Category **X** when studies have shown the risk of fetal harm clearly outweighs any potential maternal benefit from the drug. **Drugs in this category should not be used by pregnant women.** Approximately 5% of prescription drugs fall in this category.

Animal Studies: When pregnant rats were treated with warfarin, a significant number of their fetuses developed fetal hemorrhages, particularly involving the brain. In contrast, the untreated control group showed no evidence of fetal hemorrhage.

Human Studies: Since the first report of warfarin embryopathy (a cluster of birth defects) in 1966, a large volume of studies has accumulated which has identified a variety of birth defects associated with the use of this drug in the first trimester of pregnancy. These defects include underdevelopment of the nose, central nervous system defects, eye defects, underdeveloped extremities, and neonatal respiratory distress because of upper airway obstruction. In addition, an increased incidence of stillbirth, prematurity, and fetal hemorrhage has been associated with the use of this drug by pregnant women.

Warfarin can cause major or fatal hemorrhage. It is contraindicated in women who are or may become pregnant. Why? Because the drug passes through the placenta and not only may cause fatal hemorrhage to the fetus in utero, but also cause a variety of birth defects.

Helpful Hints:

1. For the pregnant woman who needs anticoagulation therapy, heparin is probably a better choice for anticoagulation since it doesn't cross the placenta and has not been linked to birth defects in contrast to warfarin, which has.

2. This drug weakly interacts with grapefruit and grapefruit juice, which can cause harmful, and even life-threatening, side effects. Before taking this drug with grapefruit juice, or before consuming grapefruit or grapefruit juice during the day while taking this drug, first read the section "Grapefruit Juice–Drug Interactions Can Make You Sick" in the appendix of this book. Then

discuss this with your pharmacist or the health-care provider who prescribed this drug.

Remember: All pregnancies have a background risk of about 3% for a major birth defect, even when mom doesn't take a drug of any kind. If you are pregnant or planning a pregnancy, always let your doctor know before taking any drug, prescription or non-prescription, or herbal remedy.

Y

ADDITIONAL DRUG AND ITS FDA PREGNANCY RISK CATEGORY

Since this additional drug is uncommonly used in pregnancy, it is listed by generic name along with its FDA Pregnancy Risk Category without more detail:

Yellow Fever Vaccine - C

Z

ZIDOVUDINE

Brand Names: Retrovir, Combivir

Drug Use: This drug is approved by the FDA for the treatment of HIV infection in combination with other anti-HIV drugs. It is especially effective in reducing maternal to fetal transmission with few, if any, adverse effects in newborns.

Pregnancy Risk Category: C

> **Category C rating:** The FDA assigns a drug to Category C for one of two reasons: (1) Studies show evidence of fetal harm when using the drug in pregnant animals, but no controlled studies have been done using the drug in pregnant women, or (2) Studies using the drug in pregnant animals have not been done, and studies of pregnant women using the drug are insufficient to reach a conclusion. Thus, the drug should only be used if the potential benefit for mom is greater than the potential risk of fetal harm, which, in many cases, is unknown. Approximately 50% of prescription drugs fall in this category.

Animal Studies: When pregnant rats and rabbits were treated with this drug, there was no increase in developmental anomalies in their offspring.

Human Studies: A controlled study for the prevention of maternal-fetal HIV transmission showed congenital abnormalities occurred with similar frequency between neonates born to mothers who received zidovudine and neonates born to mothers who received a placebo.

If possible, therapy should begin after 14 weeks of pregnancy if the immediate initiation of therapy can be delayed and won't adversely affect mom's health by doing so.

Helpful Hints: To monitor maternal-fetal outcomes of pregnant women exposed to Retrovir, an Antiretroviral Pregnancy Registry has been established. Physicians are encouraged to register patients by calling 1-800-258-4263.

Remember: All pregnancies have a background risk of about 3% for a major birth defect, even when mom doesn't take a drug of any kind. If you are pregnant or planning a pregnancy, always let your doctor know before taking any drug, prescription or non-prescription, or herbal remedy.

• •

ZOLPIDEM

Brand Name: Ambien

Drug Use: This drug is approved by the FDA for the short-term treatment of insomnia.

Pregnancy Risk Category: B

> **Category B rating:** The FDA assigns a drug to Category **B** for one of two reasons: (1) Studies show no evidence of fetal harm when using the drug in pregnant animals, but no controlled studies have been done using the drug in pregnant women, or (2) Studies show evidence of fetal harm when using the drug in pregnant animals, but controlled studies using the drug in pregnant women do not show evidence of fetal harm. Approximately 21% of prescription drugs fall in this category.

Animal Studies: When pregnant rats and rabbits were treated with this drug, no adverse fetal effects were noted.

Human Studies: There have been no studies in which pregnant women were treated with this drug and the results compared to women not treated with this drug. No reports identifying adverse outcomes in pregnant women using this drug have been reported.

Remember: All pregnancies have a background risk of about 3% for a major birth defect, even when mom doesn't take a drug of any kind. If you are pregnant or planning a pregnancy, always let your doctor know before taking any drug, prescription or non-prescription, or herbal remedy.

ADDITIONAL DRUGS AND THEIR FDA PREGNANCY RISK CATEGORIES

Since these additional drugs are uncommonly used in pregnancy, they are listed by generic name along with their FDA Pregnancy Risk Category without more detail:

Zalcitabine - C

Zaleplon - C

Zanamivir - C

Ziconotide - C

Zileuton - C

Ziprasidone - C

Zoledronic Acid - D

Zolmitriptan - C

Zonisamide - C

Appendix

ACE INHIBITOR DRUGS IN PREGNANCY

The ACE inhibitor family of drugs is commonly used to treat high blood pressure. These drugs include the following by generic name with their brand name in parentheses:

Benazepril (Lotensin)

Captopril (Capoten)

Enalapril/Enalaprilat (Vasotec oral and injectable)

Fosinopril (Monopril)

Lisinopril (Zestril and Prinivil)

Moexipril (Univasc)

Perindopril (Aceon)

Quinapril (Accupril)

Ramipril (Altace)

Trandolapril (Mavik)

The labels for these drugs have long included a **Black Box Warning** that women who become pregnant should be taken off ACE inhibitor drugs as soon as possible to avoid exposing the fetus in the second and third trimesters, when they are known to cause fetal birth defects, especially related to the kidneys. These drugs are assigned two Pregnancy Risk Categories: **C** when taken during the first trimester of pregnancy, and **D** for the last six months of pregnancy.

Now, a more recent study has raised doubt about the safety of these drugs even when taken during the first trimester of pregnancy. The uncontrolled study, published in 2006, showed that babies whose mothers had taken an ACE inhibitor during the first three months of pregnancy had an increased risk of birth defects when compared with babies whose mothers did not take any drugs for high blood pressure.

The FDA has not changed the first trimester Pregnancy Risk Category of C for these drugs. However, it has urged providers to take this information into account when prescribing one of these drugs for women of childbearing age. The FDA has also reiterated the need for providers to discontinue an ACE inhibitor as soon as possible if a patient taking one of these drugs becomes pregnant.

ANTIDEPRESSANTS IN PREGNANCY

1. Studies show that antidepressants increase the risk of suicidal thinking and suicide itself in children, adolescents, and young adults. Yet, depression itself is the most important cause of suicidal thinking and suicide. Anyone considering using these drugs must balance these two realities with the need to treat depression and bring it under control.

2. On May 2, 2007, the FDA proposed new warnings about suicidal thinking and behavior in young adults who take anti-depressant medications. The

proposed labeling changes apply to the entire category of antidepressants and include:

- Warnings about increased risks of suicidal thinking and behavior in young adults ages 18 to 24 during initial treatment (generally the first one to two months).

- Language stating that scientific data did not show this increased risk in adults older than 24.

- Language stating that adults ages 65 and older taking antidepressants have a decreased risk of suicidal thinking and behavior.

- Emphasis that depression and certain other serious psychiatric disorders are themselves the most important causes of suicide.

Steps for Consumers

- If you are currently taking prescribed antidepressant medications, you should not stop taking them.

- Notify your healthcare provider if you have concerns.

Antidepressants Involved in FDA's New Label Warnings. (Brand name is followed by generic name in parentheses.)

Anafranil (clomipramine)

Asendin (amoxapine)

Aventyl (nortriptyline)

Celexa (citalopram hydrobromide)

Cymbalta (duloxetine)

Desyrel (trazodone HCl)

Effexor (venlafaxine HCl)

Elavil (amitriptyline)

Emsam (selegiline)

Etrafon (perphenazine/
amitriptyline)

Lexapro (escitalopram
hydrobromide)

Limbitrol
(chlordi-azepoxide/
amitriptyline)

Ludiomil (maprotiline)

Luvox (fluvoxamine
maleate)

Marplan (isocarboxazid)

Nardil (phenelzine sulfate)

Norpramin (desipramine
HCl)

Pamelor (nortriptyline)

Parnate (tranylcypromine
sulfate)

Paxil (paroxetine HCl)

Pexeva (paroxetine
mesylate)

Prozac (fluoxetine HCl)

Remeron (mirtazapine)

Sarafem (fluoxetine HCl)

Seroquel (quetiapine)

Serzone
(nefazodone HCl)

Sinequan (doxepin)

Surmontil (trimipramine)

Symbyax (olanzapine/
fluoxetine)

Tofranil (imipramine)

Tofranil-PM (imipramine
pamoate)

Triavil (perphenazine/
amitriptyline)

Vivactil (protriptyline)

Wellbutrin (bupropion
HCl)

Zoloft (sertraline HCl)

Zyban (bupropion HCl)

· ·

FOLIC ACID ANTAGONIST DRUGS IN PREGNANCY

The folic acid antagonist family of drugs limit the effectiveness of folic acid, making it more likely that a baby born to a mom taking one of these drugs might have a serious birth defect, such as an open spine. The following list of commonly prescribed folic acid antagonists listed by generic name, includes drugs used to treat epilepsy, mood disorders, high blood pressure, infections, and cancer:

Carbamazepine	Primidone
Cholestyramine	Sulfasalazine
Lamotrigine	Triamterene
Methotrexate	Trimethoprim
Phenobarbital	Valproic acid
Phenytoin	

In one study, pregnant women who took a folic acid antagonist during the first trimester—when all of the organs are forming—more than doubled the risk of birth defects in their unborn babies. Meanwhile, neural tube defects, such as an open spine, and other malformations of the brain increased by more than six times after exposure to one of these drugs.

Since many of the drugs on this list are anticonvulsants—drugs used to treat epilepsy—it may be important to continue the drug throughout pregnancy for seizure control. If that's the case, this may require increasing the recommended amount of folic acid taken daily from .4 mg (the amount normally found in a multivitamin tablet) to as much as 4 mg, or 10 times the daily dose. It may also be possible to switch anticonvulsants to a safer medication that is not a folic acid antagonist. These decisions require close consultation with your doctor, preferably before becoming pregnant.

GRAPEFRUIT JUICE–DRUG INTERACTIONS CAN MAKE YOU SICK

In the late 1980s, scientists discovered that grapefruit juice contains natural substances called furanocoumarins (fur-an-o-coo-mar-ins). These substances suppress the activity of certain enzymes (proteins which regulate chemical reactions) found in the wall of our intestines. The job of these enzymes is to begin breaking down a drug before it is absorbed into our bloodstream. When these natural substances suppress the activity of these enzymes and hamper them from doing their job, less of the drug is broken down, leaving more of it available for absorption into our blood stream. **As a result, the blood level of the drug may be higher than normal, leading to a stronger clinical effect and stronger side effects.** In some cases, this has resulted in serious, sometimes life-threatening, toxic effects on the patient.

Note: To call these "grapefruit juice–drug interactions" seems somewhat misleading. Why? Because the natural substances in grapefruit juice interact with the intestinal enzymes first (not the drug) and affect enzyme activity. The suppressed enzymes then interact with the drug.

The first described case of a grapefruit juice–drug interaction occurring in a child was reported in the European Journal of Pediatrics in December 2000. An eight-year-old girl with Familial Mediterranean Fever (A hereditary inflammatory disorder that affects people who live around the Mediterranean Sea) showed serious signs of colchicine intoxication while taking the drug. The signs and symptoms involved her intestines, heart, nervous system, and blood. But when her doctors realized she had been drinking large amounts of natural grapefruit juice, they asked her to stop. Her toxic signs and symptoms disappeared.

The possibility that a drug will interact with grapefruit juice varies from drug to drug and person to person, depending on several factors:

- Individual genetics
- Type of drug

- Drug dose
- Amount of grapefruit juice consumed
- Timing of drug and grapefruit juice consumption

Fortunately, most drugs do not have a clinically important interaction with grapefruit juice.

The natural substances in grapefruit juice that interact with intestinal enzymes are found in grapefruit itself, white or pink, and in all grapefruit juice regardless of brand or whether the juice is fresh, pasteurized, or made from concentrate.

Q: Is it safe to drink grapefruit juice after a certain amount of time has elapsed between drug doses?

A: Research has shown that grapefruit juice–drug interactions may occur up to 72 hours after consuming grapefruit juice. So if you are taking a drug that is known to interact with grapefruit juice in a clinically important way, there are only two things you can do to avoid the problem:

- Switch to an equally effective alternative drug that doesn't interact with grapefruit juice.
- Stop drinking grapefruit juice and consider switching to orange juice or some other juice or liquid that doesn't interact with the drug you are taking.
- Always consult your doctor when making this decision.

Q: Which drugs interact with grapefruit juice in a clinically important way?

A: Researchers have tested hundreds of drugs for grapefruit interactions and divided the drugs into four categories:

- Strong interactors
- Moderate interactors

- Weak interactors
- None interactors

Researchers then decided that weak interactors and none interactors were unlikely to interact with grapefruit juice in a clinically significant way. But, if you re-read the case above involving the eight-year-old who was sick from colchicine intoxication, and we tell you that colchicine has been identified as a weak interactor, you might conclude that even weakly interacting drugs can have clinically significant effects if the patient consumes enough grapefruit juice, or is a child, or both.

Here are the drugs that are strong, moderate, and weak interactors (listing is generic name with brand name(s) in parentheses):

Drugs That *Strongly* Interact with Grapefruit Juice:

Amiodarone (Cordarone, Pacerone)

Buspirone (BuSpar, Ansial, Anxiron, Buspisal)

Celiprolol (not available in USA)

Diazepam (Valium, Diastat)

Halofantrine (Halfan)

Lovastatin (Mevacor, Altocor)

Simvastatin (Zocor)

Drugs That *Moderately* Interact with Grapefruit Juice:

Albendazole (Albenza, Eskazole, Zentel)

Artemether (Paluther)

Atorvastatin (Lipitor)

Azelnidipine (Calblock)

Carbamazepine (Tegretol, Biston, Calepsin, Epitol)

Cilnidipine (Atelec)

Cisapride (Propulsid)

Erlotinib (Tarceva)

Felodipine (Plendil)

Fexofenadine (Allegra)

Manidipine (Vascomin)

Nicardipine (Cardene)

Nisoldipine (Sular)

Nitrendipine (Cardif, Nitrepin)

Rupatadine (Rupafin, Rupax)

Terfenadine (Seldane)

Vinblastine (Vinblastine Sulfate)

Vincristine (Oncovin)

Drugs That *Weakly* Interact with Grapefruit Juice:

Acebutolol (Betoptic, Sectral)

Acetaminophen (Tylenol)

Alfentanil (Alfenta)

Alprazolam (Xanax)

Amlodipine (Norvasc, Amvaz)

Amprenavir (Lexiva, Telzir)

Budesonide (Entocort EC)

Caffeine (Cafcit, Fastlene, Lucidex, Nodoz)

Chloroquine (Avalen)

Cilostazol (Pletal)

Clarithromycin (Biaxin, Claridor, Claripen)

Clozapine (Clozaril, Fazaclo)

Colchicine (Colchicine)

Cyclosporine (Gengraf, Neoral, Restasis)

Desloratadine (Clarinex)

Dextromethorphan (Benylin, Robitussin)

Diclofenac (Cataflam, Diclon)

Digoxin (Lanoxin)

Diltiazem (Cardizem, Tiazac)

Domperidone (Motilium)

Efonidipine (Landel)

Enalapril (Vasotec)

Erythromycin (E-Mycin, Erythrocin, Ilosone)

Estradiol (Estrace)

Ethinylestradiol (Estiny)

Etoposide (Etopophos, Toposar)

Fentanyl (Duracesic, Fentora)

Fluvastatin (Lescol)

Fluvoxamine (Luvox)

Indinavir (Crixivan)

Itraconazole (Sporanox)

Lansoprazole (Prevacid)

Levothyroxine (Synthroid)

Losartan (Cozaar)

Methadone (Dolophine)

Methylprednisolone (Medrol)

Midazolam (Versed)

Morphine (Avinza, Kadian)

Nicotine (Commit, Nicoderm)

Nifedipine (Procardia, Adalat, Nifediac)

Nimodipine (Nimotop)

Omeprazole (Losec, Prilosec, Zegerid)

Pitavastatin (Livalol)

Pranidipine (Acalas)

Pravastatin (Pravachol)

Praziquantel (Viltricide)

Prednisone (Deltasone)

Primaquine (Primaquine)

Quazepam (Doral)

Quinidine (Quinora)

Quinine (Quin-Tab, Quinidex)

Repaglinide (Prandin)

Rosuvastatin (Crestor)

Saquinavir (Fortovase, Invirase)

Scopolamine (Scopace)

Sertraline (Zoloft)

Sildenafil citrate (Viagra)

Tacrolimus (Prograf)

Talinolol (not available in USA)

Theophylline (Elixophyllin, Quibron, Theolair)

Triazolam (Halcion)

Verapamil (Calan, Verelan, Covera, Isoptin)

Warfarin (Coumadin)

If you are taking any of these drugs with grapefruit juice, or taking any of these drugs and consuming grapefruit juice or grapefruit during the day, check with your doctor to determine if it's safe.

Source: Center for Drug Interaction Research & Education, University of Florida. www.cop.ufl.edu/fdic

NON-STEROIDAL, ANTI-INFLAMMATORY DRUGS (NSAIDS) IN PREGNANCY

The non-steroidal, anti-inflammatory family of drugs (NSAIDs) listed below by generic name are commonly used to reduce the inflammation and pain associated with arthritis, rheumatoid arthritis, and osteoarthritis:

Aspirin

Celecoxib

Diclofenac

Diflunisal

Etodolac

Fenoprofen

Flurbiprofen

Ibuprofen

Indomethacin

Ketoprofen

Ketorolac

Meclofenamate

Mefenamic Acid

Meloxicam

Nabummetone   Salsalate

Naproxen   Sulindac

Oxaprozin   Tolmetin

Piroxicam

When taken in the third trimester of pregnancy, NSAIDs have produced the following effects:

- Persistent pulmonary hypertension in the fetus, which means high blood pressure in the lungs. This potentially life-threatening condition causes breathing problems at birth, the need for respirator support, and has led to death.

- Decreased fetal kidney function, resulting in kidney failure, a lack of amniotic fluid, crowding in utero, failure of the lungs to fully grow before birth, and life-threatening breathing problems at birth.

- Infection and perforation of the newborn intestine, leading to spillage of infected material into the abdomen and the need for emergency surgery.

- Bleeding in the newborn brain.

These potential effects apply to all NSAIDs, whether purchased by prescription or over-the-counter without a prescription. They also explain why NSAIDs have been assigned a **D** pregnancy risk category when taken in the third trimester of pregnancy, meaning this family of drugs should not be used by pregnant women in the third trimester except under the rare circumstance when the potential benefit for mom, who is encountering a serious health problem, outweighs potential fetal risk.

. . . .

TAKING ACETAMINOPHEN: THE GOOD AND THE UGLY

Acetaminophen, the active ingredient in Tylenol, is probably the most popular drug for treating fever and pain in the United States.

- Acetaminophen is found in more than 90 prescription drugs and over-the-counter products, including narcotic pain relievers and cough-and-cold remedies.

- Acetaminophen is generally considered safe and is the recommended pain and fever reliever in pregnancy. But, if you take too much and overdose, it can be toxic to your liver. Herein lies the problem, especially if you are pregnant and two lives are at stake.

- Acetaminophen is the leading cause of acute liver failure in the United States. In some cases, the overdose is intentional, while in others, the overdose is unintentional.

- **Intentional cases** of acetaminophen-related acute liver failure are due to attempted suicide, amounting to roughly half the cases.

- **Unintentional cases** are usually due to unintentional overdosing. Why? Because patients didn't realize they were taking more than one drug containing acetaminophen.

- In 2006 alone, the American Association of Poison Control Centers implicated acetaminophen in nearly 140,000 poisoning cases (an average of 383 cases per day, nationwide), in which more than 100 patients died. The drug is responsible for more emergency room visits than any other drug on the market.

- Acetaminophen's toxic effect on the liver is directly related to the amount of acetaminophen consumed daily. Experts have set the maximum safe daily dose of acetaminophen at 4,000 mg per day. The directions on a bottle of Tylenol Arthritis caplets say to take 2 caplets every 8 hours, not to exceed 6 caplets per day. Each caplet contains 650 mg of acetaminophen. Thus the total daily recommended dose is 6×650 mg or 3,900 mg, which is 100 mg less than the maximum safe daily dose of 4,000 mg.

- Obviously, if you are taking another medication that also contains acetaminophen, you will easily exceed the maximum safe daily dose, increasing your risk of liver damage and acute liver failure. The following case example illustrates this point.

Case Example: You are 36 weeks pregnant and broke your arm yesterday when you fell on the ice. Fortunately, your unborn baby did not suffer any ill effects from the fall. After the doctor placed your arm in a cast, she prescribed Vicodin, two tablets every six hours, for pain. Unknown to you, Vicodin contains 5 mg of hydrocodone and 500 mg of acetaminophen per tablet. As instructed, you are taking 2 tablets every 6 hours for a total of 8 tablets per day. This equals 4,000 mg of acetaminophen daily (8 tablets $\times$ 500 mg/ tablet equals 4,000 mg), the maximum safe daily dose.

You come down with a cough, stuffy nose, chills, a fever, and ache all over. So you drag yourself to the corner drugstore and buy a bottle of Sudafed PE, Severe Cold pills, which contain 3 active ingredients: a decongestant for your stuffy nose, a cough suppressant for your cough, and acetaminophen for your fever and aching. Each pill contains 325 mg of acetaminophen. The directions say to take 2 pills every 4 hours, up to a maximum of 12 pills per day. If you follow those directions, you will be taking 12 × 325 mg of acetaminophen per pill for 3,900 mg daily. Adding this amount to the 4,000 mg of acetaminophen you are already taking for your broken arm, the total daily dose of acetaminophen will be 7,900 mg, almost double the safe daily dose of 4,000 mg.

The message? Never take more than one drug at a time that contains acetaminophen, pregnant or not. If unsure, read the labels carefully, ask the pharmacist when you purchase the medicines, or call your doctor.

Source: Cleveland Clinic Journal of Medicine, Vol. 77, No. 1, pages 19–27, Jan. 2010.

Prescription & Non-Prescription Drugs Containing Acetaminophen

Prescription Drugs:

Narcotics: Darvocet-N 50 & 100 Tablets; Esgic Tablets or Capsules; Esgic-Plus Tablets; Fioricet Tablets; Fioricet with Codeine Capsules; Hycomine Compound Tablets; Hydrocet Capsules; Lorcet-HD Capsules; Lorcet 10/650 Tablets; Lortab 2.5/500 Tablets; Lortab 5/500 Tablets; Lortab 7.5/500 Tablets; Lortab 10/500 Tablets; Lortab Elixir; Midrin Capsules; Norco Tablets; Percocet Tablets; Phenaphen with Codeine No. 3 Capsules; Phrenilin Forte Capsules & Tablets; Roxicet Tablets, Caplets, and Oral Solution; Sedapap Tablets 50/650; Talacen Caplets; Tylenol with Codeine #2, #3, & #4

Tablets; Tylenol with Codeine Elixir; Tylox Capsules; Vicodin Tablets; Vicodin ES Tablets; Vicodin HP Tablets; Wygesic Tablets; Zydone Capsules; Zydone Tablets.

· ·

NON-PRESCRIPTION DRUGS:

Cold & Flu Medications: Alka-Seltzer Plus Cold and Cough family of medicines; Benadryl Allergy/Cold Tablets; Children's Cepacol Sore Throat Formula Liquids; Comtrex Deep Chest Cold & Congestion Relief Liquigels; Comtrex Maximum-Strength Multi-Symptom Acute Head Cold & Sinus Pressure Relief Tablets; Contac Severe Cold & Flu Caplets Maximum Strength; Coricidin D Decongestant Tablets; Coricidin HBP Cold & Flu Tablets; Coricidin HBP Nighttime Cold & Cough Liquid; Dimetapp Cold and Fever Suspension; Drixoral Cold & Flu Extended-Release Tablets; Robitussin Cold, Cough & Flu Liqui-Gel medicines; Sudafed Severe Cold & Cough medicines; Theraflu Maximum Strength Nighttime Flu, Cold, & Cough Hot Liquid & Caplets; Theraflu Flu, Cold, and Cough medicines; Triaminic Severe Cold & Fever medicines; Triaminicin Tablets; Children's Tylenol Cold and Flu medicines; Infants' Tylenol Cold medicines: Tylenol Cold medications/Tylenol Flu medications; Tylenol Flu Nighttime Maximum Strength Gelcaps; Vicks 44M Cough, Cold & Flu Relief; Vicks DayQuil medicines, Vicks NyQuil medicines.

Pain Relievers: Aspirin Free Excedrin Geltabs and Caplets; Excedrin Extra-Strength Tablets, Geltabs, and Caplets; Excedrin Migraine Caplets and Tablets; Tylenol Extra Strength Adult Liquid Pain Reliever; Tylenol Arthritis Extended Relief Caplets; Tylenol Extra Strength Gelcaps, Geltabs, Caplets and Tablets; Infants' Tylenol Concentrated Drops; Tylenol Regular Strength Caplets and Tablets.

Sleep Aids: Excedrin PM Caplets, Geltabs, and Tablets; Tylenol PM Extra Strength Pain Reliever/Sleep Aid Caplets, Geltabs, and Gelcaps; Unisom with Pain Relief.

Menstrual Pain: Lurline PMS Tablets; Maximum Strength Midol Menstrual; Maximum Strength Midol PMS; Maximum Strength Midol Teen; Teen Midol Caplets.

Allergy/Sinus: Benadryl Allergy/Sinus medicines; Drixoral Allergy/Sinus Extended-Release Tablets; Sine-Aid Maximum Strength Sinus medications; Sinulin Tablets; Sinutab Sinus Allergy medications; Sudafed Sinus Caplets & Tablets; Tavist Sinus Caplets and Gelcaps; Tylenol Allergy Sinus Maximum Strength medications; Children's Tylenol Sinus medicines; Children's Tylenol Sinus Medicines; Tylenol Severe Allergy medication; Tylenol Sinus, Maximum Strength Geltabs, Gelcaps, Caplets, and Tablets.

Source: Knoll Pharmaceutical Company, 2000.

References

Borgelt, L.M., O'Connell, M.B., Smith, J.A., Calis, K.A. Women's Health Across The Lifespan: A Pharmaco-therapeutic Approach. American Society of Health-System Pharmacists, Bethesda, MD, 2010.

Briggs, G.C., Freeman R.K., Yaffe S.J. Drugs in Pregnancy and Lactation: A Reference Guide to Fetal and Neonatal Risk, Eighth Edition. Lippincott, Williams & Wilkins, Baltimore, MD, 2008.

Center for Drug Interaction Research & Education. University of Florida. www.cop.ufl.edu/fdic.

Daily Med: Current Medication Information. A Service of the U.S. National Library of Medicine. www.dailymed.nlm.nih.gov/dailymed/about.cfm.

Goldbart, A., Press, J., Sofer, S., Kapelushnik, J. Near fatal acute colchicine intoxication in a child. A case report. European Journal of Pediatrics; 159 (12): 895–897, Dec. 2000.

Martin, R.J., Fanaroff, A.A., Walsh, M.C. Neonatal-Perinatal Medicine: Diseases of the Fetus and Infant, Eighth Edition. Mosby. Philadelphia, PA, 2006.

McEvoy, G.K., Editor-in-Chief. AHFS Drug Information 2010. American Society of Health-System Pharmacists, Bethesda, MD.

Medline Plus. A Service of the U.S. National Library of Medicine. www.nlm.nih.gov/medlineplus/drug information.html.

Milunsky, A. Your Genetic Destiny. Perseus Publishing, Cambridge, MA, 2001.

PDR Concise Drug Guide for Obstetrics & Gynecology, First Edition. Thomson Reuters, Montvale, NJ, 2008.

PDR Drug Guide for Mental Health Professionals, Third Edition. Thompson Reuters, Montvale, NJ, 2007.

Pickering L.K., Editor. Red Book: 2006. Report of the Committee on Infectious Diseases, 27th Edition, Elk Grove Village, IL, American Academy of Pediatrics, 2006.

Sanders, C.S., Editor. Structural Fetal Anomalies: The Total Picture, Second Edition. Mosby, Philadelphia, PA, 2002.

Schaefer, C., Peters, P., Miller, R.K., Editors. Drugs During Pregnancy and Lactation: Treatment Options and Risk Assessment, Second Edition. Elsevier, Burlington, MA, 2007.

Schilling, A. and Colleagues. Acetaminophen: Old Drug, New Warnings. Cleveland Clinic Journal of Medicine. Vol. 77 (1): 19-27, Jan. 2010.

Stevenson, R.E., Hall, J.G., Editors. Human Malformations and Related Anomalies, Second Edition. Oxford University Press, NY, 2006.

Things to Consider When Prescribing Medications That Contain Acetaminophen. Knoll Pharmaceutical Company, Mount Olive, NJ, 2000.

Brand Name Index of Profiled Prescription Drugs

A

Abitrate—see clofibrate

Accupril—see quinapril

Accutane—see isotretinoin

Acetadote—see acetylcysteine

Actimmune—see interferon, gamma

Adalat—see nifedipine

Adderall—see amphetamine

Adenocard—see adenosine

Adoxa—see doxycycline

Adrenalin—see epinephrine

Adriamycin—see doxorubicin

Advair—see salmeterol

B

C

D

E

Effexor XR—see venlafaxine

Elavil—see amitriptyline

Elimite—see permethrin

Empirin—see aspirin

Entocort EC—see budesonide

Epitol—see carbamazepine

Epivir—see lamivudine

Epogen—see epoetin alfa

Eskalith—see lithium

Evista—see raloxifene

Excedrin—see aspirin

F

Feldane—see piroxicam

Fioricet—see butalbital

Flagyl—see metronidazole

Flexeril—see cyclobenzaprine

Flonase—see fluticasone

Flovent—see fluticasone

Floxin—see ofloxacin

Focalin—see dexmethylphenidate

Folic Acid—see folic acid

Fortamet—see metformin

Fosamax—see alendronate

Fungizone—see amphotericin

G

Gantrisin—see sulfisoxazole

Garamycin—see gentamicin

Gemcor—see gemfibrozil

Gengraf—see cyclosporine

Genoptic—see gentamicin

Gentacidin—see gentamicin

M

Macrobid—see nitrofurantoin

Magnesium Sulfate—see magnesium sulfate

Marezine—see cyclizine

Marzine—see cyclizine

Mebendazole—see mebendazole

Medrol—see methylprednisolone

Mefoxin—see cefoxitin

Meprobamate—see meprobamate

Mestinon—see pyridostigmine

Methotrexate—see methotrexate

Methyldopa—see methyldopa

Methylin—see methylphenidate

Mevacor—see lovastatin

Miacalcin—see calcitonin salmon

Micronase—see glyburide

Midamor—see amiloride

Mobic—see meloxicam

Monopril—see fosinopril

Motrin—see ibuprofen

Mucomyst—see acetylcysteine

Myambutol—see ethambutol

Mycelex—see clotrimazole

Mycelex-3—see butoconazole

Mycostatin—see nystatin

Mysoline—see primidone

N

Naproxen—see naproxen

Narcan—see naloxone

Neggram—see nalidixic acid

Neo-Merazole—see carbimazole

Neoral—see cyclosporine

O

P

Q

Quinidine—see quinidine

R

Rebetol—see ribavirin

Reglan—see metoclopramide

Regonol—see pyridostigmine

Relafen—see nabumetone

Restoril—see temazepam

Retrovir—see zidovudine

Rhinocort Aqua Nasal Spray—see budesonide

Rifadin—see rifampin

Risperdal—see risperidone

Ritalin—see methylphenidate

Robitussin—see dextromethorphan

Rocephin—see ceftriaxone

Roferon-A—see interferon, alfa

Ryzolt—see tramadol

S

Sandimmune—see cyclosporine

Sansert—see methysergide

Seconal—see secobarbital

Sectral—see acebutolol

Serevent—see salmeterol

Serophene—see clomiphene

Serzone—see nefadozone

Silphen—see dextromethorphan

Simemet—see levodopa

Sinequan—see doxepin

Singulair—see montelukast

Solu-Medrol—see methylprednisolone

Soma—see carisoprodol

Soriatane—see acitretin

T

U

Unasyn—see sulbactam

Unisom—see doxylamine

Unithroid—see levothyroxine

Urecholine—see bethanechol

V

Valium—see diazepam

Valproic—see valproic acid

Vanadom—see carisoprodol

Vanceril—see beclomethasone

Vancocin—see vancomycin

Vasotec—see enalapril

Velosulin—see insulin

Vicodin—see hydrocodone

Vincristine—see vincristine

Vioxx—see rofecoxib

Virazole—see ribavirin

Visken—see pindolol

Vistaril—see hydroxyzine

W

Welchol—see colesevelam

Wellbutrin—see bupropion

X

Xalatan—see latanoprost

Xanax—see alprazolam

Xifaxan—see rifaximin

Xylocaine—see lidocaine

Xylocaine Topical—see lidocaine

Z